Praise for *The Speckled Monster*

"An arresting and surprisingly entertaining portrayal of one of the world's great medical triumphs." —*The Arizona Republic*

"An intriguing story of a timely topic." —*BookPage*

"A timely, gripping, and often exciting account of the efforts of two people, both survivors of smallpox, to combat the disease . . . This is an outstanding medical thriller that both informs and inspires." —*Booklist*

"Carrell makes these historical figures come alive . . . A fascinating read." —*Library Journal*

"For those who take their medicine with an air of mayhem." —*Kirkus Reviews*

D0725901

Jennifer Lee Carrell holds a Ph.D. in English and American literature from Harvard University. A writer for *Smithsonian* magazine, she has taught in the history and literature program at Harvard. She lives in Tucson, Arizona. This is her first book.

The Speckled Monster

❧ A ☙

HISTORICAL TALE OF BATTLING SMALLPOX

Jennifer Lee Carrell

A PLUME BOOK

PLUME
Published by the Penguin Group
Penguin Group (USA) Inc., 375 Hudson Street, New York, New York 10014, U.S.A.
Penguin Books Ltd, 80 Strand, London WC2R 0RL, England
Penguin Books Australia Ltd, 250 Camberwell Road, Camberwell, Victoria 3124, Australia
Penguin Books Canada Ltd, 10 Alcorn Avenue, Toronto, Ontario, Canada M4V 3B2
Penguin Books India (P) Ltd, 11 Community Centre, Panchsheel Park,
New Delhi - 110 017, India
Penguin Books (N.Z.) Ltd, Cnr Rosedale and Airborne Roads, Albany, Auckland 1310,
New Zealand
Penguin Books (South Africa) (Pty) Ltd, 24 Sturdee Avenue, Rosebank, Johannesburg 2196,
South Africa

Penguin Books Ltd, Registered Offices: 80 Strand, London WC2R 0RL, England

Published by Plume, a member of Penguin Group (USA) Inc.
Previously published in a Dutton edition.

First Plume Printing, February 2004
10   9   8   7   6   5   4   3   2   1

 REGISTERED TRADEMARK—MARCA REGISTRADA

LIBRARY OF CONGRESS CATALOGING-IN-PUBLICATION DATA
Carrell, Jennifer Lee.
The speckled monster : a historical tale of battling smallpox / by Jennifer Lee Carrell.
p. ; cm.
Includes bibliographical references.
ISBN 0-525-94736-1 (hc.)
ISBN 0-452-28507-0 (pbk.)
1. Smallpox—History—Popular works.
[DNLM: 1. Smallpox—history.   2. Smallpox Vaccine—history. WC 588 C314s 2003]
I. Title.
RA644.S6C37   2003
614.5'21'09—dc21
2003000137

Printed in the United States of America

For Johnny

CONTENTS

PART THREE. HELL UPON EARTH

AFTERMATH

ACKNOWLEDGMENTS

IN the long, serendipitous chain of events that brought this book into being, three people took big risks on an unknown writer: Brian Tart, editorial director at Dutton; Noah Lukeman, literary agent extraordinaire; and Jack Wiley, senior editor emeritus of *Smithsonian Magazine*. For the privilege and joy of writing this book, as well as for deep funds of patient guidance, I am greatly indebted to all three of them.

At Dutton, Amy Hughes also offered editorial insights with sharp perception and easy grace, and Anna Cowles smoothed the process at every turn.

Dr. John Oliphant provided expert research on the Royal Navy as well as eighteenth-century London more generally, and, at the eleventh hour, Richard J. Bell, graduate student in American History at Harvard University, produced wonderfully detailed research on Cambridge and Harvard in 1721. Rupert Baker, library manager at the Royal Society, and Michael Bosson of Harrowby MSS Trust both provided help above and beyond the call of duty. Professor Isobel Grundy of the University of Alberta, Canada, was astoundingly generous with her unpublished research on Lady Mary, as well as with encouragement; Professor Susan M. Fitzmaurice of Northern Arizona University shared her transcriptions of Edward Wortley Montagu's unpublished letters. The library staffs at the Harvard Archives, the Massachusetts Historical Society, the New England Historic Genealogical Society, the Boston Public Library's Rare Books Department, the American Antiquarian Society, the Royal Archives at Windsor Palace, the Royal Naval Museum in Portsmouth, England, and the Commonwealth of Massachusetts all provided useful information and guidance.

I conducted most of the research, however, in libraries open either to the public at large, or to scholars with bona fide reasons to use their collections. In particular, I am grateful to the Arizona Health Sciences Library, the Tucson-Pima Public Library, and the University of Arizona Library in Tucson, Arizona; the Francis A. Countway Library of Medicine, the Harvard Archives, the Houghton Library, and the Widener Library of Harvard University; and the British Library, the National Portrait Gallery's Heinz Archive and Library, the Public Record Office, and the Royal Society Library in London.

Clive Coward of the Wellcome Trust Medical Photographic Library; Caroline Jennings of the Bridgeman Art Library; James Kilvington of the National Portrait Gallery, London; Susan Danforth, curator of maps and prints at the John Carter Brown Library; David Cobb, curator of the Harvard Map Collection; and the staff at Art Resource all helped to locate relevant images.

Lady Mary's unpublished poems appear by kind permission of the earl of Harrowby (Harrowby MSS Trust). Her published works are reprinted by permission of Oxford University Press. Cotton Mather's *Angel of Bethesda* is quoted with permission from the American Antiquarian Society. Quotations from the *Boston Gazette* are reprinted from Readex Microprint's Early American Newspapers Series with permission from Readex. Zabdiel Boylston's letter to Benjamin Colman is quoted with permission from the Massachusetts Historical Society. The Royal Society's papers are quoted with permission from the Royal Society, and the Sloane MSS are quoted with permission from the British Library.

Kathy Allen, Charlotte Lowe Bailey, Dan Shapiro, Kristen Poole, Martin Brueckner, and my mother, Melinda Carrell, read and reread the manuscript and offered many suggestions for improvement. My father, Bill Carrell, gave it a physician's critical eye. Derek Pearsall sent Dryden's smallpox poem my way.

My debt to my husband, Johnny Helenbolt, is boundless.

INTRODUCTION

IN Georgian London, Lady Mary Wortley Montagu sweeps out of a palatial bedroom in a swirl of satin and silk, her three-year-old daughter in tow. The servants are impassive as she floats by, but in her wake their faces pinch in disgust and their eyes meet in knowing glances. *"Unnatural,"* hisses the nurse to a maid. Ignoring them, she descends the grand staircase like the duke's daughter she is, but at the tall doors to the street, she pauses. She has grown accustomed to the delicate razors wielded in the plumed, powdered, and diamond-frosted high society of aristocrats and artists: countesses and poets once proud to claim her acquaintance now make ostentatiously absurd claims to parade out of any room she enters. But even that is less harrowing than what happens in public. She sets her shoulders and nods to the footmen, who swing open the doors. As she steps into the street, heads turn, and people begin pointing and jeering.

Just as the door closes on the safe haven of her coach, a servant in silver livery hands her a tray of carefully stacked notes: even as some mothers teach their children to taunt her, others send footmen day and night to beg for her presence. When they find her away from home, they fan out through the winding lanes of London to track down her carriage, wherever she may be.

In colonial Boston, Zabdiel Boylston rides down a muddy street; his black slave Jack follows on a mule, packing a satchel full of the tools of Boylston's trade: he's a general surgeon and an apothecary, or pharmacist. He's never been to college, but the townspeople call him "doctor" anyway, in honor of his skill. After years of practice, and before that, years of apprenticeship with his father, he's the most trusted medical man in town. A recent arrival from Scotland, William Douglass, is beginning to protest, however: Dr. Douglass may be eleven years younger than Boylston, but after studying at no fewer than four European universities, he has earned a proper medical degree. His peacock pride is infuriated by the mere presence of this untrained competitor for his fees, and even more so by the trust the provincial fools of Boston put in him.

So far, Boylston has paid no mind to Douglass's sneers: he cares little for tradition or titles. What he cares about are honest hard work and results.

That was before the recent outbreak of smallpox, however. Now, like Lady Mary, Boylston is hooted at and splattered intentionally with filth whenever he steps into the street. For fear of lynch mobs, his wife and friends beg him not to go out after dusk, but the stealthy knocks keep coming, followed by urgently whispered requests: *Will you come now, before it's too late?*

Always, he gives Jack the nod, puts on his coat, and goes out.

This is a tale of two smallpox-haunted cities and the two unlikely heroes, both outsiders to the elite ranks of the medical profession, who began the fight against that terrible disease in the Western world in the 1720s. Lady Mary Wortley Montagu and Zabdiel Boylston were not scientists; their struggles against smallpox were not systematic or even logical, according to the medical knowledge of the day. Their crusades against the "speckled monster" of smallpox were deeply personal.

Beyond speaking English, Lady Mary and Boylston had almost nothing in common. Lady Mary was the daughter of one of the British Empire's wealthiest and most powerful dukes, and the wife of one of its wealthiest private subjects. Shuttling between palatial London townhomes and grandiose country estates, she had been surrounded by opulence almost since birth. She was a study in contrasts: celebrated since childhood as a small, black-haired beauty, she cared more for rapier duels in the world of the mind than fame in the world of fashion. She spent hours reading romances and travel adventures in her father's plush library, and she loved biting word-play and wild flights of the imagination. Very early, she began scribbling her own stories. She was a Georgian Scheherazade who had the habit of telling her life's story as a fairy tale, but her heroines, like herself, were not docile princesses meekly awaiting rescue—though in the age's spirit of mockery, she christened one of them Princess Docile. Lady Mary's heroines were rebels who got themselves into trouble.

She was also one of the greatest letter writers to grace the English language. Even in hurried or teasing notes, she tells stories, deftly sketching scenes and dialogue and catching quirks of character. Thankfully, many of her correspondents recognized masterpieces when they saw them and saved her letters. She herself edited the letters she wrote home during her travels to Turkey, arranging for their publication after her death.

Her diary has a more frustrating history. Begun when she was young, it grew to many volumes: if it had survived, it would offer a woman's early eighteenth-century rival to the chatter of Samuel Pepys, whose diary remains one of the most entertaining and encyclopedic descriptions of late seventeenth-century life in London. Unfortunately, Lady Mary's diary, like a great deal of women's writing from that period, was burned by her loving family, for the sake of preserving reputations, hers included. All that remains of her journals are the memories that her granddaughter, Lady Louisa Stuart, retained of having read a few of the volumes many years before, set down in writing in 1837 as "Biographical Anecdotes of Lady M. W. Montagu."

In high contrast, Zabdiel Boylston wrote only when necessary. Boylston was a third-generation colonist who had grown up hunting, fishing, farming, and doctoring on the fringes of a vast wilderness half the world away, in the western hamlet of Muddy River, Massachusetts. Now known as Brookline, his birthplace was tiny and provincial even by the standards of the booming frontier port where he would eventually make his home: Boston, then sandwiched between the sea and the seemingly endless American forest.

To Boylston, words were tools to be used sparingly. He had learned his profession not from books but from long practical apprenticeship with his physician father. In 1726, certainly at the behest of the Royal Society and possibly at the request of the Princess of Wales, he told his side of the story in *An Historical Account of the Small-Pox Inoculated in New England*, including his case notes for inoculations performed in Boston in 1721 and 1722. It is a deliberately dry format, careful and concise; even so, a wry wit shines through. Though capable of humor, he was for the most part laconic, stubbornly upright and independent—an early incarnation of the American frontier hero.

Boylston and Lady Mary shared one crucial experience, as even a fleeting glance at their scarred faces could have told: they had both won vicious battles against smallpox. They knew firsthand the horror of a disease that could turn people into grossly swollen, groaning monsters barely recognizable as human, bubbling with pus and reeking with the sickly-sweet smell of rotting flesh. They knew the agony of skin that felt sheeted in flame, and a mouth and throat so full of sores that some victims died of thirst rather than endure the pain of swallowing. That lone shared struggle turned out to be enough to make them change the world—at the same time and in the same way, though unknown to each other.

In telling this tale, I have tried to remain faithful to its two heroes, not only as historical figures but as storytellers. In honor of Lady Mary's love of a well-told story, I have done my best to lift dry, briefly outlined scenes back into drama, relying on evidence from elsewhere to add details of sight, smell, and sound; food, clothing, and furniture; medical beliefs and scientific facts; music and poetry; even weather. Where history reports dialogue indirectly or leaves it merely suggested, I have returned it to full conversational life—while keeping as close to what was actually said as possible, often by borrowing known words from similar situations. I have drawn connections left implied by timing or juxtaposition. At times, the narrator speaks with the words and phrases of Lady Mary, Boylston, and their cohorts—not always set apart in quotation marks—to allow the reader to look at the world through their eyes, as well as to look *at* them, like marvelous butterflies pinned beneath museum glass.

The notes, in the form of short essays at the back of the book, are in honor of Boylston—and all those who like their certainties sharply demarcated from surmise, or who just enjoy the tension and spring between history and story.

For all our current fears, we are inestimably lucky to live in a world in which the threat of smallpox has shifted from ordinary to extraordinary. Paradoxically, in the absence of smallpox as an everyday enemy, it is hard to realize just how lucky we are. Sheer numbers may help. By the time the disease was vanquished in 1977, it had become far and away the most voracious killer ever to stalk the human species. With a victim count in the hundreds of millions, smallpox has killed more people than the Black Death and all the bloody wars of the twentieth century put together.

The eradication of smallpox from nature remains one of the greatest victories of modern medicine. Across the 1960s and '70s, doctors and health workers by the hundreds of thousands hunted the disease down in its last hiding places in Asia and Africa, driving it relentlessly toward extinction by a "scourged earth" policy. By lure, education, bribery, and finally by force, they vaccinated everyone within reach of the variola virus that causes smallpox.

In essence, doctors destroyed smallpox by destroying its habitat. Like vampires, variola quickly dies in the glare of sunlight; it cannot, under normal circumstances, survive long outside the human body. Using vaccination to turn every vulnerable member of the species into uninhabitable territory, doctors eventually exterminated variola from nature. In April

1978, a World Health Organization field office declared victory in a brief telegram sent winging from Nairobi to headquarters in Geneva: "Search complete. No cases discovered. Ali Maow Maalin is the world's last known smallpox case." Maalin had sickened and recovered in Somalia in the fall of 1977, though it would take until May 1980 for the World Health Organization to certify the proclamation of its Kenyan field office. Whichever endpoint you choose, the long war was over.

As Jonathan Tucker has described in *Scourge: The Once and Future Threat of Smallpox*, only two samples of the virus are known to survive, deep-frozen in maximum-security prisons in Russia and the United States—prisons that threaten to become Pandora's boxes.

Amid celebrations of victory and growing fears of a future breakout, whether accidental or deliberate, the equally dramatic origins of the long fight against smallpox have lingered in the shadows. Edward Jenner, who developed and propounded vaccination in the 1790s, is often credited as the founding father of immunology. But Jenner, more accurately, forced a quantum leap in the fight against smallpox; he did not start it.

Jenner's vaccination introduced the cowpox virus (called "vaccinia," from *vacca*, Latin for "cow") into the body through small pricks in the skin, the body's first and best shield against disease. Though related to smallpox, cowpox is a minor ailment, one most healthy human bodies (as well as healthy bovine bodies) can easily conquer. In mustering troops against vaccinia, however, the body also goes on high alert against its lethal cousin variola, the smallpox virus (whose name derives from the Latin adjective *varius*, meaning "spotted"). When and if variola tries to sneak into a vaccinated body, it's killed off before it can establish any strong footing, much less a stranglehold.

Jenner's contribution was to find a virus related to, but far less dangerous than smallpox with which to put the body's immune system on alert. Introducing virus into the skin in order to produce smallpox immunity, though, had already been in practice in the British Empire for seventy-five years: but the old form of inoculation—then called "engrafting" and now called "variolation"—used live smallpox virus. The danger in doing so, of course, was that it could produce full-blown smallpox; patients undergoing inoculation could also spread the disease, triggering an epidemic.

When variolation worked, it produced no more than a mild case of the disease in a patient kept safely quarantined. Except at the point where the virus had been force-fed into the body, it left no scars. Even this relatively gentle encounter with the disease, though, granted the one great gift of surviving smallpox: complete and permanent immunity.

Vaccination, on the other hand, put the patient at far less risk of serious complications, and removed altogether the risk of spreading smallpox. It also, however, delivered a lesser gift: temporary and, in some cases, only partial immunity. It was less absolute, but vaccination's shield would prove to be more than strong enough.

Before 1798, when Jenner published his first vaccination paper, however, variolation for all its risks was not merely the best, but the *only* means of protection against smallpox. In the throes of epidemics that could kill as many as one in three victims, and leave many others grotesquely scarred or blinded, the roughly one-in-a-hundred odds of dying from variolation often looked very good.

Neither Lady Mary nor Boylston invented inoculation; they were crucial catalysts rather than inventors. At the beginning of the eighteenth century, European medicine was helpless against the disease, but loath to admit it. Recognizing that failure, Lady Mary and Boylston were willing to look elsewhere for relief.

The paradox of using smallpox to fight smallpox was not a product of methodical Western science. Its discovery and development lie hidden in the unrecorded history of the folk medicine of the Middle East, the Caucasus, and Africa. Many people around Lady Mary and Boylston sneered not only at their lack of training, but at their willingness to pay serious attention to rumors coming from even more absurdly "ignorant" sources: Ottoman women and African slaves.

In the 1720s, Louis Pasteur's germ theory lay another 140 years in the future, and the mechanisms of disease were as yet little understood. No one knew *why* inoculation might work; they only gradually became certain that it *did* work. Observers did know two important facts about smallpox, however. They knew that the disease was virulently contagious, and suspected that it was passed by breathing "bad" air somehow infected by victims, or by the presence of victims' clothing and bedding. Secondly, it was already common knowledge that those who had survived smallpox were forever after immune: with smallpox, there was no double jeopardy.

This is a history of long ago, but the quarrels that erupt through this story are still very much with us. Inoculation was controversial for the same reasons that smallpox vaccination remains controversial: it is dangerous— though the degrees of danger are greatly different. In all kinds of inoculation—variolation, vaccination proper (with the vaccinia virus), flu, polio, measles—doctors *make* patients a little bit sick, at least locally, in order to keep them healthy on the whole. Or so they hope.

But all vaccinations carry risks: some percentage of patients will have adverse reactions, or prove to have no ability to fight the disease they've been exposed to, and will sicken seriously and possibly die. With smallpox vaccination, the risk of death is one or two in a million for primary vaccinations, and one in four million for revaccinations. For variolation, it ranges between one in fifty to one in a hundred. No one, now, is going to say that one-in-fifty odds are an acceptable risk. In a world without smallpox, neither are the one-in-a-million odds of the old vaccine—which is why the United States began phasing it out in 1972.

But what of a world in which smallpox is a maybe? When that "maybe" could result in a global pandemic that could kill millions within months if not weeks? Precisely how much of a maybe makes the odds of vaccination worthwhile?

It is one thing to argue about numbers, another entirely to argue about your own children, as both Lady Mary and Boylston discovered.

In the end, their tale is a history of hope: through the hatred, dying, threats, and shouting there is always visible a defiant will to live, to learn, and to love. That, as much as anything else, is what has made this tale of two heroes and a terrible disease worth the telling.

How difficult a thing it is, to set Truth in a clear light in this case to the satisfaction of an unbelieving world.

—*Zabdiel Boylston*

I am going to write a history so uncommon that in how plain a manner so ever I relate it, it will have the air of a romance.

—*Lady Mary Wortley Montagu*

⊰ PART ONE ⊱

London

❧ 1 ❧

Two Marys

EARLY in December 1694, an assassin emerged from the streets of London to sneak westward across the park, slip unseen through the halls of Kensington Palace, and attack the beautiful and beloved young queen.

Six years before, it had taken a revolution to put Mary and her Dutch husband, William of Orange, on the British throne, but on this wintry day her attacker was neither counterrevolutionary nor common robber. Nothing more than a tiny protein-coated and exuberantly proliferant tangle of DNA, it was the virus now known as variola major. Its identification would take another two and a half centuries, but in 1694 the disease it triggered was already notorious. "The small pox," the English called it, to distinguish it from "the great pox," syphilis, whose strange rashes it sometimes mimicked.

Silently, without so much as a lone tickle or twinge of warning, the infection burrowed deep into the queen's body. For almost two weeks, it stayed out of sight, as the virus multiplied in the dark. Meanwhile, Mary seemed to be wrapped safe within the gilt pavilions and cupolas of her favorite pleasure house, its rooms festooned with laughter and music, swept with the rustling of silk, and gleaming with forests of the blue-and-white Chinese porcelain she loved to collect.

Then, five days before Christmas, fever exploded through her body, chased by intense flashes of pain in her head and back. Without telling anyone she was ill, she dosed herself with her old-faithful cold remedies, but by evening nothing had helped. With a smallpox epidemic raging in London, Queen Mary assumed the worst. She sent everyone who had not already had the disease away from the palace and shut herself in her innermost room. Veering between shivers and sweats, she wrote a last long letter of love and advice to the sometimes wayward king. After locking it in a little drawer in the desk by her bed, she spent the rest of the night burning her diaries and long-treasured letters, preparing to die.

Three days later, a deep reddish-purple flush crept in uneven patches across her face. Confronted with this rosy fire, the nine physicians who gathered at her bedside looked grim. They knew of two maladies that commonly produced it, and neither was good news.

"If the queen is lucky," they intoned among themselves, "it might be measles." If she were not, they knew but could not yet bear to say, it would turn out to be smallpox.

The only way to find out was to wait.

The next day, a cold and blustery Sunday, the ominous blush faded, and blisters began to rise on the queen's face, arms, hands, and feet. Despite the now inescapable diagnosis of smallpox, the physicians' hopes rose along with her bubbling rash.

"At least she does not have the purples," they told each other with relief. The mere appearance of the blisters canceled out the possibility of that horror: the rare but invariably fatal form of early hemorrhagic smallpox, which made its victims leak blood from every orifice while their bodies swelled beneath skin turned to dark purple velvet, until they died of heart failure—all before a rash of telltale pocks could ever break out.

"Then she is out of danger?" asked King William.

But the doctors shook their heads. "That we cannot yet say."

The king, who had suffered the disease in childhood and lost both parents to it, broke down and wept. He was a soldier at heart, a daring and some said brilliant commander who relished any threat that action and strategy might answer. He thrilled to direct men through the danger and chance of the battlefield, but as his wife headed into her own private war with smallpox, there was nothing he could do but watch from the far shore of immunity. He set up a camp bed inside Mary's room and refused to leave her side.

You can believe what a condition I am in, loving her as I do, he scribbled to a cousin. *If I should lose her, I shall have done with the world.*

He was not alone in his fear; nor was the queen. All that day and the next, which was Christmas Eve, courtiers and bishops pressed into the stifling sickroom. Still more milled just outside the door, while less exalted crowds gathered in hushed throngs amid the snow flurries down in Kensington High Street.

Up in the palace, the doctors held their breath and kept their voices low. Perhaps, after all, the queen would suffer only what they called "kind and distinct" smallpox—the most common and least debilitating form of the disease, in which the pocks remained relatively small and self-contained, resembling a savage case of the chicken pox. Overheard in snatches, the physicians sounded as if they were arguing over a malodorous orchard they both loathed and longed for, producing foully abundant "crops" of "limpid" blisters.

"You talk like the horned gardeners of hell," snapped the king. "Are you sure you are doctors?"

The queen's blisters, the physicians continued in soothing tones, appeared to be ripening into plump and mellow pustules. Such putrid fruit might smell like death, but it heralded a far better chance for survival than any other form of the disease.

On Christmas morning, the blisters on the queen's face began to change, flattening and spreading into rosy spots. "Measles, after all," said someone in quiet triumph. But not quiet enough: before the others could protest, the words were snatched up, stretched out, and tossed through the streets as news that the queen was clear of smallpox and out of danger. Cheers and hat tossings erupted through the city and the nearby countryside.

The doctors, however, had not been quite so optimistic, nor had they been unanimous in this opinion of measles. Just as some predicted, the red spots proved not to be a new rash. By evening, it was clear that they were the old blisters in the process of sinking until they were once again level with the surface of the queen's skin, buried but visible like vials of poison beneath glass. Watching helplessly, the doctors felt their hearts sink as well. The sores darkened to purple and black; they were outlined with rings of red like burning coals.

That night, it seemed as if the queen's invisible foe were clamping her chest in a vise; her breathing grew labored, and she began spitting up blood. The next morning, a gentle probe with a lancet revealed what the pessimists had feared most: her sunken sores had filled with blood. She was also bleeding into her urine and from her vagina.

"Why are you crying?" she asked the crowd hovering around her bed. "I am not very bad." They were brave words, but no one believed her. It was no longer possible to deny that she had come down with possibly the most monstrous of the several forms of this terrible disease that doctors then regularly distinguished: flat or crystalline or bloody pox, they called it. Late hemorrhagic smallpox.

In the hours that followed, the queen's face swelled as her mouth, nose, and throat filled with so many blisters that they ran together into one raw sore, making it agony to eat, drink, or speak. Blood seeped from around her eyes and through her gums. Her nose bled uncontrollably, and she began to vomit and shit blood. From her breath and body oozed a sickly-sweet stench of decay so thick that at times even her most devoted nurses fled the room, retching. The slightest brush against her peeled skin away in strips, leaving her shivering like a creature flayed alive.

With a torturer's cruel cunning, the disease did not touch the queen's mind even as it ravaged her body. She was conscious until very near the end, inescapably aware of her transformation from beauty to beast. Late on the evening of the eighth day, she drifted into oblivion; she died at just past midnight on the twenty-eighth of December, only thirty-two years old. To most of those watching, it seemed a blessed release.

They feared, however, that the king would go mad with grief.

The queen missed deliverance by the slim margin of a single generation.

As she lay dying in Kensington Palace, a rebellious five-year-old—also named Mary—was already kicking against the stiff skirts and even stiffer proprieties in which her family sought to encase her. Most of her days were spent miles away from the dangers and diseases of London, under the wide sky of the Wiltshire downs. For her health, she was trotted out from the rambling Jacobean manor house of West Dean and up into the downs to take the air in demure and ladylike fashion. Up there, though, she ignored the rules of the polite world that lurked in her grandmother's house below. To the end of her days, she remembered racing as fast as her small legs would carry her, straining to reach the great golden bauble of the sun and pluck it from the sky before it set in the west.

Mary Pierrepont had been christened in London, in St. Paul's Church, Covent Garden, in May 1689, just one month after the coronation of William and Mary in Westminster. The infant was named in honor of her mother, who bore the same first and last names. Her first name was also a nod to the new queen, whose rise to power the baby's family had backed.

The honorific "Lady" was fastened to her first name before she reached the age of two, when her father, Evelyn Pierrepont, succeeded not one but two childless older brothers dying young, to become the fifth earl of Kingston; his vast estates amounted to his own petty kingdom.

When Lady Mary was three and a half, her exhausted mother died from complications following the birth of her fourth child within three years and eight months. Along with her two younger sisters, Lady Evelyn and Lady Frances, and her new baby brother, William, Viscount Newark, Lady Mary was bundled into the country, into the cold care of their father's mother.

Only a few memories flared up from the dim years between the death of Lady Mary's mother and that of her forbidding grandmother, when she was nine. Of her quest to catch the setting sun, she later wrote: "A fine thing truly, if it could be caught," adding with an adult sigh, "but experience soon shows it to be impossible." Her childhood self admitted no such defeat. When the sun lay out of reach, she chased the distant lumbering spire of Salisbury Cathedral, though the faster she moved, the faster it, too, ran away from her. Let other children play with shells and smooth stones, baby dolls and hobbyhorses: Lady Mary was born with a stubborn yearning for seemingly impossible glory.

Several years later, to the hollow clop of horse hooves, the grind and spatter of coach wheels bouncing from pavement to muck, and the shouts of coachmen yelling for passersby to give way, a crowd of young men drifted like a bright perfumed flurry of confetti into a small tavern under the sign of the Cat and Fiddle. It stood in Sheer Lane off the Strand, just north and west of the Temple Bar, the stone gateway that once marked the western boundary of the single square mile that was the ancient City of London proper.

The flashier men amid this crowd wore knee-length coats, breeches, and waistcoats (or vests) of jewel-colored velvet trimmed with gold buttons, silver lace, and fur. Long and luxuriously curled wigs framed their faces, while high, boxy heels displayed ankles and calves wrapped in silk hose. Battles had long since been won with gunpowder, but they still wore swords, and most of them still knew how to use them. They were followed about by as many bowing servants as they could afford; for a few, this amounted to a small private army.

To suppose these men nothing more than an impotent flock of overbred, empty-headed peacocks, however, would be a serious mistake. They were ferociously talented and even more ferociously ambitious. One day soon, they would run Britain; already, they could be dangerous. They could also be charming and extraordinarily witty.

The proprietor of the place, Mr. Christopher Cat, was pouring wine and passing platters heaped with the savory mutton pies, flavored with thyme, nutmeg, and onion, succulent with butter and currants, that made his establishment famous. This excellent man had long since christened his even more excellent pies with his nickname, Kit Cat. Now, the name of both man and meat pie was attaching itself to the fledgling club that met at his tavern.

At these once-a-week gatherings, a sprinkling of dukes, earls, and lesser lords discarded enough of the brittle niceties of rank to mingle freely with gentlemen soldiers and politicians, doctors and lawyers, painters, poets, and playwrights. There was even one man of their company "in trade," as they said a little dubiously of merchants: their host was the round-faced, jovial Jacob Tonson, publisher and bookseller of many of the day's finest volumes.

The lure that drew men of such disparate rank together was politics: to a man, they were Whigs, which meant that by the touchstones of the day, they were liberal. While they believed in the rightness and necessity of a monarch, they also fervently believed that the king must share real power with Parliament. A decade earlier, it had been these men, along with their fathers and uncles and brothers, who had engineered the Glorious Revolution that had set the current king and his poor late queen on the throne.

At present, however, the men munching mutton pies at the Cat and Fiddle were not discussing politics. They were discussing women.

Dr. Samuel Garth stood, swept aside his red cloak, and raised his glass to a countess:

She o'er all hearts and toasts must reign,
Whose eyes outsparkle bright champagne.

To shouts of laughter and approval, everyone drank. Once each year, the company met to cast ballots on the subject of beauty. Those ladies voted London's fairest of the fair had their names inscribed with a diamond on a drinking glass. Then they reigned as "Venuses of the Feast," the celebrated subjects of the club's toasts for the entire ensuing year.

These earthly goddesses were never present. Instead, their absent eyes, lips, and lovely cheeks, their wit and Whiggish politics, were put forward as excuses for the men to drink deep among an exclusively male and increasingly raucous company. The Kit-Catters spent at least as much time celebrating Bacchus, god of wine, as they did praising Venus and her capricious son Cupid.

Charles Montagu, Lord Halifax and king of the quick rhyme, took a turn:

Fair as the blushing grape she stands,
Excites our hopes and tempts our hands.

From across the table, the earl of Kingston eyed Halifax lazily. "I know of one lady," he said, "who outshines your whole list like Romeo's Juliet, trooping among crows."

Next to him, Thomas, Lord Wharton, banged down his bowl of wine. "Name her, my Lord Lady-Love," he challenged. "Or do you mean to keep her to yourself until you can make a small rearrangement to Caesar: *I saw, I conquered, I came?*"

Amid jeers and groans of laughter, Kingston smiled. Unlike Wharton—who, it was rumored, had proved devil enough to take his pleasure with a woman on an altar—Kingston groomed a reputation as an elegant and envied rake. His friends did not feel the need to lock up their wives and daughters when he came to call.

"He's luring us into folly, more like it," roared Dr. Garth. "Meaning to make laughingstocks of us by linking us to some draggle-tailed Drury Lane drab."

No amount of catcalling, however, could get Kingston to reveal the lady's name. In the end, his fellows rejected his nomination.

"On what grounds?" demanded the earl.

"No one else has ever seen the lady," shot back Lord Halifax.

"Then you shall see her!" cried Kingston.

Moments later, several footmen scurried into the street and swarmed onto the earl's coach, which sped away. Emerging at the bottom of the lane, the coachman turned his back on the foul open sewer of the Fleet Ditch to the east and clattered west down the thoroughfare of the Strand. A hundred years earlier, when Queen Elizabeth ruled the land and Shakespeare ruled the stage, great lords had lined this street with their palaces that bore their names. As the wealthy had drifted westward in search of ever-receding quiet and sweet country air, though, the old mansions had dwindled, some falling down, some divided, most replaced by shops. Now, though the Strand might be narrow and crowded by the standards of Louis XIV's Paris, it was nonetheless one of the most extravagant shopping boulevards in Europe. Bay windows curved into the street, teasing passersby with fragrant and fragile luxuries from all over the globe: silk stockings and silver, fringed gloves and feathered fans, linens, lace, china, and the newfangled curiosity of tea.

The earl's servants ignored it all. Trotting through the chaos of Charing Cross, the coach turned down Pall Mall and up St. James's cutting across to the quiet splendor of Arlington Street. At last, it drew to a stop at a palatial town house perched on the eastern edge of the Park.

The footmen in their liveried finery were admitted without fanfare, but once inside, their message produced a flare of French displeasure from Madame Dupont: a tavern was at no time any place for a lady, and by the time they managed to deliver her, it would be full night.

The earl's message, however, was not a request; it was a command. Under Madame Dupont's disapproving eyes, maids hurried to pull a flounced petticoat down over the lady's shift and cage her torso in a satin brocade bodice stiff with slivers of whalebone. At her waist, their fingers flew as they attached the matching gown that swept down around the floor in a heavy three-quarter circle, leaving a gap in front for the embroidery and lace of the petticoat to show. The long train they fastened up behind in a voluptuous bustle. They dressed her hair into a high tower topped with pleated lace that fell down her neck in a long cascade, and they pinned diamonds deep into the curls, where they winked and glimmered with coy grace.

Ensconced like a silken sugarplum in the earl's gilt coach, she peered out at the wonders of London crowding around her as the company sped back the way they had come. Carrying wax-dipped torches, footmen jogged in a long train on either side, so that the coach seemed to float through the gloom within its own magical globe of golden light. Through this halo flowed a parade of workers swarming home, shopkeepers shuttering windows, peddlers hawking the last of their pears and nuts from handcarts. Herds of bullocks and sheep trotted toward slaughter, and heavy trundling wagons carted coal. She glimpsed pickpockets, ballad singers, and pockmarked beggars missing eyes and limbs; she saw swords drawn, fists bunched, and mouths twisted into leers. Once in a while, she glimpsed the icy disdain of another fine lady in a coach and six.

The earl's coach never slowed until it drew up to the sign of the Cat and Fiddle. A footman lifted her safely over the filth of the street to the threshold of the tavern. She was announced, the doors were thrown open, and firelight heavy with the scents of red wine, roast meat, and men doused in musk and civet spilled across her satin slippers.

Silence settled through the room as Kingston took her by the hand and presented her to the astonished company. Tiny and fine-boned as a wren, with dark hair and dark eyes that sparkled with precocious intelligence, she was indeed beautiful, but the Lady Mary Pierrepont, Kingston's eldest daughter, was also a little girl: ten, at a guess, and surely no more than twelve.

Two years earlier, on New Year's Day in 1699, Lady Mary's grandmother Pierrepont had died. With her grandson set to inherit the earldom of Kingston, she left her fortune to her granddaughters. The proud heiress of the Evelyns of West Dean, she bequeathed the bulk of her fortune to seven-year-old Lady Evelyn, who had been destined for it since her christening. To docile little Lady Frances, she left the handsome sum of £1,000 toward a dowry. To Lady Mary, quite contrary, she left nothing at all.

Her grandmother's death, though, gave Lady Mary something far more valuable than cash: escape to her father's famously magnificent household. While Lady Evelyn was shuttled off alone to priggish Aunt Cheyne's, presumably to learn the finer points of being an Evelyn, even if only by first name, the other three children stayed together. Like tides drifting after the moon, they began following the seasonal pull of their father. Instead of shuttling between their grandmother's house in West Dean and Aunt Cheyne's in Chelsea, they now spent summers up north at Kingston's grand country estate of Thoresby House—an architectural cousin of Hampton Court and Chatsworth—on the edge of Robin Hood's old haunt of Sherwood Forest, outside Nottingham. From the Christmas holidays through the daffodil-fringed days of spring and early summer, they lived in his town house at the edge of the park, in one of the most fashionable neighborhoods west of London.

As a result, Lady Mary danced through her father's field of vision more frequently than before, at an age when she might have seemed both a pretty toy and a partner in mischief; from then on, she lived within easy reach of his whims.

That same year, the Kit-Cat Club had first skittered through London gossip. Its fame as a stronghold of Whig loyalties, however, was forged in the shadow of catastrophe, a year and a half later.

Queen Mary's death had left King William a childless widower, due to be succeeded by his wife's younger sister, Princess Anne. Following her marriage to Prince George of Denmark, Anne had at first seemed bountifully, blessedly, mind-bogglingly fertile, but by 1700, after seventeen pregnancies, only one sickly child remained alive. On this son, William, duke of Gloucester, the Whigs had pinned all their hopes for the future of the Stuart dynasty.

On June 24 of that year, Gloucester's eleventh birthday party was drawing to a close amid the sparkle of fireworks and the snap of military parades at Windsor Castle, when he felt a flush of heat and complained of a headache, sore throat, and chills. Two days later, the velvety purple rash of hemorrhagic smallpox crept across his skin. Three days after that, he was dead.

His mother was inconsolable. The Whigs, with cold political judgment unclouded by personal sorrow, were just plain stunned. Rampaging through a child's birthday party, smallpox had once again swatted its way into the councils of the great, to shift the course of history.

In smaller towns, smallpox was an all-or-nothing terror: there were either no cases, or a full-blown epidemic. But with half a million souls thronging together along the banks of the Thames, London was large enough for smallpox to fester as an ever-present threat. For the most part, the disease stalked through the city's overcrowded, unsanitary tenements, plucking at the children of the poor. Every so often, though, it would throw its head back and roar, storming through the streets to fell young and old, rich and poor, alike. In 1694, Queen Mary had been one of 1,683 dead and upwards of 10,000 ill; in 1700, smallpox was not quite that strong, but it was strong enough: the child duke of Gloucester was one of a thousand dead.

To the Whigs who had put him in line for the throne, Gloucester was the one who mattered most. In their eyes, he had been the last acceptable heir to the House of Stuart.

In the weeks following Gloucester's death, rumors muttered that King William would bring his dead wife's half-brother James, Prince of Wales, back from his long exile in France. A Roman Catholic who idolized the absolute monarchy of the French Sun King, Louis XIV, the exiled prince was nobody's notion of an ideal heir, but in King William's eyes, he was family. To the Whigs, he spelled disaster. Twelve years earlier, they had ousted the prince's petulant fool of a father, King James II, from the throne in a brief and nearly bloodless coup d'état dubbed the Glorious Revolution. Passing over the prince, they had handed the throne to the more promising—and Protestant—couple, William of Orange (the ousted king's nephew) and Mary (the ousted king's eldest daughter). The prince, feared the Whigs, had spent those twelve years honing his grudges against them to glinting hatred. Suddenly, thanks to smallpox, the once glorious revolutionaries had everything to lose. All across London, Whigs of all walks of life huddled together in taverns like the Cat and Fiddle, in coffeehouses and drawing rooms, to take comfort in each other's company and debate what might best be done about the succession.

After a year of wrangling, on June 12, 1701, Parliament passed the Act of Settlement, debarring the Prince of Wales—and all other Roman Catholics—from the throne. As previously arranged, Mary's younger sister Anne would succeed King William. After Anne, Parliament proclaimed it would toss the crown high over France and send it spinning toward Germany, to the tidy town of Hanover and the waiting head of the dowager electress Sophia.

The granddaughter of England's first Stuart monarch, old King James I, Sophia was Protestant, willing to share power with Parliament, and trailed by robust male heirs in two succeeding generations: both Protestant, and both named George. Furthermore, Sophia and the first of these Georges had already survived smallpox. Apparently, the House of Hanover had escaped not only their Stuart cousins' weakness for the Roman religion, but their well-known susceptibility to smallpox.

In London, as both smallpox and the storm it had brewed up over the succession melted away, men who had drawn together against the growing dark found they still liked each other in the clear light of day. Their numbers swollen, their loyalties cemented, the Kit-Catters kept meeting, but released from dread, their debates circled back to the delicious subjects of wine, women, and song.

So it was that Lady Mary's entrance into the Cat and Fiddle caught Lord Halifax open mouthed and midpoem on the wonders of yet another famous beauty, who just happened to be the elder sister of one of Lady Mary's friends. Shining with delight, Lady Mary stepped into the silence and spoke:

Even great Lord Halifax's skill
Before such beauty must fall still.

Across the room, he raised one eyebrow, and took up her verse, raising his glass once more and picking up where she had left off:

To gaze in awe at Venus' face,
Caught in Virtue's strong embrace.

He gestured first to the lady's husband and then turned to Lady Mary with the great teasing flourish of a full court bow, as if she were the dead queen come again.

That was fine: it gave her more time to think. By the time Halifax rose again, she had him. She nodded first to him and then curtsied to Sir Godfrey Kneller, the court portrait painter. Last spring, she and her friend had been to Sir Godfrey's studio to watch him paint the lady in question; Lady Mary had seen Lord Halifax there. She looked around the men gathered around her, leaning in to catch her words, and felt her heart swoop up to the ceiling with joy:

With so much justice, so much art,
Her very picture charms the heart.

Kingston was staring at Lady Mary as if a pet monkey had spouted Shakespeare. Glancing from daughter to father and back, the company regained its gallantry. The roar of approval was deafening as the men declared her the undisputed queen of the Kit-Cat Club.

Fêted and petted, fed candies and sips of wine, she was whirled from one member to another. Halifax claimed her first and presented her to Sir Godfrey. She met Will Congreve, whose new comedy, *The Way of the World*, was the latest rage on the stage; he handed her on to Dr. Garth and the poet Arthur Mainwaring. Her father's closest friend, Charles Howard, earl of Carlisle, was there, along with John Vanbrugh, the playwright who also played architect with enough panache to design Carlisle's opulent palace, Castle Howard. She tried not to look shocked by the hotheaded republican Charles Spencer, who insisted she call him plain "Mr." rather than "Lord" (though within a year he would succeed without protest to his father's earldom of Sunderland). Toward the back, she met a young member of Parliament named Robert Walpole. One day, he would transform the position of first lord of the treasury into the recognizably modern office of the prime minister; now he just focused his slightly scruffy charm on making Lady Mary laugh.

"Pleasure," Lady Mary recalled later, "was too poor a word to express her sensations; they amounted to ecstasy: never again, throughout her whole future life, did she pass so happy a day." As if she had plucked both the sun and the moon from the sky, now she knew not only what she wanted: she knew she could get it. For the rest of her life she strove to shine at the center of rapt circles of brilliant men.

❧ 2 ❧

THREE REBELLIONS

LADY Mary's Kit-Cat triumph proved hard to equal. Her brother Will obligingly thought her the best of all possible girls, but one little boy tumbling about her feet hardly constituted an adoring circle of brilliant men. She made do, for a while, with girls.

In Arlington Street, she scrambled nine feet up to giggle over the garden wall with the Brownlow girls next door—until Miss Nelly leaned on a loose brick and took a long tumble. Thereafter, their visits were strictly constrained to formal affairs of footmen, coaches, and straight-backed chairs prickling around the edges of a drawing room. Without the *haut goût*—the high spice—of danger, as she called it, Lady Mary soon bored of the Brownlows.

In London and up north at Thoresby House, she christened her friends with extravagant names from her favorite romances, listing them painstakingly on the inside cover of the blank book into which she copied her best poems and stories. She named herself Clarinda and her friend Jane Smith Hermensilda; they were trailed by Melecinda, Florice, Belvedira, Aminta, and Artemisa, among others. Only her stubbornly realist little sister, Lady Frances, insisted on being listed under her actual name, F. Pierrepont.

Out in the wider world, smallpox subsided to a small threat, sputtering fitfully in corners. With the invincible arrogance of youth, Lady Mary ignored it. There were myriad other more interesting dangers: the king, for instance, was killed by a fall from his horse. *The king is dead*, cried his adopted people in 1702. *Long live Queen Anne*.

For the most part, Lady Mary's girlhood rolled gently on, the days—as she put it in one of her tales—threaded with silver and gold. She never forgot her dream of brilliance, though. In its pursuit, she made herself a rebel three times over, punctuating the tranquility of her young life with the burst and spatter of fireworks.

Her first rebellion was to write. Her second was to learn. And her third was to love.

She never found out who betrayed her.

At fourteen, she had meant the tale of her father as a kind of homage, carving and polishing it with more care than she had lavished on any other piece of writing; nevertheless, she would never have so much as hinted its existence to him. Her enemy did more than hint. What the earl of Kingston heard filled him with such fury that he did not wait to send for his daughter; he raged through the gilded magnificence of Thoresby himself, ignoring the painted company of laughing cherubs and Caesars in triumph slipping past him on the walls.

The earl was fast, but the servants' hissing current of gossip was faster. By the time he threw open the door to his daughters' rooms with a crash and sent Lady Frances, their French governess Madame Dupont, and several maids scuttling into the hall, Lady Mary had obliterated two of her poems beneath blots of ink.

Tamping his fury down to an icy hauteur, he stepped inside. He had not yet dressed; his purple velvet morning gown and sable-trimmed cap heightened the strangely delicate pink of his wide cheeks, full jowls, and long, faintly hooked nose. There was nothing delicate, however, about his wrath. Lady Mary sank to her knees and kissed his hand in the ritual court greeting he always demanded from his children.

"I have heard that you are a meddling minx," he said, letting his diamond ring needle her cheek.

She caught her breath. Her favorite reading had long been the fiction and poetry *à clef*, "with a key," that filled her father's library shelves: tales that masked real-life adventures of love under false, florid names, all nestled in fantastic settings like jewels set in spun sugar. Half the fun of reading them was working out the puzzle of who was who. Recently, she had discovered they were even more fun to write.

She had first tried writing about herself, intensifying her girlish infatuation with Jane Smith into a full-blown romance. Transforming herself into the male shepherd-poet Strephon, Lady Mary dedicated the whole volume to "the beauteous Hermensilda." But Jane, daughter of the speaker of the House of Commons, had shed her part as Hermensilda and abandoned Lady Mary to become a maid of honor to Queen Anne. In any case, most of their adventures had to be heavily embroidered or invented altogether, although they had made the part about carving their names in the ancient oaks of Sherwood Forest satisfyingly real. So Lady Mary cast a connoisseur's eye upon the amorous adventures of her father: full of everything a romance reader could want, except possibly pirates or a bandit king.

"Where is this book?" he demanded, his black eyes hooded with menace.

Slowly, she held it up to him.

He took it between finger and thumb, pursing his full lips. "What have you put in it?"

Her chin went up. "Love and wit." Only a week ago, carving the roast as hostess at her father's table, she had heard Mr. Congreve proclaim these the only fit subjects for the drama.

Contempt cascaded over her. "What can an ignorant slip of a girl like you possibly have to do with love and wit?"

A flush crept up her neck to her cheeks and faded away again.

He opened his fingers, dropping the book to the floor in front of her like some dead, broken-winged thing. She heard another clatter and glanced down. A knife lay atop the book.

"In a few moments I intend to read it cover to cover," said her father. "If I find so much as the shadow of a trespass into disrespect, the whole book will burn. So I suggest you remove any trace of folly."

Hot tears spilled down her cheeks, but her father said nothing more. Under his pitiless gaze, she picked up the knife and slit out twenty pages.

"Burn them," he said as she finished.

She gasped, but the look on his face made her gather up the scattered leaves and cross to the fire. One by one, the pages slipped into the flames, bursting into brief crackling glory before curling away into black nothingness.

"Bring me what is left," he said behind her.

Sitting cross-legged in Madame Dupont's armchair, he read for what seemed like hours, whipping the pages as he turned them, while Lady Mary stood in the center of the room, trying not to wring her hands or suffocate on fear and her own fury. Outside on the terrace, a peacock wailed like a lost soul.

"There are one or two pretty rhymes here," said Kingston at last, standing up. "In a womanish way." Stashing the book under his arm, he stalked to the door.

At the threshold, he paused. "You do not dream of seeing your follies in print, I hope?"

Polite tradition held that aristocrats published only by circulating their work anonymously in manuscript; ladies did not publish at all. "No, my lord," she said, glaring at the floor.

There was a short silence, broken by the book itself as Kingston sent it whizzing across the room toward the fire. Lady Mary stumbled forward just in time, thrusting her hand into the burning heat to scoop up the book before it could land atop the coals.

"I have made you a lady, mistress Mary," said her father with distaste. "See that you deserve the courtesy of that title." He whirled about and strode from the room.

She fled across the floor to her writing desk, smoothing a hand across the book's thick vellum cover. She knew a better use for her father's odious knife. She picked it up and sharpened a quill. Opening her book, she riffled through the pages until she found one of the last remaining blank spaces. Then she dipped her pen into ink and squeezed a new poem into the emptiness:

> 'Twas folly made me fondly write:
> For what have I to do with love and wit?
> I own I trespass'd wickedly in rhyme,
> But, oh, my punishment exceeds my crime.
> My follies though on parchment writ
> I soon might burn and then forget,
> But if I now both burn and blot,
> By me they cannot be forgot.

Still seething, Lady Mary turned to the reverse of the title page and wrote, *I question not but here is very many faults, but if any reasonable person considers three things, they would forgive them: 1. I am a woman, 2. without any advantage of education, 3. all these was writ at the age of 14.*

As soon as possible, she acquired another book, gripping it like a weapon bound in fine-grained leather. Knowing the irritation it would cause her father, she dropped her mask of male authorship and titled her new book as if for print, carefully inscribing the first page:

> *The Entire Works of*
> *Clarinda*
> *London*

She couldn't alter her age or her sex, but her education she could do something about. For two years in her midteens, Lady Mary spent six hours each day burrowing into the black leather chairs that lurked in the stately hush of her father's library at Thoresby. Whenever Madame Dupont looked in, she saw the girl lost in romances and travel tales: giddy things, no doubt, but at least they kept the little hoyden quiet.

As soon as Madame went away again, Lady Mary turned back to the contraband books that she kept hidden in a cubbyhole in a little-used corner: a Latin grammar and dictionary.

Under Madame Dupont's strict care, Lady Mary's education focused on French, riding, dancing, and carving with precision and delicacy the immense roasts proper to a lord's table. These were the skills that would please a man in a wife, thought Dupont; conversing in Latin on the finer points of philosophy and poetry was what a man's friends were for.

But Lady Mary did not care to please a man, she meant to please herself. Boys like her brother were carefully escorted across the sacred ground of the classics; breaking into the ivory tower by herself, Lady Mary ranged freely through its treasures. Later, she would come to appreciate Virgil and Horace. Those much-worshiped monuments, though, were not what lured her in.

Whatever her father might say, her will to learn had everything to do with both love and wit. She tunneled her way into Latin in search of the unbridled, violent loves of Ovid's *Metamorphoses*, unadulterated by translation: Jove consuming Semele in bright, burning fire; Daphne scraping Apollo's fingers as her smooth skin scurfed into tree bark and she took root as a laurel rather than yield to his lust; Acis' crushed body flowing into a bloody river for the sake of Galatea's love; mutilated and trembling Philomel escaping her brother-in-law's repeated rapes, flying free at last in the shape of a nightingale.

Despite Dupont's dim view of educated women, Lady Mary's scholarly accomplishments soon attracted her most tenacious lover.

She met Edward Wortley between tea and cards in the apartments of his sister Anne. He was enchanted by the rarity of a lady with a taste for classical poetry; Lady Mary was enchanted by the rarity of a man who appreciated that hard-won taste. He offered to help her in her studies; she pretended to need it.

A few days later, a parcel arrived for her. The scents of brown earth and new ink slid in magic-carpet curls from the paper as she unwrapped it; within gleamed the leather and gilt of a superb edition of Quintus Curtius' Latin history of Alexander the Great. It was the perfect gift: quietly admiring her command of Latin, appreciating her love of books, and beckoning her into long, exotic hours of armchair travel. Nor had Mr. Wortley neglected gallantry. Facing the title page, a poem unfurled compliments in a neat, spidery hand: Alexander would have "laid his empire down" and made "polished Greece obey a barbarous throne," it declared, had Persia only managed to show the conqueror beauty like Lady Mary's.

Eleven years older than Lady Mary, Edward Wortley Montagu—or Wortley, as he preferred to be known—was heir to the lion's share of Newcastle's coal mines. In business, he was as pitiless and gritty as his coal; in politics, he had already won grudging respect for prickly integrity. A Whig member of Parliament, he spent his happiest hours in debate with men of searing wit. His closest friend was the satiric journalist Joseph Addison, just then making waves as one of the main writers of a new paper, *The Tatler*; he also counted Addison's paunchy, black-wigged Irish-born associate Richard Steele—the paper's editor and chief writer—and William Congreve among his close acquaintance. Through Wortley, Lady Mary glimpsed reentry into the world of brilliant men, this time welcomed as an adult rather than a petted child.

Her visits to Anne grew more frequent, and more stilted. Soon, the unfettered girlish laughter in Anne's letters evaporated as well, replaced by a stiff courtliness: she and Lady Mary still wrote, but the correspondence, like the friendship, became a charade. Anne was still writing out and signing the letters, but her brother was composing them, and Lady Mary knew it; her replies, though addressed to Anne, were meant for Mr. Wortley.

Her father had no inkling of their dalliance.

A few years earlier, as Lady Mary had neared seventeen in the spring of 1706, her thirteen-year-old brother Will left for Cambridge, taking a great part of her day-to-day laughter with him. That December, Queen Anne elevated Lady Mary's father in the peerage, moving him up a rank as the marquess of Dorchester; the title of earl of Kingston instantly descended to his son. Meanwhile, Lady Mary and her friends underwent transformations of a different sort, blooming into eminently marriageable ripeness. She had been in no hurry to marry, however, and on that subject, father and daughter agreed. Far from being willing to squire his daughter through the company of eligible wits that he graced with his presence, Dorchester wanted her out of the way, while he cast lascivious eyes on her acquaintance, for himself.

In 1708, when Lady Mary was nineteen, he bought Berrymead Priory, a big old house set in fragrant gardens in Acton, three miles west of London. Conveniently close to town, the place was still far enough away to serve as sweet escape whenever clouds of sickness and stench thickened the city air. Smallpox had shaken off its long fitful sleep, and was once again scattering its blisters across London with ominous if not quite epidemic thickness.

Having worked his way up in the peerage, however, Dorchester did not intend to allow smallpox or any of London's other pestilential fevers—typhus, typhoid, influenza—to muck through his family. The house in Acton was part of his plan to secure the new title for future generations. It was also useful, he discovered, whenever he wished respite from his offspring's inquisitive eyes.

To Lady Mary, Acton had seemed more a place of exile than safety. Then she found that she, too, could make use of a shield from inquisitive eyes: in February 1710, Anne Wortley died, glassy eyed and shivering with fever. Wortley lost his favorite sister and Lady Mary her best friend; they had both lost safe cover for their flirtation. Just shy of twenty-one, Lady Mary was not to be deterred. Within a month, she dared what tight-lipped and tighter corseted conventions of virtue decreed unthinkable, and her father would never forgive: she took up the pen to write Wortley directly. Soon, their correspondence bloomed into the deliciously forbidden drama of a secret courtship.

From the beginning, she was clear about what she wanted and what she could offer: *I can esteem, I can be a friend,* she wrote, *but I don't know whether I can love.* She proposed a tranquil meeting of minds, a rational relationship based on shared interests, calmed by country life and enlivened with travel.

That was not nearly enough for Wortley. *I love you,* runs the subtext of most of his letters, *and I despise myself for it.*

They wrote often and at length, hurling hidden pages of sniping argument at each other. They met furtively and infrequently at luxury shops in the New Exchange on the Strand, walking in and out of church, and driving in stately circles around the ring in Hyde Park. There, the women who hawked oranges and sweets to famished young lords and ladies also ferried pretty messages between coaches, tying love letters around their oranges with bright ribbon, for a price.

In April, Wortley looked for Lady Mary several days on end in the park, but did not find her. One of the orange women he had employed earlier as go-between found him though. "Fair lemons and oranges!" she shrilled as she approached. "Cherries just ripe," she added in a lower register, though he saw none among her offerings. Brushing by him with skirts pinned up in a bustle as bright—if not quite as clean—as the fruit in the wide flat basket she balanced on her head, she whispered in his ear: "The young lady sends to say that Betty can see as she gets a message." By the time he processed this offer, she was swinging her mocking hips away down the lane.

He caught up with her and dashed off a querulous note.

Three days later, his friend Richard Steele forwarded him a reply. *This is left tonight with me to send to you. I send you no news because I believe this will employ you better. Your most obedient servant,* he scrawled on the outside, his smirk nearly visible in the ink.

Wortley tore open the letter. It was not from Lady Mary; it was from the orange woman, Betty Laskey:

> *Dear Sir,*
> *I ask pardon for my presumption, but the occation that happened makes me take this liberty. My Lady Mary gave orders to write to let you know she received your two letters this day. The very time you went away she went to Acton and is very ill of the measles, and is very sory she could not write sooner.*

Wortley's skin prickled with apprehension. The red-spotted rash, high fever, and swollen eyes of the measles were dangerous. Even if Lady Mary survived, she might well emerge from the sickroom blind. Another, far worse fear, though, sputtered at him from the dark corners of the room: In the early stages, measles was easily confusable with the worst kinds of smallpox. Some doctors held that the purples—hemorrhagic smallpox— was a foul double brew of disease, "smallpox and measles mingled." Others used the measles as a safe haven, a diagnosis to cling to until all hope was past, as if they might ward off the smallpox by refusing to name it.

Measles was rife that spring, but the smallpox was worse. By May, the city was spiraling into the worst smallpox epidemic England had ever seen, its spotted tracks visible at every turn. Laborers who could not afford to be ill trudged about with pocks still ripening, and newly recovered urchins roughhoused in the streets, sowing the last late scabs—or "seeds"—from the soles of their feet and the palms of their hands into the dust and the puddles. Everywhere were the coffins: new made and stacked high on carts, in single-file quick procession to the churchyards. One morning, Wortley had nearly collided with a woman hurrying by with a tiny coffin not two feet long tucked under her arm; he could still smell the raw scent of new-cut wood. She had glanced up at him, but her face was empty: no sorrow, no rage, just emptiness.

However proudly the doctors, apothecaries, and quacks might point to their successes, the only real safety lay in already having survived the scourge, as Wortley had. But Lady Mary, as he well knew, had not.

He was being womanish, he told himself. Excitable. His father and grandfathers had reserved such reeling fears for the worst visitations of the plague. But the plague, taunted a voice in his head, had not been seen in epidemic strength in London in forty-five years—since 1665. Smallpox, some warned, was taking its place as the scythe of an angry God.

Outside the window, a deep bell tolled another victim to the grave; beyond that he heard a rumbling of heavy wheels. For a moment he wondered whether the dead-carts of the plague had returned to trundle through the night, stacking corpses like kindling and dumping them in open pits ringed with bonfires. He shook himself; surely the smallpox could never sow its dead as thick as the plague once had. He flicked the curtain aside and saw a cart carrying the living: a woman and two wailing children. He breathed a sigh of relief.

Then she turned her eyes up to his and he stepped back and froze. Her face was thick with yellow pocks; so were the children's. The despair in the woman's eyes sent a cold wind knifing through his belly. In a moment, the cart was gone, trundling west, no doubt, toward the pest house of Westminster. But in his mind, the images of the pocks lingered, glowering like embers in the dusk.

Shuddering, he let the curtain fall closed and returned to the letter:

> *Betty tooke a great deal of troble goeing often to Acton to see for a letter, but Lady Mary could gett no conveniency to write. She gives her love and respects to you, but if it is not expressed as is proper you'l excuse it as from whence it comes instead of my Lady.*
>
> *Lady Mary desires you to direct your letter for Betty Laskey at the Bunch of Grapes and Queen's Head in Knightsbridge. She had not time when Betty gave her the letters to read them. She signs her name to this for I shewed it her.*
> *April 17th 1710*
> *M.P.*

Wortley spent a bad night, tossing and pacing. He had lost his favorite sister—his poor Anne—only two months before; he could not bear to lose Lady Mary too. At dawn, he sat down to draft her a letter.

Though last night I was perfectly well till I saw the letter signed by you, he wrote, *I am this morning downright sick. The loss of you would be irretrievable; there has not been—there never will be—another Lady Mary.*

He took a breath and reined himself in.

You see how far a man's passion carries his reflections. It makes him uneasy because the worst may possibly happen from the least dangerous distempers.

He meant, no doubt, to be comforting, but his own fears kept creeping through. It was a thousand to one, he wrote, that he would next hear of her recovery. He could not keep from wondering, though, what might happen if the news were not so fine. She might lose her complexion or her sight, he mused. With this, the demon whispers in the dark slid sideways into his letter: Both the measles and smallpox could cause blindness, but only smallpox was notorious for ruining faces with permanent, stomach-twisting scarring.

Assuring Lady Mary that his love would weather all possible ravages of disease, Wortley's love twisted back into jealousy: *I should be overjoyed to hear your beauty was very much impaired, could I be pleased with anything that would give you displeasure, for it would lessen the number of your admirers, but even the loss of a feature, nay of your eyes themselves, would not make you seem less beautiful to—*

He never finished the draft. Overcome, he dashed off a clean copy of his letter, and Betty headed back to Acton.

Two days later, Wortley still had received no answer; in the city, the care-fully counted and reported death-count for smallpox soared up toward one hundred per week. He could not step out to head for a coffeehouse or the theater without passing two or three funeral corteges—strangely tense and more hurried than stately, the mourners' ranks thinned by fear to ragtag, blank-faced huddles. Once, crowds had parted in the midst of the Strand to reveal a man covered with pocks stumbling down the street, crying with hunger, but every time he veered toward a shop, its door banged shut. At one, a pail of scraps was shoved through a doorway, along with a harsh cry, *Take it and be gone.* But before he could fetch it, some boys snatched it up and began pelting him. Howling, the man had limped away down the street, with the boys circling at a distance.

I entreat you not to let another day pass, he begged Lady Mary. *Send one line to let me know you do not grow worse.*

Her reply, when it finally came, arrived through a different channel than the one he had used. About the smallpox she remained obstinately silent. She confirmed, however, what the London gossip mill had been whispering to him but he had refused to believe except from her pen: Her fever and her spots sprang from the measles. She would live, and keep both her color and her sight. In the matter of Betty Laskey, however, she could not keep her temper; the rest of the letter was blistering. *Your indiscretion has given me so much trouble, I would willingly get rid of it at the price of my fever's returning,* she snapped. *You employed the foolishest and most improper messenger upon earth.* Betty was certainly attentive, but she was also as rapa-cious as a raven and about as discreet as one croaking in a field full of ca-naries. Lady Mary denied that she had ever had anything to do with the woman, much less given her a commission to carry messages, and told Wortley that he had been a fool to let himself fall for such an obvious con game.

Wortley refused to see anything amiss with his means of approach; in his eyes, Lady Mary owed him great thanks for taking such pains to get through to her. He hired Betty again to tell her so.

How could you think of employing that creature? Lady Mary shot back. *She has made everything public to every servant in this house. Imagine the pretty pickle I am in.*

She yearned to return to London to sort things out in person, but smallpox dashed her hopes. Margaret Brownlow, one of the girls next door with whom Lady Mary had once giggled over the garden wall, was sitting amid clouds of white satin, sewing her trousseau, when she was seized with shivering and sweats. By evening, red flecks were drifting thickly across her, marking the spots where the pocks would rise. Up and down Arlington Street, windows shuttered and doors slammed as if by themselves. Those who could crammed into coaches and sped west to clean air. The less fortunate passed by the Brownlow house with faces averted and feet skimming at a quick patter, pressing themselves against the opposite side of the lane.

While Arlington Street panicked, Lady Mary fretted out in Acton. *I have just now received a letter,* she wrote Wortley in morose irritation, *that tells me a Lady is fallen dangerously ill of the small pox over against our house.* It was the first time she had deigned to name the disease. *I am to stay here till all danger of infection is over.*

The danger did not appear likely to pass anytime soon. Dr. Garth and his fellow physicians were stretched skin thin across shivering nights and stench-filled days, tending to ten and then twenty thousand ill. Londoners trembled in church, weeping through sermons proclaiming God's just punishment on a wicked world. They repented their manifold sins and then fled out to buy amulets and astrological signs against the scourge. Quacks and mountebanks swarmed out to feed on the panic, plastering their bills for marvelous cures on every street corner and house post. IN-FALLIBLE PRESERVATIVE FROM THE INFECTION! SOVEREIGN CORDIALS AGAINST THE CORRUPTION. THE ONLY TRUE ROYAL ANTIDOTE AGAINST THE SMALLPOX AND ALL OTHER INFECTIONS! At their best, they did no more good than a glass of water—but no more harm, either, grumbled Dr. Garth. At their worst, they preserved patients from the smallpox by dispatching them with poison first.

Lady Mary had other worries. Her father at last noticed the bright flutter of Betty, and the correspondence with Wortley that the orange woman's presence marked like a flag. For the sake of his own honor, Wortley was forced to propose marriage; for the sake of his daughter's honor, Dorchester was forced to entertain the notion. Far from apologizing for his indiscretion, Wortley insinuated that Lady Mary had leaked news of the correspondence on purpose. On the brink of being forced into the alliance she had so longed for, she was no longer sure she wanted him.

One door down from her father's town house, smallpox silenced another set of longed-for wedding chimes, even as shrieks of mourning slipped through shuttered windows and rose from the chimneys. For days, Mrs. Brownlow had been anointing Meg's face every hour with thick layers of cream, painting it on with a feather to soften the scabbing pocks and save her daughter's complexion, but nothing helped. Meg's skin stretched taut over pools and geysers of pus; she died smelling of sour milk and sweet rottenness, swollen beyond all recognition. Deep into negotiations to marry her to the marquess of Lindsey's heir, Meg's family rocked briefly in grief. Then they dried their eyes, hunched their backs against disaster, and went on with their plans very nearly as before, smoothly substituting the name of Meg's sister Jane where the contracts had once read "Margaret."

Still out in Acton, the news made Lady Mary shiver. In the making of a great match, fathers spent months and years negotiating the exchange of children for cash, titles, lands, and political support or protection. The future of whole families was what mattered: particular children were expendable. Death, her father observed tartly, was an acceptable reason for failing to marry as one's family directed. Wayward desire was not.

Lady Mary still yearned to return to London, but as soon as she was movable, Dorchester banished her still farther west—"over the hills and far away," as she put it—to West Dean, the half-forgotten home of her early childhood. *I know not whether you can make me happy,* she concluded to Wortley; *you have convinced me you can make me miserable.*

That summer, as smallpox deaths mounted into the thousands, she wandered alone through the Wiltshire woods, staring glumly at the fish in the streams and wishing for more interesting company. She tried to content herself with translating the stoic philosophy of Epictetus and asking the bishop of Salisbury to critique it. In letters to friends, though, she dropped all pretense of stoicism. *Men are vile inconstant toads,* she scrawled.

Early in August, Wortley wrote to tell her that the marriage negotiations had broken off. Her father, he complained, was insisting that he entail the lion's share of his property upon a hypothetical eldest son: the accepted practice for keeping an inheritance intact, preventing future generations from splintering it to nothingness. Wortley had no problem with the notion of keeping an inheritance whole, but argued that it was irrational to settle everything on an unborn heir who might or might not turn out to deserve it. He preferred to keep the power to bestow his wealth as he saw fit, according to the proven merits of his offspring. It was not a question of valuing her, he told Lady Mary: *I know too high a rate can't be set upon you.* But her father had done just that—and having found a price that Wortley was unwilling to pay, Dorchester was gleefully exploiting it.

To revitalize his spirits and mend his fragile pride, Wortley stalked off to Belgium, to the original Spa. He had not given up all hope of a resolution, however. He begged Lady Mary to write often, care of Richard Steele. *For I know that when you write,* he scribbled, *you shine out in all your beauty.*

As August spilled into September, which stretched into October, her letters fluttered through Steele's door and stacked up on his desk. Arriving on the continent, Wortley had called a sudden truce with business, politics, and especially love, and asked Steele to hold all his mail—but neither Wortley nor Steele deigned to tell Lady Mary so. So she waited. Near the end of October, as the smallpox epidemic loosened its grip of terror on London, Lady Mary received the letter she had been longing for since summer. Tangled with anger and eagerness, she withdrew to her chamber to read it, but instead of tenderness, she found a mean-spirited rant, disagreeing in nitpicking detail with everything she had written.

Mockingly, she translated his letter back to him: *Madam, you are the greatest coquette I ever knew; the only happiness you propose to yourself with a husband is in jilting him most abundantly.* Filling with indignation, she resumed her own voice. *You are unjust and I am unhappy,* she wrote. *'Tis past— I will never think of you more, never.*

Wortley could not so blithely dismiss Lady Mary from his mind. After Christmas, he wrote to present his grievances once again. She wrote back in self defense, and soon they were once again sparring via smuggled correspondence. What other man, she exclaimed to Frances, would attempt not to flatter but *argue* her into love, backing his points with quotations from the classical poet he graciously ceded to her as "your admired Virgil"?

"What other woman," retorted Frances, "would find such churlishness charming?"

"He has all the qualities of an upright man," protested Mary.

"And no single quality of an amiable one," sniffed Frances.

Their father judged Wortley neither upright nor amiable, and saw to it that Lady Mary was carefully watched. Private meetings became next to impossible; in public Wortley disdained melting into her throng of suitors. From a dignified distance, he watched her dancing at Dr. Garth's ball, flushing with pleasure at Mr. Handel's newfangled Italian operas, and relishing the scandal of a bigamy trial in the House of Lords. Little by little, he convinced himself she was in love with someone else. But he could not discern with whom.

Lady Mary had irritations other than Wortley's jealousy to think about.

With her sister Lady Frances and some girlfriends, she formed a clandestine club called the Sisters in Affliction. In defiance of the marriage-market haggling of their fathers, they declared themselves predestined for Paradise, code for husbands who would also make handsome and passionate lovers. They dedicated themselves to rejecting Hell—threatened husbands who filled them with revulsion or fear—and they urged each other to believe that some gray neither-here-nor-there state of Limbo—marriage to men of convenient wealth and emotional neutrality—was possible. It was not only girls who faced such trials, however, as Lady Mary discovered all too well that spring.

Having thwarted the marriage she wished for, Mary's father now set about condemning poor Will to Hell, marrying him to a fatuous fifteen-year-old heiress whose lone asset was to arrive in the family towing one of the largest fortunes in England.

One evening in April, Lady Mary was serenaded in Acton by a group of young rakes, Wortley's prime suspect among them. After singing under her bedroom window, her suitors had all been invited into the drawing room for punch. The party then moved on to the house of a duchess, where they danced till dawn.

The next morning, a footman brought her a single letter sitting on a silver tray.

At last I am ready to confess my errors, wrote Wortley. *I retract all I have said of you and ask your forgiveness*. His fair words cloaked a foul message: He declared he had at last discovered who her other lover was. Worse still, in a pretense of willingness to assist in furthering her new affair, he offered to take this information to her father.

I wish you all possible happiness, she replied acidly, *and myself the quiet of never hearing from you more*.

Carving at her father's table up at Thoresby that summer, Lady Mary heard the news that had set all of Europe to trembling. On April 17, the very day she had received that infernal letter from Wortley, Emperor Joseph I, the great hope of the Hapsburgs in both the Holy Roman Empire and Spain, had expired of the smallpox in Vienna, swathed in twenty yards of sweat-drenched scarlet cloth. Three days earlier, Louis, eldest son of King Louis XIV and therefore the grand dauphin of France, had died of the same disease, shivering in a drafty room outside Paris.

Their doctors belonged to the opposing camps of the hot treatment and the cold, Dorchester and his cronies surmised. Fearing above all else that the emperor's pocks might fail to ripen, his conservative doctors had no doubt turned the sickroom into a dark crimson hothouse, draping not only His Imperial Majesty but the bed, windows, and walls in the warm color of red, which ancient tradition held would open pores and lure the pus out into pocks. If that weren't enough hocus-pocus, the windows were probably shut, the fire stoked up, and the patient buried beneath quilts and blankets. None of it to any effect, grumbled Lady Mary's father, but to increase the imperial misery. The dauphin's doctors, on the other hand, appeared to have worried far more about the poison ripening in too much abundance than failing to ripen. Rumor had it they'd done their best to chill the effervescence they feared was boiling in Louis's blood by allowing no bedclothes beyond a light coverlet drawn up to the prince's waist. They had thrown the windows open wide and quenched the fire in the grate too.

Neither treatment, griped Dorchester, was worth the paper a single quack bill could be printed on—much less the mountains of gold that royal physicians extorted for such tortures. Moderation, observed Dr. Garth, is what is called for, neither roasting patients nor freezing them. "A miracle," retorted her father, "is what is called for. None of you has the least notion of what to do in the face of smallpox, save to scrape to yourselves tidy fortunes in fees for your ignorance." His rant over, Dorchester spun the conversation toward the politics of the French, Imperial, and Spanish successions, all three now redirected by the smallpox just as the British succession once had been.

Lady Mary listened with only half an ear. Smallpox might rearrange the chessboard of Europe as many times as it pleased; at twenty-two, she was still far more entranced by the subjects of love and wit. Wortley had been unforgivably rude, but he had also been right: there was someone else. In imagination and intellect, in his love of music and words, Lady Mary's Paradise was her match. Unfortunately, he was also far beneath her in rank and fortune. He was not—and never could be—for her, and she knew it. In the summer of 1711, though, love was still a delicious game. Full to brimming, she painted her glory and agony in long letters to her fellow Sister in Affliction, Philippa Mundy. The world glowed with an inner fire when her beloved was present; it lost all savor and color when he was not. Hunts, balls, and races crowded her days, but how dull they all were, she sighed, unless Paradise was by.

The discovery that her father was negotiating a marriage for her dissolved this flippant ennui. There was nothing particularly wrong with the Honorable Clotworthy Skeffington, son and heir to Viscount Massereene. On the other hand, there was nothing particularly right with Clodworthy Clotworthy either: he cared nothing for poetry or theater, music or dancing. He would rather listen to his dog snore than to a Latin oration, she exclaimed, and he would have a much better chance of deciphering the dog. The heart of the matter was not his middling looks, his middling character, or even his widely different notion of the finer things in life. It was simply that with the sweet touch of Paradise floating in her mind, the thought of Skeffington so much as brushing her sleeve gave off a faint but unmistakable fire-and-brimstone whiff of Hell.

2 November 1711

I am glad, dear Phil, that you begin to find peace in this world. I despair of it, God knows. The devil to pull and a father to drive, and yet—I don't believe I shall go to Hell for all that, though I have no more hope of Paradise than if I was dead and buried at a thousand fathoms. To say truth, I have been these last ten days in debate whether I should hang or marry, in which time I have cried some two hours every day, and knocked my head against the wall some fifteen times. 'Tis yet doubtful which way my resolution will finally carry me.

For you, if you do abandon hopes of the pretty Paradise you once placed your heaven in, however, may you find another flowing with milk and honey, as charming, as enchanting, and every way worthy of such a lovely Eve.

She paused to stare at the letter that had streamed of its own accord, as it seemed, from her pen. Knowing she would not manage so much as one complete sentence in an interview with her father, she decided to write him a letter as well. Though she wrote to Philippa with the ease of a falcon wheeling in flight, she worked over the missive to Dorchester for days. In what she hoped was just the right tone of submissiveness, she begged to be excused from the proposed marriage. In atonement for refusing his choice, she offered never to marry at all.

He did not deign to send an answer; he sent for her instead, to explain her impertinence in person.

Lined by a gauntlet of footmen, the doors to her father's study yawned open. He was standing near his desk in a golden fall of autumn light. She took a step forward to offer the usual obeisance, but he stopped her with a look. He waved toward her letter, floating alone on the dark gleaming sea of his desk. "What is this aversion you refer to, daughter?"

She tried to speak, but no sound would rise from her throat.

Dorchester leapt into movement, pacing swiftly in front of the long windows. Presently, he said, "No doubt you have some other fancy in your head." He stopped and glanced back at her. "Before you refuse the settlement I have provided for you, daughter, let me be clear: I will never negotiate a treaty with anyone else." He beckoned to her, and she felt her feet slipping across the floor, dragging her to stand before him. "Especially not with that frozen-souled miser Wortley," he said softly. "I will not have my grandchildren reduced to beggary." He bent close; she could smell the cinnamon on his breath and the sweet-sour odor of his body beneath a thick masking scent of musk. "Is it Wortley?"

She shook her head no.

He stepped back, his eyes narrowing. "Then who?"

"No one, my lord," she stammered. "I would prefer to live singly."

"If you are founding your hopes on my death," he said, "you will find yourself mistaken. You will get nothing but a pittance. Enough to keep you out of the poorhouse if you live in a cottage and conserve candle wax."

"Yes, my lord."

Her very meekness infuriated him. "Do I not have the right to dispose of you as I see fit?" he shouted, swiping her letter from the desk and whirling around to face her once more.

Between them, the letter eddied and tossed, spiraling toward the floor.

"Yes, my lord," she said again. "But am I to have no say whatsoever in my own destiny?"

For a moment, it looked as if he might backhand her, but he turned away to stare out the window at the yellowing leaves; somewhere, they were already burning them. He clasped his hands so tightly behind his back that his knuckles blanched. "I am no Calvinist," he said at last, grinding out the words. "Make your own choice: marry Massereene's heir, or live out your life as country-cloistered spinster."

"May I consult the family?"

"Ask the family," he spat. "Ask your friends. Ask the man in the bloody moon. But consider your answer carefully: I will call for it this winter in London." He seated himself and drew out another a set of papers: obviously the draft of her marriage contract. "Meanwhile, you may spend Christmas here alone, to see how you like it. Now get out."

Clinging to the notion that any chance to escape Skeffington was a victory, Lady Mary laid her choices before the rest of the family in the drawing room the next day, as a steely rain needled the windowpanes.

"You are such a little romantic, Mary!" cried Lady Kingston from the tea table, whose control she had greedily assumed as the ranking lady of the family. She had also taken the familial liberty of dropping Mary's "Lady." Lady Mary, however, could not bring herself to address her brother's insipid limpet of a wife as Rachel. She did her best not to address her at all.

She looked hopefully at Frances instead, but Frances shook her head. "I am sorry you will ruin yourself," she said primly. "But if you will persist in being so unreasonable, I cannot blame Father, whatever he may inflict on you."

"What is so wrong with Skeffington?" asked Lady Kingston. "He will make you a viscountess."

"I do not love him," frowned Lady Mary.

"But there is no necessity of loving," exclaimed Lady Kingston, setting her cup down with a definitive click. "Consider the best marriages from one end of town to the other: You will find very few women in love with their husbands, I assure you. Yet many are happy."

Kingston rose. "There, madam, I must agree with you. Thankfully, your equation works equally well the other way round." He bowed and strode from the room.

"You see?" cried Lady Kingston. "Civility is all that is required."

The rain disappeared, and in the last scattershot spears of light, Will found his sister on the rise where she had once taught him to chase the setting sun, just as she had long before down in Wiltshire. Without a word, he took her hand. They both gazed in silence at the fiery globe sinking in the west, but neither made any move to sweep it from the sky.

When it had disappeared, leaving behind the silvery green scent of rain and a sky washed pink and orange, Will cleared his throat. "If it would be of service to you, I will tell Father the hardship he is putting on you. You have only to say the word."

She looked up at him, startled as always that he had somehow escaped little boyhood. When had he grown taller than she? When had he learned such courtliness? But he was nineteen: not yet of age, but a man nonetheless, already married, with a child on the way.

"It will do me no good—nor you either," she said. "He'll just disinherit you."

"He can't," said Will with a wry smile. "Caught fast in his own favorite trap of entail."

She smiled back, in spite of herself. "Perhaps not disinherit. But he can make your life hell."

"He has already delivered me there," he said, looking steadily off into the distance. "Mary," he began, scanning her face, "might there be . . . is there any other man—of smaller fortune, perhaps—who might make you happy?"

"It is impossible, Will," she whispered, squeezing against the lump in her throat. "He is impossible."

He took both her shoulders in his hands. "However much Father is against it," he said with fierce gallantry, "I will assist you in making you happy after your own way. You have only to ask."

The rest of the family left to spend the Christmas holidays in London, leaving Mary and Frances behind at Thoresby, confined to the few small rooms that were all that their father would heat. She took refuge in her correspondence with Philippa.

> *12 December 1711*
>
> *Your obliging letters, Dear Phil, are some consolation to a poor distracted wretch of wretches. 'Tis yet dubious whether I go to Hell or no, but while I delay between doubting and choosing, here I stay, spending the irretrievable days of youth in looking upon withered trees and stone walls. A decayed oak before my window, leafless, half rotten, and shaking its withered top, puts me in mind every morning of an antiquated virgin, bald, with rotten teeth, and shaking of the palsy. I find I have a mortal aversion to being an old maid.*
>
> *Adieu. Don't forget your quondam Sister in Affliction. Write often, long and comforting letters, to your poor, distressed, yet ever faithful friend.*

Dorchester let his daughters stew till the middle of February, sending the coach to fetch them back to London just in time to help with preparations for another wedding: Aunt Cheyne had arranged for their sister Evelyn to marry John Leveson-Gower, Baron Gower, on March 13.

She had thought herself resigned to Hell; then she glimpsed Paradise at the wedding. A few days later, when Dorchester summoned Lady Mary to give her final answer, her certainty surprised them both. "I prefer a single life, my lord, if you would be pleased to allow it."

"Pleasing me," he retorted, "is only to be done by obedience."

That afternoon, he sent a footman to her room. "Your father sends his regards, my lady, and the consequences of your answer," he said, depositing a small valise in her hands with an ostentatious bow. "His Lordship suggests that you pack."

Standing alone in the middle of her chamber, she opened the valise. In the bottom was a note in the hand of her father's secretary. *You will shortly be confined where you may repent at leisure*, said its neat lettering. *Consider this case sufficient to hold all you need for your new life.*

She began to shiver as if the case had held all the cold that Thoresby's unheated stone walls had gathered in thirty years of winter; it seemed to pour forth through her bones in a glacial flood. Later that evening, she wrote her father again, this time in a wavering hand: *My aversion to the man you propose is too great to be overcome. Married to him, I shall be miserable beyond all imagining. I am, however, in your hands. You may dispose of me as you think fit.*

So pleased was Dorchester with this surrender that he strode to her chamber to embrace her as the prodigal daughter returned, allowing her to kiss his hand good-night. From then on, he proceeded as if she had given eager consent.

At the beginning of June, a letter arrived from Lady Jekyll. Inside lay a tightly folded enclosure in a hand Lady Mary had not seen for over a year, and had never expected to see again. *I have been grieved for some time to hear you are to be confined to one you do not like*, mourned Wortley. She agreed to meet him, though only to disabuse him of his error. She could marry or not as she pleased, she assured him.

Almost immediately, the two picked up wrangling where they had left off: about where to meet (Lady Jekyll's, Sir Godfrey Kneller's, or her Italian tutor's), whether she cared enough for him (yes), whether her father could be induced to reopen negotiations with him (no). Wortley was no Paradise, but he was not Hell either. By mid-July, Lady Mary began to glimpse a middling path to escape.

To Wortley, she wrote: *Were I to choose my destiny, I had rather be confined to a desert with you than enjoy the highest of rank and fortune in a court with him I am condemned to.* Still, she did not want to overstate the case. *I am sincere enough to acknowledge*, she added, *there are parts of your humor I could wish otherwise.*

To Philippa, she was more candid.

> *My dear Phil,*
> *My adventures are very odd. I see no probable prospect of my ever entering charming Paradise, but since I cannot convince him of the necessity of what I do, I rack myself in giving him some pain. I may go into Limbo if I please, but 'tis accompanied with such circumstances, my courage will hardly come up to it. In short I know not what will become of me. This is the real state of my heart, which is now so much perplexed and divided that*

I change resolves every three minutes. You'll think me mad, but I know
nothing certain but that I shall not die an old maid, that's positive.
    Limbo is better than Hell.

The decision to elope more or less made, the lovers still found plenty to
dicker about: where and when it would take place, even whether it was best
to abscond in a coach and six, or a coach and pair. Lady Mary did not think
it necessary to tell Wortley that she had not yet said good-bye to Paradise.
She did inform him, however, that she would not make the smallest move
before consulting her brother in Acton. Only when Will promised his support did she go forward.

Come next Sunday under the garden wall, at ten o'clock, she wrote on Monday, August 11. *It will be dark, and it is necessary it should be so.*

Sensing treachery, her father descended upon Acton. Dorchester knew
nothing for certain, but his interrogations of the household convinced him
his suspicions were right. After a terrifying interview, he dismissed Lady
Mary under guard to her chamber, with a command that she was not to
come out again, except to step foot in his coach the next day. She wrote
Wortley in a panic, telling him that their plans had been foiled. *I shall be
sent back to West Dean*, she wailed, *never to come from thence but to give myself
to all that I hate.* Much later, with the rest of the house asleep, she smuggled
out another message: She would creep out onto the balcony between six
and seven o'clock in the morning. If he could, Wortley should contrive to
fetch her then. It would be their last chance.

Shivering as if the birds' morning songs were slivers of ice, she waited
the whole promised hour, but Wortley did not come.

Later that morning she was hustled into her father's coach, escorted by
her brother and a dour old maid of her father's choosing, who made it impossible for Will and Mary to talk. Thundering west, Will never said a
word, but held her hand. She watched him watching the miles streaming
by, a small smile playing around his mouth. Its quicksilver curve seemed
the only tilt of happiness in the whole of a cold, hateful world.

At the inn that night, she discerned his amusement: tipped off to their
route, Wortley had taken a room as another guest. She did not see him that
night or all the next day, though she was aware that he was doggedly trailing their party.

The second night, with her suspicious maid snoring away in the next
chamber, Lady Mary sat up sleepless with her brother. Near midnight, he
excused himself; a minute or two later, the door reopened, but the man it
admitted was not her brother. It was Wortley, wrapped in preposterous
black.

Her anxiety splintered into giggles. "I used to yearn for a bandit king," she said, drawing him to a looking glass, "but I never dreamed he would turn out to be you. If any robbery is committed tonight, you will be taken up for it."

"We have no time for games," he said, grabbing her hand and drawing her through the dimly lit hall and down the stairs. The courtyard was empty but for one mare placidly munching its bit amid torches that were sputtering out.

"Where is the coach?" she whispered.

He made no answer, but mounted the horse, reaching back for Mary. She took a step back.

"Come," he said, motioning impatiently. "There is a parson ready to marry us less than fifteen minutes away. We will be back before anyone suspects we are missing."

In the flickering dark, she seemed to grow half a foot. "What do you mistake me for, Mr. Wortley?" she hissed. "A dairymaid? I am not going anywhere until you provide decent conveyence."

He stared at her for an instant, and then dismounted and stalked back toward the inn.

"Where are you going?"

"To ask your brother if I may borrow the only coach in the house," he said tersely.

She slipped in front of him. *"You cannot be serious."*

"Do you have another proposal?" he asked coldly.

"Involving my brother will force him either to cover his tracks by using me very ill when we return—to the point of beating me black and blue, you understand—or to live in my father's disgrace forever. What sort of return for his kindness would that be?"

"Your father will reconcile himself to us, once the thing is done."

"The thing?" Anger soared inside her. "You do not know him as I do. If you take me, you must take me with nothing but the clothes on my back." She turned on her heel and headed back into the inn. "Adieu. I am entirely yours, if you please."

She saw him no more that night. The next day, her father's coach delivered her to West Dean. A week after that, on the twenty-seventh of August, she went for a walk in the garden with Will; he came back to the house alone, saying that she had wished to walk on.

She never returned. Instead, she slipped through a gate and stepped into a coach manned by no fewer than six footmen. As Wortley wished, they drove to Salisbury in silence, lest they bicker on the way to the altar.

He stared straight ahead with a grim look on his face; Lady Mary watched her former life recede out the window and wept.

The moment Lady Frances heard that Mary was missing, she stoked the fire and began piling it with her sister's journals and bundles of carefully kept letters. Lady Mary was beyond help, but Lady Frances meant to protect herself, Will, and everyone who had ever been an accomplice in the affair. As Lady Mary had predicted, Dorchester's fury was boundless. He cut her off entirely, refusing so much as to hear her name spoken in his presence.

Lady Mary took pains to display unconcern. As soon as possible, she sent Frances a chatty letter from Wortley's home outside York. *I thought to find Limbo*, she gushed, *but I have entered Paradise.*

That position, however, was a front almost from the start. For several years, Wortley had been outraged by his failure to possess her; in possession, he could not bear to be near her. It did not help that he had discovered, after the wedding, that Paradise had been his rival right up until that last flight. In disgust, he turned about-face and ran the other direction, keeping as much distance as possible between them by moving between his London bachelor's quarters over a shop off the Strand, his father's house outside York, and his family's coal-mining business near Newcastle. Lady Mary would not admit she had made a mistake, but by January 1713, she was strongly advising Philippa to choose family over romance.

For all Wortley's jealous fears, she had not cuckolded him. With impeccable timing, she produced a son and heir nine months after the elopement, on May 16. He was christened Edward Wortley Montagu, Jr. Wortley stayed in town for the whole length of her lying-in, the six-weeks court that new mothers presided over from their beds, from which they were not allowed to rise. It was the longest period they had yet spent together. The very morning she was free, she found him in his study, packing.

"So much for conjugal bliss," she said icily from the door.

"You would do well to control your sentiments," he said tersely. "They are nothing but affectation."

"Affectation!" she cried. "A pious prude in love with her stableman, Mr. Wortley, could not be more outraged by her own passion than you are."

They quarreled, and Wortley departed abruptly, leaving Lady Mary to wander about London all afternoon like a soul adrift. *You have not been gone three hours*, she wrote that evening, *and I have called at two people's doors. Without knowing it myself, I find I am come home only to write to you. The late rain has drawn everybody to the Park. I shall pass the whole evening in my chamber, alone, without any business but thinking of you, in a manner you would call affectation, if I should repeat it to you.*

Her eyes sore from hay fever, dim light, and crying, she left off at dusk and went early to bed. The next morning, she awoke early to find Frances pushing hollow-eyed into her bedchamber.

"What is it?" gasped Mary, her stomach dissolving into cold fear for Mr. Wortley.

"It is Will," said Frances. "He has been taken with the smallpox."

❧ 3 ❧

A DESTROYING ANGEL

MY brother has the small pox, Lady Mary scrawled numbly at the bottom of the letter she had written to Wortley the night before. *I hope he will do well.*

She would never have been allowed near the sickroom, since she had not had the disease herself. Still in her father's disgrace, however, she was barred even the comfort of holding vigil with the family. Pacing through her tiny rooms alone with dread coiling tightly about her heart, she had to await the few terse messages Lady Frances could smuggle out and finagle whatever else she could from Dr. Garth.

When word came at last, she sifted between the lines for hope: *My brother,* she wrote Wortley, *is as well as can be expected. But Dr. Garth says 'tis the worst sort, and he fears he will be too full, which I should think very foreboding if I did not know all doctors (and particularly Garth) love to have their patients thought in danger.* She refused to admit that her brother, not yet twenty-one, had already been pronounced beyond remedy. Six days later, on July 1, he died.

The howl that rose through her mounted in waves until she thought she must burst. Fists to mouth, she strangled her grief into a silent scream that she poured into her journal: Will had been her best and only natural friend, standing by her even as she found herself banished from the rest of her family for the sake of a man whose desire had frozen to disdain. His death left her worse than alone.

She had never seen the smallpox at work, but she had heard plenty about it and saw its scarring tracks everywhere. Spotted and blown like a carcass left in the sun, Will began to haunt her dreams. In her waking hours, her fears veered in the direction of Wortley: *Your absence increases my melancholy so much I fright myself with imaginary terrors, and shall always be*

fancying dangers for you while you are out of my sight. . . . I am afraid of every-
thing. There wants but little of my being afraid of the smallpox for you, so unrea-
sonable are my fears, which, however, proceed from an unlimited love. If I lose
you—she broke off and fought for control—*I cannot bear that* If, *which I*
bless God is without probability, but since the loss of my poor unhappy brother, I
dread every evil.

Never again would she dismiss smallpox as a mere irritation. From then
on, it surged dark and terrible in her imagination as her own private demon.

A week after her brother's death, her husband had still finalized no plans to
come south. Terrified for her new son and herself, Lady Mary fled north.
While she stayed near York, searching for a suitable house, Wortley kept
his distance, residing in bachelor's quarters in the tiny borough where he
was campaigning for a seat in Parliament. He insisted that she make all decisions about where and how they would live and grew irritated when she
consulted him, even by letter. Then he questioned all her choices: of
house, of coach and horses, of servants.

Wortley would have preferred the Sheffield area, but she chose the Ital-
ianate elegance of Middlethorpe Hall, just south of York. Shifting between
Middlethorpe and London, Lady Mary whiled away a lonely year playing
with her son and bickering long-distance with Wortley, who continued to
flee every scene as soon as possible after her entrance.

The following summer, this dull run of affairs was punctured by two
deaths and a wedding. At the end of May 1714, the dowager electress
Sophia died in Hanover at the age of eighty-four, leaving her son George
as Queen Anne's heir. Two months later, on July 20, Lady Mary's sister
Lady Frances married John Erskine, earl of Mar, an unprincipled Scottish
spendthrift fifteen years her senior. It was an inexplicable match—except
as political insurance for Dorchester: Mar was a power among the Tory
ministers of state. Lady Mary caught no whiff of the proceedings until too
late to urge rebellion on her sister; she was not even in town when the cer-
emony took place. A week later, the queen fell ill. She had a rosy red rash,
said the whispers; perhaps the scourge of smallpox had struck her family
yet again. It had not, but that reprieve failed to improve her health. On
August 1, 1714, Queen Anne died.

Up in York, Lady Mary saw George I proclaimed king amid fireworks,
pealing bells, and rumbling fears of rebellion in favor of James Francis Edward Stuart, once the Whigs' nemesis as the exiled Prince of Wales and
now the chief challenger to George's claim for the throne. The Pretender,
the Whigs branded him. His followers they called Jacobites—after Jacobus, the Latin form of James.

With the kingdom on the edge of riots and his wife and child in direct path of Jacobite armies rumored to be massing in Scotland, Wortley remained in London, awaiting the new king. In the middle of September George arrived from Hanover to claim his new crown, and Wortley saw his star rise, along with the Whigs generally. He even began to gain ground in reconciling himself to Lady Mary's father; by October 1, she could finish a letter to him saying, "My duty to Papa." The Jacobite rebellion failed to materialize, but consumed by London politics, Wortley ignored his wife.

I cannot forbear any longer telling you I think you use me very unkindly, complained Lady Mary, still alone up in York in November. *I parted with you in July, and 'tis now the middle of November. As if this was not hardship enough you do not tell me you are sorry for it. You write seldom and with so much indifference as shows you hardly think of me at all. You never enquire after your child.*

At last, Wortley stirred himself to make arrangements for Lady Mary and their child to join him in London. *I have taken a house in Duke Street*, he wrote, *near both the park and your father's house.*

She wrote back in a dither. The houses in that street were damp and falling down, she said. In particular, she hoped he had not taken the house of his cousin, Mr. George Montagu, nephew and heir to Lord Halifax, her long-ago partner in rhyme.

Wortley retreated once again to silence. Lady Mary grew frantic, as he knew she would: There was a particular terror about the house in question.

To Mr. Edward Wortley Montagu, to be left at Mr. Tonson's, Bookseller, at the Shakespeare's Head over against Catherine Street, in the Strand, London.

6 December 1714

> *Pray let me know what house you have taken, for I am very much afraid it should be the one where Mr. George Montagu lived and in which Mrs. Montagu and her child both died of the small pox, and nobody has lived in it since.*
>
> *I know 'tis two or three years ago, but 'tis generally said that the infection may lodge in blankets, etc., longer than that. At least, I should be very much afraid of coming into a house from whence anybody died of that distemper, especially if I bring up your son which I believe I must, though I am in a great deal of concern about him.*

Before she could finish this letter, another arrived from her suddenly gregarious husband. Montagu had had two houses in Duke Street, Wortley suggested. He did not bother to say which one he had let.

I have received your second letter, Lady Mary added to the bottom of the one she had already begun, *and hope by your mentioning another house of Mr. G. Montagu's that you have not taken that which Mrs. Montagu died in. I know of but one he lived in, in that street.*

This time, her fears about smallpox were neither random nor irrational. It had come to seem a time-honored tradition for pestilence to shadow the start of each new reign; previously, the epidemics of starkest memory had been the plague. With cruel irony, King George came accompanied by the scourge that had set him on the throne: the smallpox. The disease never entirely departed from London, but before the last epidemic in 1710, there had been a lull for a dozen years, long enough for Londoners to grow complacent, dismissing it as the mere inconvenience of a childhood disease. Now, only four years later, it was back at full putrid strength, sending Londoners young and old scattering before it. Perhaps, rumor muttered, the spans between epidemics would go on dwindling until London bubbled with infection year in and year out.

Once, Lady Mary had tormented Wortley by withholding information in a time of smallpox; now he took revenge in selective silence. *As to the child,* he replied, *if you do wrong about him, you will have no reason to blame me, for I desire it may be as you like best. You shall know by next post which of Mr. Montagu's two houses we have taken,* he promised. *It is certainly not that which was thought in danger of falling.*

The next post came and went, however, with no enlightenment, and Lady Mary began to despair. *I hope you'll take care to have the house all over very well aired, which I am sure is particularly damp in that situation. There should be fires made in all the rooms, and if it be the house Mrs. Montagu died in (which I hope it is not) that all the bedding (at least) be changed. Lady Mary Montagu got the smallpox last year by lying in blankets taken from a bed that had been laid in by one ill of that distemper some months before.*

Finally, just before Christmas, Wortley told her what she wanted to hear: he was not, after all, consigning her to a stew of infection. *I am very well satisfied about the house,* she replied. Even so, she decided to leave their precious son behind in York, rather than expose him to the hazards of a cold journey or cankered city air. At the beginning of the new year, she set out alone for the brave new Hanoverian metropolis of London.

At twenty-five, Lady Mary was beautiful, witty, highborn, and wealthy. She had shackled herself to a husband so cold and remote that she nicknamed him Prince Sombre, but however stingy Wortley could be emotionally, he spared nothing where his reputation was concerned. They had a fine (if possibly infected) house in a fashionable part of town, and he supplied all the gowns and jewels proper to her station. So long as she did not disgrace him, he left her at liberty to do as she pleased. Even the smallpox seemed to bow in her presence and withdraw, waning to a faint glimmer of its former terror. In January 1715, the city spread itself invitingly before her, and she determined to enjoy it.

She acquired an invitation to hear a private reading by a poet her father favored—the rising poet of the age, some said. Having achieved quick fame for his *Pastorals* and a mock epic called *The Rape of the Lock*, Alexander Pope had taken up the greatest of literary dares: He had begun translating into English rhyme the sixteen thousand ancient Greek lines of the greatest of all classics, the *Iliad*.

Lady Mary admired his verse for its muscular symmetry, but the man who stood up to read in the leather-and-gilt hush of Lord Halifax's library was as far from that description as possible. A slender four and a half feet tall, with a back twisted and humped, Pope was a victim of Pott's disease, or tuberculosis of the bone. His detractors snarled that he was a venomous and impotent hunchbacked toad; he mocked himself as "that little Alexander that women laugh at." He was edgy and his forehead was furrowed from chronic pain, but his large eyes snapped with glee.

Lady Mary knew why, for Mr. Congreve and Dr. Garth had let her in on a jest in progress. The previous fall, at Pope's first reading-in-progress of the *Iliad*, Lord Halifax had interrupted the poet several times to proclaim, "I beg your pardon, Mr. Pope, but there is something in that passage that does not quite please. Be so good as to mark the place and consider it a little at your leisure. I am sure you can give it a better turn." Afterward, Dr. Garth had dared the fuming poet to read the same passages over a few months hence, only pretending to have changed them.

Now Mr. Pope bowed awkwardly to Lord Halifax. "I hope Your Lordship will find your objections to these passages removed," he said, and proceeded to read them exactly as he had the first time.

There was a brief, expectant pause. "Nothing can be better!" Halifax exclaimed. "Now they are perfectly right!"

The smothered merriment that burst out later at the postreading celebration in the studio of Pope's friend, the portrait painter Charles Jervas, whirled Lady Mary into the heart of London's literary and artistic elite. Soon, at the challenge of Pope and "Johnny" Gay, she undertook to write a series of seven town eclogues, one for each day of the week, satirizing high society. Peccadilloes in the bedroom, vanity at the dressing table, and folly at the card table: she relished the absurdity of wealthy London's minor sins.

Poets and artists did not occupy all her time: she was also in demand in the highest circles at court. At fifty-five, the king was a handsome man with china-blue eyes, long, fine fingers, and a long nose. As a monarch, he was conscientious and demanding, though not brilliant. As a man, he was a quiet, domestic sort who liked to spend time with family and close friends; he was also a deft storyteller who liked a good, earthy joke. He did not, however, speak more than about ten words of English, and never attempted to learn. For him, German and French were enough.

In part because she could join in the French raillery, Lady Mary soon became one of very few English ladies regularly invited to the intimate supper parties hosted by the two ladies known as "the king's women": his tall, angular, and slightly gawky forty-eight-year-old mistress, Melusine von der Schulenberg, and his portly half-sister, Sophie Charlotte von Kielmansegg. The Maypole and the Elephant, as they were known to the more irreverent wits frisking about the palace.

Though Lady Mary was duly grateful for the weight of the king's eyes upon her, the parties that seemed so relaxed and homely to him seemed to her excruciatingly brittle and dull. One evening, as the Maypole made the king chuckle by snipping caricatures of his courtiers out of paper and the Elephant sparred over some obscure phrase in Mr. Locke's philosophy, Lady Mary had to clench her jaw to keep from screaming with boredom. Her only partner in small high-jinks was thirty-year-old James Craggs, fast rising in the ranks of power due to formidable talent in the council room and an equally formidable talent, it was rumored, in the bedroom. Tonight, he was late; as a result, Lady Mary had been marooned at a card table with three Germans so staid they might as well have been stuffed. Half an hour later, she gave up on Mr. Craggs and dared to contrive an escape.

"*C'est injuste,*" complained the king in his heavily German-accented French as La Schulenberg delivered Lady Mary's request to withdraw early, along with an indulgent recommendation to grant the young lady mercy. "*Absolument perfide,*" he added, gazing down at Lady Mary's black hair and creamy décolletage as she sank into a curtsy. "It is unfair, absolutely perfidious, my lady, that you should cheat me of so charming a presence in such a disloyal manner." It amused him to tease her, engaging her in inventing ever more rococo apologies. Not until he saw that she was no longer certain whether he was teasing—perhaps she had really irritated him—did he allow her to depart. Or desert, as he maintained.

Released, she flew with quick pattering steps down the grand marble staircase of Kensington Palace, her gown billowing behind like wings, brushing against the dark curlicues and leaves of the wrought-iron balustrade. She was glancing over her shoulder, as if pages even now might be chasing after her to call her back, when she ran hard into someone at the foot of the stairs.

"What's the matter?" cried a deep voice as two hands seized her. "Is the company put off?"

"Oh, Mr. Craggs," she gasped. "No. It is just that I have had prodigious trouble in coaxing the king to let me go." Up this close, he was even more handsome than generally allowed, though some affected to scorn his broad-chested exuberance as more proper to a porter than to the whipcord beauty of the ideal courtier.

"The king particularly wished you to stay?" he asked; in reply, she gave him a sly little smile.

Suddenly Mr. Craggs tossed her over his shoulder and leapt upward two and three stairs at a time. No amount of pounding on his back slowed him even a jot; in any case, she was giggling too much to do any real damage. At the arched entryway to the king's apartment, he set her down, ostentatiously kissed both hands, and disappeared without a word. Before she could so much as shake out her crumpled skirts and smooth her hair, the bewildered royal pages flung open the doors and reannounced her.

"*Ah!*" cried the king with obvious pleasure. "*La revoilà!*" She has returned!

There was nothing for it but to curtsy and rejoin the party. "Lord, sir!" she exclaimed as the king raised her up. "I have been so frightened!" Laughing breathlessly, she regaled the company with a lively rendition of Mr. Craggs's prank. Amusement played around La Schulenberg's lips, but the king's older friends gravely shook their heads; the young British were not merely undignified, they were altogether hooligans.

Just then, the pages threw open the doors yet again and announced Mr. Craggs.

"*Mais comment donc, Monsieur Craggs,*" bristled the king, laying a possessive hand on Lady Mary's shoulder, "*est-ce que c'est l'usage de ce pays de porter des belles dames comme un sac de froment?*" Is it the custom in this country to haul fair ladies about like a sack of wheat?

For an instant, Craggs was struck dumb, his expression frozen blank. Recovering, he bowed particularly low. "There is nothing I would not do for Your Majesty's satisfaction," he said smoothly.

The king decided to be pleased; after commending Mr. Craggs's courage in daring to appear ungallant for the sake of still greater gallantry, he turned away again.

"*Bloody hell!*" Craggs swore in Lady Mary's ear. "Do you possess so much as a single drop of discretion?" He had done her a great favor, he made it bitterly clear, keeping her in the king's favor; in return, she had painted him to the king as a rival.

Lady Mary colored, but said nothing. *I dared not resent it*, she wailed to her diary later that night, *for I drew it upon myself, and indeed I am heartily vexed at my own imprudence.*

The king, thought Lady Mary, was a bit of a blockhead, but she liked him for all that. His son was another matter. George, Prince of Wales, she deemed a mean-spirited prig. "He looks on all the men and women he sees as creatures he might kick or kiss—for his diversion," she sniffed to her sister. Soon, however, Lady Mary was drawing the prince's eyes as well as the king's.

One evening, the prince called his wife away from the card table to see how charmingly Lady Mary was dressed. Caroline of Ansbach, Princess of Wales, came as called, but failed to share his raptures. "Lady Mary always dresses well," she observed dryly, returning abruptly to her cards. Soon after, the prince was made aware of Lady Mary's regular attendance at his father's supper parties. Directly, despite all her fine dressing, his ardor not only cooled but curdled; he could no longer see her without taunting her as a deserter gone over to the enemy's camp: throughout the eighteenth century, Britain's kings and their heirs competed jealously for power, splendor, loyalty, and sometimes women.

As her husband soured, the princess grew noticeably more friendly.

On the ninth of August, the day after Lady Mary's sister Frances—now the countess of Mar—gave birth to their first child, the earl her husband disappeared, leaving her without money or any notion of where he might be going. On the tenth, Lady Mary's father was promoted yet again, reaching the pinnacle of the peerage as the first duke of Kingston.

Frances was sworn by her husband's family not to discuss any of her difficulties with her father, but, reduced to selling jewels, plate, gowns—everything of value—she had obviously been left penniless. The earl of Mar soon turned out to be far worse than a wayward husband: he had absconded for Scotland to head the Jacobite armies of the Pretender. The rebellion that had been festering since Queen Anne's death at last broke into the open, and the new duke of Kingston found that instead of acquiring political insurance in the form of a Tory son-in-law, he had saddled the family with one of the chief Jacobite traitors.

In mid-November, Jacobite and loyalist armies clashed in Scotland at the Battle of Sheriffmuir. The Hanoverians claimed victory, but for all its ferocious slaughter, the battle was indecisive. Inept even in treason, Mar unintentionally helped his Hanoverian foes by failing to seize any of the many advantages his army had been left with. In the following weeks, however, the Pretender himself was expected to land any day and galvanize the rebel army into a far more dangerous force. All Britain hushed and hunched down, poised to leap into the carnage of another civil war.

The anxiety of it all exhausted Lady Mary. One afternoon in mid-December, she withdrew early to her chamber. Lying in her stately four-poster bed, canopied and draped in embroidered brocade, she was unable to sleep. The chambermaid must have stoked the fire with enough coal to heat all of Sweden. Tossing and turning, she kicked the bedclothes off. Directly, she shivered and pulled them back up. At last, her head pounding and her skin burning, she rose to drink in cold air at the window, but when she stood up, the room spun. She could barely stagger to the washbasin before she began vomiting.

Still reeling, she called her maid and had young Edward and his nurse packed out of the house without waiting for daylight. By morning, her fever had dipped a little, but her back throbbed dully and her headache intensified until she thought the front of her skull must be clapping open and closed like a loose shutter in a storm. As the sun climbed in the sky, her fever turned around and soared ever higher.

Richard Mead and Samuel Garth, both royal physicians and members of the Royal Society—and Dr. Garth a longtime friend in the bargain—were sent for. But Lady Mary guessed what was wrong long before she heard their coaches halt at her door. After all her running, the demon smallpox had finally caught up with her—as it happened, very close to the same day that it had caught Queen Mary, twenty-one years before.

The two doctors tended toward agreement, though they would confirm no diagnosis before the telltale rash. They ordered her bled, to which she submitted though she detested it, and prescribed both a "gentle" vomit to empty her stomach, and a purge, or laxative, to empty her bowels. Four times a day, they poured down her throat a medicine only a half-step away from magic: two parts powdered bezoar—or ground-up "stones" of calcified hair and fiber found in animal stomachs and valued since ancient times as an antidote to poison—and one part niter, or saltpeter—one of the chief ingredients of black gunpowder. This mixture, Dr. Mead intoned, leaning on his golden-headed cane, was "to keep the inflammation of the blood within due bounds, and at the same time to assist the expulsion of the morbific matter through the skin."

Snow already blanketed the cobblestones of Duke Street below her window, but grooms padded them further with straw. Smallpox, Dr. Mead announced outside her door, was a dangerous effervescence of the blood.

Lady Mary, advised Dr. Garth, his eyes fixed upon Wortley, was therefore to be kept from any commotion, confabulation, and passion—whether grief, love, or fear—that might further stir up the poison boiling inside her.

"How is my little boy?" she begged everyone who drew near. "He is well," came the unvaried reply.

Despite the hushed tiptoeing around her bed, her mind grew restless with a strange, brilliant clarity, as if she had previously been imprisoned in a cloudy crystal ball that some unseen hand had suddenly wiped clean. She could not sleep, but the doctors refused her any opiates, so she chattered through the night, the nurses nodding off as the candles guttered in the darkness.

The next morning, the fever began to fall, though her skin was still hot to the touch. Soon, tiny red flecks no bigger than pinheads and smooth with the surface of her skin sprinkled across her forehead. Hour by hour, they flowed down her body from the top of her head to the tips of her toes, as if some fiery-eyed destroying angel stood caught out of time behind her bed, the hot wind from his wings blowing a slow-motion storm of red sand across her. Even as the flecks drifted downward, those that had appeared first began to rise into hard little bumps. They neither itched nor hurt, but when she rubbed them, they rolled like shot scattered beneath her skin. This time, no diagnosis of measles would rescue her. She most certainly had the smallpox; the only question was what kind.

The next day, the spots went on growing in size and deepening in color, gathering most densely on her face, forearms, and hands. All the while, her fever went on falling, until she felt almost well. Perversely, Dr. Mead and Dr. Garth grew graver with every visit. What they knew but did not tell her—still guarding against fear—was that her rash was already quite thick. At this early stage, that was a dangerous sign.

In the eighteenth century, as in the twentieth, doctors distinguished four main types of smallpox, though they labeled them with different names and distributed them with different logic across the branches of the smallpox family tree. Everyone who dealt with it realized that the best of this bad disease was "distinct" or "discrete" smallpox, which presented a rash scattered thinly enough so that the pocks remained separate—or distinct—with patches of normal skin in between. In "confluent" smallpox, sometimes called "coherent," the rash was so dense that across much of the body—especially the face, hands, and forearms, where it was always thickest—the pocks ran together into one huge festering sore; little to no normal skin was left. In everyday terms, these victims were said to be "very full."

The remaining two types—flat and hemorrhagic—were once often lumped together (sometimes with confluent) as "malignant smallpox." In "flat," "crystalline," or "warty" smallpox, the slow-growing blisters usually ran together, but never really rose much above the surface of the skin and did not fill with the same kind of thick yellow pus found in discrete and confluent pocks. Instead, shallow ripples spread across the skin's surface, stretched over sores buried in its deepest levels; large strips of the top layer of skin, along with the delicate coverings of most mucous membranes (inner nose, mouth and throat, anus, vagina), eventually just sloughed off. Almost three quarters of these cases were children under fourteen.

Hemorrhagic smallpox was subdivided into two kinds, "early" and "late," both marked by profuse bleeding at every orifice, as mucous membranes and blood vessels seemed to melt away. In the early type, once known as "the purples," death came before any pocklike rash broke out, though the skin transformed to dark purple velvet. In late hemorrhagic smallpox, victims survived long enough for blisters—often flat in type—to appear, but they quickly filled with blood, darkening to bruised purple and black, ringed with red. In both kinds of hemorrhagic smallpox, it was not the bleeding, but heart failure or fluid in the lungs (pulmonary edema) that proved the immediate cause of death. Nearly all these cases were adults; two thirds were women.

These malignant cases were relatively rare (just over 9 percent of the total number of smallpox cases), but they were death sentences so terrible to behold that they loomed monstrous in the imagination. Flat smallpox carried about a 3.5 percent chance of survival; in late hemorrhagic smallpox it was 3.2 percent. Early hemorrhagic smallpox had no survivors.

Eighteenth-century doctors saw these malignant types as crop failures. Flat and purple smallpox did not ripen properly, while confluent cases quickly grew overripe. Twentieth-century doctors explained all three of these serious developments as the results of differing degrees of immunodeficiency; some people with otherwise healthy immune systems inexplicably had little to no power to fight back against the variola virus. As early as the seventeenth century, it was known that such weakness in the face of smallpox ran in families—the Stuarts, for example. Pregnancy was another high-risk factor, already obvious to early doctors.

In Lady Mary's sickroom, the first days sped by in pairs. The first prerash fever had been much the most uncomfortable stage so far. As the red spots flowed down her body across the following two days, she began to feel better. With her fever still falling, she felt better still as the spots bubbled into blisters for another two days. "How is my boy?" she kept asking.

"Still unspotted," came the answer.

The same could no longer be said for her. As she watched, the red bumps filled with a clear liquid that gradually thickened to opalescent grayish white; now they began to look like large flat pimples that might be called "pocks." A ring of red circled the base of each one, while their centers sank in a small dimple.

At last she saw what the doctors had been quietly worried about: hour by hour, the pocks went on growing, running into each other until large sections of skin looked to be covered by a single marbled blister. She could not see it, but her face swelled so much that her finely carved features began to submerge, the skin pulling taut over nose, ears, chin, and cheeks; her eyes squeezed into slits. Those who did glance at her face thought she looked unnaturally old or young: the disease was transforming her into a grotesque gigantic changeling, wrapped in a tight gray caul that veiled all her features.

At last, the doctors issued a diagnosis: she had the confluent smallpox. The news skittered around London and winged north to the armies burning Scotland: *Lady Mary is exceedingly full and will be very severely marked.*

However much they irritated her, Lady Mary was lucky in having Dr. Mead and Dr. Garth at her bedside. Besides being known for compassion, they were both moderates in an age when medicine was unabashedly aggressive; in attempting to be heroic, it was more often horrific.

A very few practical men had begun systematically observing their patients and describing symptoms that clustered into specific maladies. The most eminent physicians of the day, however, were abstract philosophers who snipped and stretched experience to fit theory, in their case a modified version of the ancient Greek theory of the four humors. Good health, in this system, was a perpetual circus act, balancing ever-shifting quantities of blood, black bile, green bile, and phlegm, as well as the oppositions of hot and cold, moist and dry. Imbalances tipped people into the morass of sickness; restoring a patient to health meant bringing them back into balance.

To do so, doctors tried to relieve whatever the body was producing in too much abundance by either repressing or removing it, while nurturing the growth of whatever they judged to be lacking. It was the relief side of this equation into which medicine had long put most of its efforts and its faith—though *relief* proves a bizarrely inopportune word for their ministrations.

Any and all possible bodily emissions were sometimes thought necessary to force. The most commonly practiced "evacuation" was bloodletting: slitting veins open at the wrists, arm, groin, or in serious cases, the jugular, to let poisons escape with the blood. If all else failed—or, in the delicate cases of infants, right at the beginning—doctors applied leeches to the temples or behind the ears. They also induced sweating, salivating, and blistering, and they administered clysters, or enemas, and ferocious laxatives and diuretics. An unholy array of emetics produced immediate and sometimes prolonged vomiting. Many, if not most, of the medicines they put into a body were designed to send something else shooting out of it, making eighteenth-century medicine a leaky, spraying, spewing art.

It was an art, furthermore, divided into three territories with jealously—though often unsuccessfully—guarded boundaries. Physicians were university men with medical doctorates. High (and highly expensive) priests of the mysteries of diagnosis, they solemnly prescribed treatments but rarely provided them, though things were changing in progressive and ruthlessly practical places like Edinburgh, or the University of Leiden over in Holland. In London, any procedure, such as bloodletting, that involved cutting was still by law the purview of the surgeons—historically, a specialized branch of the razor-bearing brethren of barbers, with whom they shared a guild until 1745. In contrast to the learned doctors, a surgeon was a mere "Mr." who learned his trade by apprenticeship. The men who concocted the potions and powders that physicians prescribed were the apothecaries, or pharmacists. Scurrying through the cracks in this system was an army of panacea-peddling quacks, mountebanks, and empirics.

Wealthy patients not only paid all three of the proper medical professions to dance attendance at their sickbeds: as a kind of status symbol of conspicuous consumption, they consulted multiple physicians. Poorer people made do with surgeons, apothecaries, local wisewomen or nurses, and the potions of the quacks: and were often better off for it.

Lady Mary was neither stifled with blankets, nor frozen with drafts of the bitterly cold December wind. Instead, her room was kept as pure and cool—but not frigid—as possible. She was fed a meager diet of oatmeal and barley-gruel. In the beginning, the cooks were directed to boil preserved figs, plums, and tamarinds with her gruel, to keep her "open and cool." To drink, she had mild diuretics: small-beer "acidulated" with orange and lemon juice, and sweet German wine thinned with water.

Every two or three days, the surgeon arrived to bleed her: to relieve the poison boiling over in her blood. Even this was moderate. Some physicians, sniffed Mead, were terrified to bleed at all, while others could not be stopped: when the virtually unkillable King Louis XIV of France had had smallpox, he was bled ten or eleven times in a matter of weeks.

A week after she had fallen ill, her fever was almost down to normal. Bored with illness and still fretting over her child, she claimed she felt fine, but the doctors would not let her get up. Across the next four days, the gray liquid inside the pocks went white and congealed to beeswax-yellow pus; the rosy rings around their bases faded. Still, though Lady Mary would not have thought it possible, the pocks went on growing. Her distended skin began to hurt. The sores glued her upper lip to her now bottle-shaped nose, and her face grew blank and bored as her features disappeared beneath the swelling. Her peglike fingers could no longer wield a pen. Her mouth, too, was filled with sores, along the tip and sides of her tongue, the roof of her mouth, and the back of her throat. Just as it became agony to swallow, saliva gushed out in rivers.

For a while, she managed the single rasping word, *"Boy."* Then even that was scraped from her, and the world collapsed into a narrow battle to survive.

On the eighth day of the rash, the tenth of her illness, her period gushed out early, ruining the sheets in a flood more like a hemorrhage. Her fever spiked back up to the heights it had reached in the first two days. Worst of all, some of the pocks began to burst, emitting a cadaverous stench.

Like the queen before her, she had made a quick, cursed journey from beauty to beast, no longer fit to delight the eyes of a king. She might be too sick to know it, but others were riveted from one end of the kingdom to the other: *Poor Lady Mary Wortley has the small pox,* gossiped James Brydges, earl of Carnarvon, to a friend fighting in Scotland, *just as it began (to her great joy) to be known she was in favor with one whom every one who looks on cannot but love. Her husband, too, is inconsolable for the disappointment this gives him in the career he had chalked out of his fortunes.*

"With a pair of good eyes like Lady Mary's, being marked is nothing," Lady Loudoun scoffed to her husband, also with the army in Scotland. Complexions, she commented archly, could be bought.

Eleven days in, Lady Mary entered the critical stage of confluent smallpox. In places, strips of skin peeled away; elsewhere, boils erupted as secondary infections attacked the raw, stagnating wounds. A brown crust crept over her whole body; from under the scabs leaked pus stained rust with blood. What little was left of her skin felt sheeted in flame as her temperature jagged even higher, hovering between 103° and 105°—though they did not then measure temperatures so exactly, relying on touch. She slid in and out of delirium. Most ominously, her breath began to rattle in her chest. In confluent smallpox, it was this secondary or "suppurative" infection caused by reabsorbing all that pus—or else pneumonia triggered by the infection of the airways—that killed.

For two days across Christmas, whispers slid through the drawing rooms: Lady Mary would die.

While she fought for her life, the whole kingdom held its breath and peered northward, wondering about its own survival: on December 22 up in Scotland, the Pretender landed at last.

For Lady Mary, the crisis receded as suddenly as the disease had sprung forth. Just before dawn on the fifteenth day, her fever broke. *"My son,"* she whispered, as the world settled back into place around her. "Safe," began the nurse, but that was enough. Lady Mary sank into a deep, healing sleep.

Slowly—maddeningly slowly—the scabs dried and began to fall off. By the end of the first week of January 1715, the swelling was subsiding and the rattling of her breath was gradually growing mute. Most of the dark crust that had covered the rest of her body had crumbled away, though the dark-brown "seeds"—or imbedded scabs—of smallpox still lay buried in the palms of her hands and soles of her feet. She would live; that was now clear. What kind of life might be in store for her, though, was not.

They had veiled the mirrors on her walls and dressing table when she first fell ill, and no one had as yet made any offer to uncover them. By the twisted red pits that now mottled her still swollen hands and arms, she was not sure if she wanted them to.

Curiosity and dread plucked her mind this way and that. At last, she asked her maid to bring her a hand mirror and then sent her away again. Reclining on a couch, her face hidden beneath a silken mask, she could see frost dancing in filigreed designs across the tall windows. Snow thinned daylight to a pale, downy blue; even so, the light made her eyes ache.

She kept the mirror carefully reversed, playing fitfully with the light that careened off its surface and shattered against the far wall. On that same wall gleamed the portrait that Sir Godfrey Kneller, the finest painter in the kingdom, had finished of her only a few months ago. In his hands, the ivory sheen of her gown set off the creaminess of her face, breast, and hands. As a matter of course, he had caught the likeness of her delicate features; more mysteriously, he had also caught the shine of intelligence in her eyes, and wicked merriment in the pointed arch of her brows, inherited from her father.

She would not look like that, anymore. "It would make a man weep to see what she was then, and what she is like to be, by people's discourse, now": so the diarist Samuel Pepys had mourned in 1668, standing before two portraits of Frances Stewart, duchess of Richmond and breathtakingly beautiful mistress of King Charles II. He had gone in his coach to stare at the paintings four days after the whispers had scuttled through London that Richmond—like Lady Mary more recently—was "mighty full" with the smallpox. The duchess would live, they murmured, but "wholly spoiled."

Only a little more than a month ago, another king had been casting his eye upon Lady Mary, and the whole world seemed to lie in raptures at her feet. From what she had gleaned lately, that would no longer be the case. When she asked Dr. Garth about her face, he had set aside his frown and pronounced with forced cheer that she would again be fair, but she hadn't trusted him since her brother died. Others who had clustered around her bed, clucking sympathetically, had been more circumspect.

She slipped off the mask and twirled the mirror around.

The face she saw was unrecognizable. Though the swelling had gone down since the worst of the crisis, her fine, long nose was still bottle shaped, her lips thickened and cracked. Her eyelids were puffy and her eyelashes had all fallen out. The last time she had glanced in a mirror, her skin had glowed like translucent ivory; now she saw deep, twisted craters stained a splotchy reddish brown, as if someone had slapped over the face she knew a thick, poorly modeled mask of discolored, clotted papier-mâché. At least Mr. Wortley, she thought bitterly, would be satisfied. Once, he had wished she might lose her complexion so that she might also lose some of her admirers; smallpox had finally granted his wish.

She called her maid back and handed her the mirror. "Take that picture out of my sight," she said, nodding at the Kneller. *Before I tear it*, she thought—though, really, it would take a full-fledged knife-throwing brawl to make the face once again match its disfigured original. As the maid staggered away with the painting, Lady Mary did what she always did in distress: she rose, crossed to her desk, and picked up a pen.

> *How am I chang'd! Alas, how am I grown*
> *A frightful spectre to myself unknown!*

For almost a hundred rhyming lines, a new eclogue spilled through her pen, full of self-mockery. Once, she had spent hours at her dressing table, deep in happy debate about the fall of curls and the exact placement of beauty patches. Opera tickets, perfume, Japanese lacquer, and flowers had all been strewn at her feet. Statesmen, soldiers, beaus, wits, gamblers, and country squires had vied for a kind glance; she had herself paused on her way out the door, to appreciate the figure in her mirror. But "now," sighed Lady Mary, "beauty's fled, and lovers are no more."

But it was not just that admirers had fled, she mused; her enemies were stepping out of the shadows to take their place. When it was thought she would die, someone showed another of her eclogues to the Princess of Wales, whose court it lampooned. As it became clear that Lady Mary would live, her enemies crowed over what this impolitic bit of poetry might do to whatever shreds were left of her court career. "She will be pitted but not pitied," tittered the many ladies who despised her.

Her friends had carried these insults to her like some foully titillating bouquet, expecting her to hurl sharp quills of revenge, but Lady Mary was less concerned about Caroline than the king: the face she had seen in the mirror was no delicacy to delight a monarch. Titles, offices, lands, and palaces: these were sugarplums that fell into the laps of kings' playfellows, all now slipping away like the white silk remnants of a dream. . . . Wortley would not be pleased about that, at least. But he would not be the only one watching either. She winced, knowing that the snake den of London society—friends and enemies alike—would stare in fascination as the king's attraction for her went slack and began to feather elsewhere. *Pitted, but not pitied*, indeed. Her pen began to scratch across the paper once more:

> *Cease hapless maid, no more thy tale pursue,*
> *Forsake mankind, and bid the world adieu.*
> *Monarchs and Beauties rule with equal sway,*
> *All strive to serve, and glory to obey,*
> *Alike unpitied when depos'd they grow,*
> *Men mock the idol of their former vow.*

Her reverie was interrupted by the arrival of Dorothy, Lady Townshend—as innocent, imprudent, and flittering as her brother Sir Robert Walpole was careful and cunning, and long one of Lady Mary's closest confidantes.

Dolly caught her breath as Lady Mary turned unmasked toward the door. "Oh, Mary," she cried, crossing the room to take her friend's hand. "You have lost more loveliness than I ever saw in another face."

Lady Mary sighed, set down her pen, and rang for tea. At least Dolly was honest. "'Tis certain, dearest Dolly, that I have lost what beauty I had—just when I was beginning to realize its advantages."

⇥ 4 ⇤

BIDDING THE WORLD ADIEU

"THERE is no species of fever," announced Dr. Mead, "which requires the body to be thoroughly cleared of the remains of the disease more than the smallpox." So Lady Mary's blood was let yet again, and she was purged several more times. After that, recovery called for drinking deep drafts of both asses' milk and fresh air.

It was a bitterly cold winter: the Thames froze solid enough to hold a frost fair on its strangely solid, opaque surface. Wrapped in furs, with hot stones tucked beneath her feet on the coach floor and her face protected from snow glare and curious stares alike by the silken mask she never shed, Lady Mary ventured out to share in the carnival games, puppet shows, roast apples, and fortune telling. She also began once more to entertain a chosen few of her old admirers in the safe warmth of her home: Mr. Jervas, Mr. Pope, and Johnny Gay were not allowed to see the ruin of her face, but she welcomed their undiminished adoration of her mind.

Early in February, the Pretender scuttled back to France; the earl of Mar went with him. As the fever of rebellion fizzled out, the nation, too, began to recover. In London, a few Jacobite prisoners were executed, but the king exhibited remarkable leniency for the period. Even as Parliament attainted Mar, the crown granted his wife not only safety but an income. The loyalty and goodwill of Frances's family were not to be trifled with.

Even now, Lady Mary managed to get herself into more trouble than her sister—and to do so in rhyme. The Princess of Wales had digested her acidic poem in silence, but the rest of the world could not let it go. Late in March, the disreputable pirate-publisher Edmund Curll printed it along with a few others, hinting that they were by Pope, Gay, or "a lady of quality," by which everyone understood Lady Mary. Deeming this attribution to be more scandal-mongering advertisement than discreet disguise, Pope determined to take revenge. Two days later, he arranged to meet Mr. Curll at the shop of his own publisher, Bernard Lintot. After first scolding Curll as a knave, Pope reluctantly made a peace offering of a glass of wine. It was a ruse: Pope doctored Curll's drink, and the printer spent the rest of the day and night vomiting.

Lady Mary snickered until Pope published his schoolboy prank in grotesque detail in a pamphlet titled *Full and True Account of a Horrid and Barbarous Revenge by Poison, on the Body of Mr. Edm. Curll*. Abruptly, Lady Mary stopped laughing. Though her name never actually showed up in print in connection with this fiasco, it might as well have proclaimed it with a flourish of trumpets. She did not find the cost to her reputation pleasing; Wortley was even less amused.

They did not have to face this absurd disgrace for long. On the seventh of April, the newspapers named Edward Wortley Montagu as the next British ambassador extraordinary to the Ottoman Empire—or Porte, as the empire's government, perched at the other end of Europe in Constantinople, was then called. He had accepted the next-to-impossible job of brokering peace between the Holy Roman and the Ottoman empires, just when the emperor and the sultan were glaring daggers at each other, preparing once more to unleash their dogs of war.

"*Forsake mankind, and bid the world adieu*," Lady Mary murmured to herself. To her friends' uncomprehending horror, she announced that both she and baby Edward would go along.

Preparing for her journey, Lady Mary regained her old strength and spirit, but she kept her face hidden behind the silken mask.

"You must take it off sometime, my dear," said Dolly.

"Never," said Lady Mary. Friends, admirers—even acquaintances who had glimpsed her once across the theater, she sighed in exasperation—sent remedies to erase the smallpox scars. "All marked infallible," she said, rifling through the jars, bottles, and powder papers piled higgledy-piggledy on a table in her sitting room, "which is true, so long as you are discussing failure." She picked up a few and read their labels. *Lemon juice and salt to bleach the brown stains. A syrup of white wine steeped with sheep's dung.*

"I thought that was a preventative," said Dolly.

"Prevents good taste," said Lady Mary. "Before, during, and after." She dropped the bottle back on the table and moved on. *Ointment of almond oil, chicken grease, goat tallow, and gold. Alternating face-washes of vinegar and bran-water. A jelly of camphor and calves' feet.* Snatching up a scrap of paper, she stared at it in silence for a moment, and then sank into a chair in helpless wonder. "From Mrs. Brownlow," she said, tossing it to Dolly. "Her recipe for boiling cream to an oil, with directions to anoint it with a feather. She would have sent the feather, too, but after Meg died the servants burned it."

"At least that one worked," said Dolly with a shiver. "Skulls don't have scars, leastways, not that kind of scar. I think you should investigate the Balm of Mecca. Sounds so exotic, and has nothing to do with, well—"

"Excrement," said Lady Mary. "No—it is said to be made from tears wept by a tree more aromatic than frankincense. Unfortunately, it is also as rare as the phoenix, and as dear. Half an ounce is said to be worth a whole kingdom. Mr. W will never pay."

"Kingdoms come cheap in Constantinople," sniffed Dolly.

The strangest story of all, though, came from Dr. Garth, his coach hurtling up to Lady Mary's door after a meeting of the Royal Society. Presided over by Sir Isaac Newton, the Royal Society was one of Europe's most elite gatherings of scientifically interested men, so voracious for information about the natural world that they had begun soliciting news from every nook and cranny across the globe. Two and a half years earlier, in October of 1713, reported Dr. Garth, a preposterous tale had trickled west. The Turks, it was said, protected themselves from smallpox by inserting the scab of someone else's pock into a small incision in their own skin.

Lady Mary shuddered and laughed.

"Precisely," said Dr. Garth with a nod. But several months later, the Fellows had heard the absurd story again, this time in more detail from one of their own members, Dr. Emanuel Timonius, then practicing medicine in Constantinople. "Foreign, you know," shrugged Dr. Garth. "Italian. But is a Fellow, with a degree from Oxford as well, so was deemed to merit at least passing attention." Dr. Timonius not only repeated the tale, but claimed miraculous success for "engrafting," as he called this practice of transferring the disease from one person to another. Still dubious, Sir Hans Sloane began canvassing other sources, particularly Dr. William Sherard, British consul in Smyrna. They had just heard back from Dr. Sherard, said Dr. Garth. Engrafting, or inoculation, was not practiced in Smyrna, but Sherard had heard of it.

Lady Mary leaned forward. "Heard what?"

"That is all he said," reported Dr. Garth. "Though he promised to endeavor to find out more."

At the end of May, at a glittering farewell party given in Lady Mary's honor by Lord and Lady Townshend, Dr. Garth made a beeline through the poets and the painters toward the guest of honor, still masked. Tossing aside some superfluous conversation on drama, or verse form, or possibly architecture, like so much kindling, he announced that the Royal Society had at last received Dr. Sherard's final report on engrafting.

"*Engrafting!*" protested a young poet. "What will we care about tending orchards, once we have lost the very flower of British wit?"

"A great deal, I imagine," said Lady Mary, "when you discover that this engrafting claims to prevent the flowering of the smallpox."

Around them, the crowd quieted and drew closer.

"Dr. Sherard," said Dr. Garth, "has confirmed Dr. Timonius's account, and forwarded a paper by a certain Dr. Jacopo Pylarinus of Venice, who has also practiced medicine in Constantinople."

Lady Mary cocked her head, and Dr. Garth bowed and proceeded. Both Timonius and Pylarinus, he said, claimed that an old hag would prick a patient's arm with a needle; into the blood that appeared, she would mix a tiny bit of "matter" or pus from the pock of some unfortunate sufferer of full-blown smallpox. The recipient soon contracted a mild form of the disease, suffering no more than a brief, low fever and a few shallow pocks that quickly dried up and fell off, leaving no scars. The operation was said to have originated among the Circassians, he said with a mischievous glance at the mooning young poet, whose daughters were the most exquisite of the hothouse flowers to be found in Turkish harems.

Lady Mary cut his jest short. "Why haven't we tried it?" she cried. "Why haven't *you* tried it? The Royal Society? The Royal College of Physicians?"

"Because it is an old wives' tale, my lady."

"Begging your pardon, Doctor," chimed in Lord Townshend's brother, a merchant who had spent three years in Constantinople a few years before. "But Lady Mary's question has merit. With my own eyes, I have seen two hundred people undergo the operation. Only two died."

Dr. Arbuthnot's voice sliced through the rising babble. "A new book by Peter Kennedy—a Scottish surgeon who has himself visited Constantinople—considers the reasons judiciously: in his estimation, it is fear of death on a grand scale that makes the British so timorous to try it. No one, says Mr. Kennedy, knows whether inoculation will in fact deliver the protection bestowed by a natural bout with smallpox, but we can be pretty certain that the operation will pass on the disease. It might well trigger an epidemic."

"I have read that book," said Mr. Townshend. "You have left out Mr. Kennedy's uncertainty: 'If this method is so innocent as those who practice it assert or maintain it to be,' he writes, 'it need be no more minded than giving or taking the itch.'"

"Fear!" scoffed Lady Mary. "I should rather claim greed as an excuse."

"You have put the question the wrong way round," said Dr. Garth. "It is not why haven't we tried it, but why *should* we? Only two died, Mr. Townshend says: but as I would put it, only two were killed. Why should we take such a risk?"

In answer, Lady Mary reached up and slipped off her mask; around her every other face blanched.

Slowly, her face had recovered most of its old shape. She was not, as she had feared, entirely disfigured: but her great beauty had been scraped away. Despite all the ointments and jellies and washes, her skin remained stained and pitted, as roughly scored as a nutmeg grater. Her eyelashes had never come back, changing her once merry gaze into a fierce, falconlike glare.

"To prevent this," she said.

Timonius's and Pylarinus's descriptions were duly published in the *Transactions of the Royal Society*—along with various reports about giants' bones, rattlesnakes, comets, fortune-telling dreams, and weird weather—but after an initial sensation, interest proved short-lived. As Dr. Garth predicted, inoculation was dismissed as an old wives' tale, a bit of mystical Oriental nonsense, good for a pleasant little shiver of curiosity at the bizarre and backward practices of the East, but no more.

Meanwhile, Lady Mary left her mask off and quietly laid her final plans for her family's departure. They included hiring one of Mr. Kennedy's colleagues, another Scottish surgeon named Charles Maitland, to attend the Wortleys throughout their stay in Turkey.

On the first of August, 1716, Lady Mary and Wortley, their three-year-old son and his nurse, their new Scottish surgeon, a chaplain, secretaries, lady's maid, valet, steward, two cooks, footmen, grooms, and other assorted servants in silver livery stepped up into coaches and wagons. The crowd cheered, sniffled, and waved farewell, and the adventurers waved back. Then the drivers shouted, horses leaned into their harness, wheels grudgingly poured into their work, and the new British ambassador extraordinary to the Ottoman Porte and his entourage were off.

Holding heavily scented handkerchiefs to their noses, the cavalcade ducked beneath the ornamental arches at Temple Bar, now decorated with the heads of Jacobite traitors, and crossed the bridge over the open sewer of the Fleet Ditch. Clattering through Lud Gate—the westernmost gate in the old city walls—they strained uphill into the summer-ripe throng of London. Everyone, it seemed, was trying to sell something with a song: cherries, chair mending, or chickens (alive and squawking), socks and songbirds (alive and singing), asparagus and almanacs, eels and oysters, books and brooms, milk, matches, and mops. On either side, shops like little gilded theaters wafted perfume and compliments into the street.

The ambassador's party churned past the new expanse of St. Paul's Cathedral and turned sharply south, skidding down the steep hill and across shop-lined London Bridge. Long lines of laborers and wagons piled high with produce streamed against them, pushing to get into the city. On a rise beyond the bridge, they halted to gaze back one last time. St. Paul's sleek new dome rose from the city's gables like an immense pillared egg. On every side, sun glinted off an urban forest of spires and dodged among fraying threads of smoke to spill like a shower of gold coins across the Thames, still dotted with barges and oared boats and striped with long wharves.

They did not expect to see home again for many years, but Wortley was not the sort to moon with sentiment. His business lay far to the east, in another city at the opposite edge of Europe. By far the fastest and easiest route to Constantinople lay by sea, south around Spain and then east across the Mediterranean. Determined to find some way to coax the emperor and the sultan into an unlikely peace, however, Wortley had opted for the difficulty and dangers of an overland journey in order to stop first in the emperor's favorite city of Vienna.

From the Rhine to the Main to the Danube, from the Morava to the Iskar to the Maritza, to the Golden Horn itself with the ethereal brilliant blue of the sea floating beyond, they followed the paths that water had carved across the European continent. Whenever they could, they floated smoothly and silently down the rivers. When they could not, they stepped into coaches and trundled along the banks, raced across wide plains, or toiled through mountain passes at preposterously steep angles, inching between fanged peaks draped in glaciers and snowfields like diamond necklaces laid across ermine.

On September 3, they arrived in Vienna, a pleasure hive of balls and operas, concerts and theater, as well as a den of intrigue. Its citizens had long since run out of room on the ground and had begun piling their way into the sky. All the houses reached the dizzying height of five or six stories—as if the builders, Lady Mary exclaimed, had "clapped one town on top of another." Shoemakers and tailors lived next door to great ladies and ministers of state, with no more than a thin partition dividing them. The interior furnishings of even the minor nobility's apartments, though, were as magnificent as those of sovereign princes elsewhere: moderation was no virtue in Vienna.

Before Lady Mary could be presented at court, she had to acquire a properly monumental court gown: "more monstrous and contrary to all common sense and reason," she wrote to Frances, "than 'tis possible for you to imagine." Its hooped skirt and train covered acres of ground; while the whalebone cage of the bodice and high-backed collar squeezed Lady Mary's torso into a tinier space than she had thought possible. Inconvenient, not to mention uncomfortable, she remarked, but it certainly showed the figure to great advantage.

She also had to have her hair done. Viennese ladies engaged architecturally minded hairdressers and lady's maids to build their hair into three-story towers a yard high, reinforced with gauze and ribbon and bristling with jeweled bodkins—"it being a particular beauty," scoffed Lady Mary, "to have their heads too large to go into a moderate tub." As she watched in horrified fascination, her hair was combed over a pad the same shape—but four times as big—as the rolls that London milkmaids used in balancing their wide wooden pails on their head. To Lady Mary's natural hair, the headdress architects added a great deal of false hair, plastering the mixture together with prodigious amounts of powder.

Dipping and swaying like a ship under top-heavy sail, she tottered off to be formally presented to the three empresses. Fair haired and twenty-five, the reigning empress Elisabeth Christine played cards, waited upon by two dwarfs. The black-veiled empress mother Eleanore Magdalene proved tiresome, "perpetually performing extraordinary acts of penance," sniffed Lady Mary, "without having ever done anything to deserve them." The dowager empress Amalia, however, commandeered her interest. Presiding over a shooting contest, Amalia sat enthroned in her garden, surrounded by archduchesses and maids of honor in full court dress, their Tower-of-Babel hair sparkling with jewels. All the noblemen of Vienna pressed round as spectators, but only the ladies were allowed to shoot. They took turns aiming light guns down a long alley at three targets: Cupid holding a goblet of wine, Fortune holding a garland, and a sword circled with a poet's laurels. Bestowed by the dowager empress herself, first prize was a fine ruby ring set round with diamonds, in a gold snuffbox. It went, as a matter of course, to an archduchess who happened to be not only her daughter but her namesake.

In Vienna, even adultery was both excessive and ritualized; every great lady was expected to display a husband on one arm and a gallant lover on the other. Lady Mary had many offers from young men eager fill the lover's place, but she refused them all. "She sticks to her English modes and manners," one English courtier reported to another, "which exposes her not a little to the railleries of the Vienna ladies. She replies with a good deal of spirit, and is engaged in a sort of petty war, but they all own she is a witty woman, if not a well-dressed one." Pope wrote to tease that she had "out-traveled the sin of fornication" to arrive "at the free region of adultery." He could not fathom why she should persist in wishing to "pass from that charitable court" and head for "the land of jealousy, where the unhappy women converse with none but eunuchs, and where the very cucumbers are brought to them cut."

Though diplomats on all sides wanted the British ambassador to press onward to Constantinople, King George had other ideas. He summoned Wortley to attend him in his beloved Hanover, which he was visiting for the first time since taking the British throne. So in the middle of November, the Wortley Montagus veered north.

Lady Mary despised Bohemia (now the western part of the Czech Republic), complaining that the villages were so poor that clean straw and water were "blessings not always to be found." Sometimes they traveled all night rather than stop at one of the miserable inns whose hot, crowded rooms were itchy with vermin and thick with foul scents. In Prague, she proclaimed the fashions even more absurdly excessive than in Vienna: between hoopskirts and headdresses, the women virtually disappeared. On the other hand, the city's cooks dished up the best wildfowl that she had ever tasted.

Crossing the mountains dividing Bohemia from Saxony at night, she peered out the frost-etched window and saw barely an inch of grace between the wheels and a precipice that sheered hundreds of feet into the foaming anger of the River Elbe. Silhouetted up ahead in the moonlight, she glimpsed the postilions—the men who supposedly controlled the coach by riding its horses rather than driving them—nodding off while the horses thundered into a wild gallop. Forcing the window open, she leaned out and shouted, *"Look where you are going!"* Next morning, Mr. Wortley grudgingly commended her for saving all their lives.

Stopping in Leipzig only long enough to buy material to make liveries for still more pages, as well as some "gold stuffs" for Lady Mary—all for half what it cost in Vienna, she exulted—they raced ever northward, arriving in Hanover on the night of November 23. King George loved its neat comforts, but his cramped court had long since grown peevish, despising the place as an overstuffed snippet of a city. The Portuguese ambassador counted himself quite lucky to have two wretched parlors in an inn, but the Wortley Montagus found themselves installed in the spacious luxury of the palace.

"*Ah! La revoilà!*" teased the king, indulging in their old private jest as Lady Mary was presented, but though he took little notice of any other lady thereafter, irritating the Hanoverians no end and delighting the English, she soon discerned that his affection was of a different nature than it had been. She amused him, and he wished to impress her, poor lady; that was all. "Both pitted *and* pitied," thought Lady Mary ruefully as she followed him about, professing rapture with the German ingenuity that invented superb heaters and then disguised them as China jars, statues, or inlaid cabinets. At least she did not have to feign fascination with the results, as baskets piled high with oranges, lemons, and other exotic fruit appeared upon the king's dinner table in the middle of winter. "A fruit perfectly delicious," she rhapsodized upon her first taste of pineapple.

Lady Mary's friends had all expected she would greet Hanover as an opportunity to pull out of the arduous journey; perhaps the king, too, indulged in that hope. She surprised them all. "While Mr. W is determined to proceed in his design, I am determined to follow him," she announced, stepping back in the coach. *Forsake mankind, and bid the world adieu*, she told herself.

As the Wortleys reentered Vienna, Lady Mary's friends both new and old grew seriously alarmed. Prince Eugene of Savoy, general-in-chief of the emperor's armies, warned her of killing cold on the snow-covered Hungarian plain. Others hinted at deaths far worse than freezing; Pope's letters twitched that curtain of discretion aside, dwelling openly on rape.

Hungary, Serbia, Bulgaria, and Macedonia had been killing fields for several centuries, yanked this way and that between the Holy Roman Emperor and the Ottoman sultan. Only six months earlier, Prince Eugene's army had annihilated an entire Turkish army at Peterwaradin (modern Petrovaradin, now in Yugoslavia), which lay along their route. Still celebrating that victory, the Viennese were looking forward to more. It was vengeance that inspired them, as well as policy: thirty-three years before that, in 1683, a Turkish army had thrust its way clear to the walls of Vienna, very nearly bursting through them before they were forced to retreat. Whenever the Austrians and Turks took a break from fighting, the Tatars descended to raid anything left worth stealing, while the emperor's Catholic armies turned their swords on Protestants. Thus a territorial contest between superpowers had been razored by religious and cultural differences into endemic savagery of a kind that Western Europe had rarely experienced.

As her departure neared, Lady Mary's women friends broke into tears whenever they saw her, but she made light of both their nerves and her own. To Pope, she wrote, *I think I ought to bid Adieu to my friends with the same solemnity as if I was going to mount a breach, at least if I am to believe the information of the people here, who denounce all sort of terrors to me. I am threatened at the same time with being frozen to death, buried in the snow, and taken by the Tatars. How my adventures will conclude I leave entirely to Providence; if comically, you shall hear of them.*

To Frances, she claimed that her only fears were for her son. They were not, however, dire enough to make her alter her course. Also, she was having trouble taking Prince Eugene's warnings seriously. She saw the great man often, she said, but it was as if she had met Hercules serving as a slave in women's clothing at the court of Queen Omphale. She refused, however, to elaborate on this tantalizing bit of innuendo.

Adieu, dear sister. . . . If I survive my journey you shall hear from me again.

On January 16, 1717, they slid out of Vienna. Snow lay thick over the land, but the ambassadorial party wrapped themselves in furs and set their coaches on runners to become sleighs, racing southeast across "the finest plains in the world, as even as if they were paved." Far from being terrified or even tremulous, Lady Mary was exhilarated.

At night, they lodged with governors and army officers. They were given honor guards, and bishops and nobles feasted them with wine, winter fruit, and venison. Five days later, they reached Buda, the old royal Hungarian city that has since combined with the mercantile town of Pest on the opposite bank of the Danube to form Budapest. The city and its castle lay in ruins; outside the walls a Serbian shantytown huddled in narrow rows, the odd, half-dug-out houses looking like thatched tents. With no reason to linger, they departed that same day.

Heading almost due south, they skirted the western edge of the Hungarian Plain, keeping close to the Danube. The hiss and slice of the runners, the jingle of harness and crack of whip, the snort and heave of the horses, sounded thin and brittle in a world otherwise wrapped in white silence. During the day, they glimpsed the ruins of Turkish towns in the distance, marked only by falling minarets. Nearer their path, farms and fields lay destroyed and deserted. Immense flocks of birds rose up around them, and wolves howled in the shadows of the forests that pressed down the mountains toward the river. In the few villages they passed, the sheepskin-clad villagers always gave the travelers space to warm up by their stoves and dished up abundant food, garnered mostly by hunting: wild boar, venison, and pheasant. They had been ordered to provide the ambassador's party with whatever they needed gratis, but Wortley paid them full worth—which made their hosts press ever more food on the travelers, as parting gifts. At night, the winter stars glittered overhead like shards of ice.

On January 26, they crossed the frozen river. At the hilltop fortress of Peterwaradin, they waited two days to finalize the details of their transfer from the Austrian to the Ottoman Empire and then set off with an escort of two hundred heavily armed Imperial troops. The Turks were to meet them with exactly equal numbers, exactly halfway through the no-man's-land between Austrian Peterwaradin and Turkish Belgrade.

A little ways outside town, they came upon the site of the Austrian victory that had been celebrated with such relentless joy in Vienna. Thirty thousand Turks had died in a matter of hours, and had been left to the wolves and the crows. In deep winter, the cold thinned the odor into nothingness, but the diamond shimmer of the ice only heightened the horror that enveloped the ambassador's party. For what seemed like hours, they drove in silence across a field strewn with skulls and the mangled and shredded bodies of men, horses, and camels, all frozen into a grisly, glistening tableau.

At the village appointed, their Turkish escort turned up with one hundred too many unsmiling soldiers. Hatred was far keener than the cold; no one wished to linger. Circled by turbans and scimitars, the British ambassador, his lady and son, and their retinue were soon speeding south and east, while the relieved Austrians retreated north.

Wading through thick snow, the British party's horses dragged them uphill into heavily fortified Belgrade on February 5. They expected to stay only one night, but the pasha, or military governor, sent a polite but firm invitation for them to remain until he heard from the grand vizier in Adrianople. Regretfully, that might take as long as a month. Surrounded by several hundred heavily armed soldiers, they were in no position to refuse his request. They were lodged with a qadi, or religious judge, named Achmet Bey, in one of the most splendid houses in the town.

They were awarded a whole chamber of Janissaries—the crack troops of the Ottoman army—to guard them, but whether they were being guarded from enemies or as enemies remained disconcertingly vague. The Janissaries, Achmet Bey confirmed, were slave soldiers just as Lady Mary had heard. But in their case, he said, the word *slave* was misleading: they were indeed slaves of the sultan, but the Janissaries were among the most powerful men in the empire. The wiliest and most ruthless rose to become pashas (a title for generals and governors) or even the sultan's chief executive officer, the grand vizier himself.

"They owe loyalty to nothing and no one but the sultan," said Achmet Bey, "and sometimes, they force that formula in the other direction." Seized as young boys from among the empire's non-Muslim population— mostly Balkan Christians, he said—they were marched to Constantinople, where they were circumcised, converted, and mercilessly trained. Lady Mary tried to pity them, but whenever she glimpsed them through the door, their scorn dried her pity to dust.

Their host spent much of the day in his library, but he supped with the ambassador and his lady every evening. Unaccustomed to the free ways of Western women, he delighted to spend hours sitting cross-legged on cushions with Lady Mary, discussing poetry, religion, and philosophy. She began by telling him—in Italian, the language they shared—a Persian tale she had read in French; he paid her the compliment of assuming she was cultured enough to have learned it directly from the source, and went on to stir her with the bright delicacy and searing sensuality of Arabic and Ottoman love poetry. At her request, he taught her the rudiments of Arabic grammar and scansion; at his, one of the ambassador's secretaries taught him the Roman alphabet. Lady Mary sparred with him in lively debates about their differences in religion and day-to-day life, especially the confinement of women in harems and veils. "There is but one advantage in it," he teased her. "When our wives cheat us, nobody knows it."

He both entertained and educated her with inexhaustible grace, but still, she yearned to be back on the road and moving. To Pope, she chalked it up to the weather: colder than it had ever been anywhere but Greenland, she groused. Despite the hardworking stove, the windows kept freezing up on the inside. Faintly audible between the lines of her letter was a hum of nerves pulled taut, and a stubborn refusal to acknowledge the whisperings of inadmissible fear.

At last, three weeks later, official summons to Adrianople arrived. Assured that the route was plague free, they headed for the town of Nissa (modern Nis, in Yugoslavia). Their guard of Janissaries swelled to five hundred: against the thieving Serbs, they were told. For seven days, they traveled at breakneck speed through narrow mountain valleys, with dark fir forests pressing down on all sides. The horses foundered and died in their traces, or stumbled lame; in compensation, their peasant owners were beaten for slowing the company down. Lady Mary wanted to empty her pockets in payment, but Wortley stopped her: the aga, or general, of their Janissaries would only take the money as soon as it left her hands.

When they came to villages, the Janissaries seized whatever they fancied, no matter how ill the peasants could spare it or how little sense it made in terms of husbandry. "Lambs just fallen, geese and turkeys big with egg: all massacred without distinction," she mourned. Watching this grinning cruelty, but helpless to stop it, Lady Mary wept tears of rage every day.

At one village, their second cook fell ill; the Janissaries would have left him to freeze alone on the road, but their surgeon, Mr. Maitland, insisted upon staying behind with him. They would catch up, he assured Lady Mary in his Scottish burr, as soon as the man recovered. As long as the ambassador did not threaten to slip from their grasp, the Janissaries were indifferent. Lady Mary pressed the surgeon's hand in gratitude, and the Wortleys sped on. After a brief stop in Nis, they pushed up and over yet another range of peaks and rumbled down to the city of Sofia (now the capital of Bulgaria) on the banks of the River Iskar, in the midst of another large and beautiful plain. There, she had the luxury of one free day.

As if she might wash all the anger, horror, and fear away, at ten o'clock in the morning she summoned a Turkish-style coach and headed, informally and incognito, for the hot baths for which Sofia was famous.

The *hamam* or bathhouse was a pale cluster of domes like opaque bubbles that had settled into the ground. In the outer dome, Lady Mary slipped off her shoes and tipped the portress a crown. An interpretress and two maids in tow, she ducked inside.

Small round skylights pierced the high marble curve of the ceiling, so that the air itself, moist and faintly redolent of sulfur, gleamed faintly with the sheen of pearl. A sinuous Turkish melody wound languidly through the vault overhead. In the center of the tiled room, four scented fountains of cool water plashed and sang, arcing into basins that spilled smoothly into streams running into inner rooms. Around the edges of the room ran two sofas: not Western couches, but built-in ledges of marble, one set above the other like a wide stair, the lower spread with crimson carpets and cushions. Reclining on these, braiding each other's ebony and honey-gold hair with pearl ribbon, drinking the bittersweet earth of thick Turkish coffee and the sweetened fruit juice called sherbet, lounged two hundred women.

For a moment, all movement ceased. Long before, Lady Mary had startled the Kit-Cat Club into silence for being dressed up like a lady. Now, it was simply for being dressed: save Lady Mary and the servants stepping in behind her, every woman in the room was naked.

The Turkish ladies recovered first. Unfolding themselves from the attentions of their slaves, they approached her cooing with delight: *Uzelle, pek uzelle*, they murmured over and over: "Charming, very charming."

They drew her farther into the room and tried to help her out of her clothes, but thankfully, they had a little trouble with the flaring jacket and fitted waistcoat of her riding habit. At last, though, she let a black-haired young beauty who was also the highest-ranking lady among them slide the jacket from her shoulders and reach in with slender fingers to unbutton her waistcoat.

At the sight of her tightly laced stays beneath, all the Turkish ladies blanched and stepped back aghast, but curiosity and civility soon drew the black-haired lady back again. "Englishmen," she informed her companions after inspecting the boned corset, "lock up their wives in little boxes shaped like their bodies." Inch by inch, the others crept near. European women, they all assured Lady Mary through her interpretress, were to be pitied for being such slaves as to be kept prisoner in their own clothing; no man of the East would dream of such barbarity.

Lady Mary shed no more than her jacket and waistcoat; unwilling to endure the sight of more savagery, her hostesses pressed her no further. All around her, though, women sat, knelt, and walked with a majestic grace that made her think of Milton's Eve, clad in nothing but proud honor. They were beautiful in face and slender of body, and their long, lustrous falls of hair were unlike anything she had seen among the rarely washed, oft powdered and pomaded heads of Europe. But what entranced her more than anything else was the shining expanse of smooth skin, all of it unmarred, as she was all too aware that hers was, by the red pits and twists of smallpox scars.

She left earlier than she would have liked: she had only one day to play tourist and thought a visit to the ruins of Justinian's church should not be passed up. The ruins were a disappointment; she longed to return to the baths, but Mr. Wortley and the Janissaries were relentless. Their cavalcade left the next morning, toiling up and over the last mountain range that blocked their way to Constantinople.

Every step toward Turkey swathed her more luxuriously in a warm Mediterranean world scented with lemon, wild thyme, and cedar. Vines grew wild over the hillsides, and the very air was spiked with paprika and mint, softened with olive oil, and sweetened with honey. Cypress speared the sky and music twined like serpents swimming through the trees. Lithe, long-haired boys danced, sunlight rained gold upon an infinite carpet of flowers, and everywhere shone the color blue. From the dome of the sky, to smooth jewel-stones set in gold, to the tiles poured across walls, the Ottomans washed their world in the intense brilliant blue still known simply as "Turkish," in its old French form: turquoise.

On March 24, they at last reached Adrianople (modern Edirne), the jewel of western Turkey and Sultan Achmet III's favorite home away from the splendors of Topkapi Palace in Constantinople, as well as the staging ground for invasions of Austria. As the sultan found it pleasing to be in Adrianople that spring, so did all his ambassadors. The Wortleys were housed in one of the grand signior's palaces on the banks of the Maritza River. As Wortley impatiently awaited his audience with the sultan, Lady Mary sat day after day in a marble kiosk in the garden, listening to the dance of the river and sipping sherbet or coffee as nightingales sang in the cedars. Poetry was everywhere: fine ladies at their looms made her think of the *Iliad;* Greek children playing upon Pan pipes and adorning lambs with flower garlands brought to mind the pastoral worlds of romance.

"Mr. Wortley," she murmured aloud to no one, "you have brought me at last to Paradise."

Still, the ivory curves and twining limbs of Sofia glimmered in her mind. How was it that two hundred ladies could let their robes slide away without revealing the least sign of smallpox?

With the perfectly recovered second cook in tow, Mr. Maitland caught up with the ambassador's party in Adrianople late one night a week after his employers' arrival. Lady Mary was greeted with this joyous news when she awoke the next morning—and also with the information that the man's illness had not been a bad cold. He had gone down with the plague.

"If you ask me, Cook's illness was nothing more than a Turkish hoax— an excuse for a leisurely jaunt through the mountains," grumbled Lady Mary to the surgeon when he came to pay his respects. "I thought the plague killed everyone by the village-load, but I glimpsed him flailing knives in the kitchen just an hour ago, fat and jolly as ever. Are you quite sure that plague was the problem?"

"Yes, my lady," said Mr. Maitland.

"You are proving yourself an even more miraculous healer than Dr. Arbuthnot and Mr. Kennedy claimed. . . . But I tell you, in the matter of marvelous medicine, I am quite catching up with you, Mr. Hare, and if you are not careful, I shall speed by like the plodding but patient old Tortoise. In your absence, I have been investigating this inoculation business."

He groaned.

"Don't be dismal. It sounds quite promising. Except that they do go on about 'engrafting' and 'transplantation' distressingly like the king talking up his orchards of pineapples and oranges—a sure way to ruin the taste of pineapple, if you think about it too long. I hope you have a strong stomach: I should like your help in delving into the matter farther. Locate this Dr. Timonius, for example, and sound him out."

"Yes, my lady."

⊰ 5 ⊱

My Dear Little Son

Adrianople
April 1, 1717
  Dear Papa,
  My deepest duty to Your Grace and the Duchess.

Lady Mary ground out an entire wearisome paragraph of obsequiousness. It was worth it: she knew her father could not resist the bright lure of her kowtowing, and she very much wanted him to read on.

> *Those dreadful stories you have heard of the plague have very little foundation in truth. I own I have much ado to reconcile myself to the sound of a word which has always given me such terrible ideas, though I am convinced there is little more in it than a fever, as a proof of which we passed through two or three towns most violently infected. In the very next house where we lay, in one of 'em, two persons died of it. Luckily for me I was so well deceived that I knew nothing of the matter, and I was made to believe that our second cook who fell ill there had only a great cold. However, I left our doctor to take care of him, and yesterday they both arrived here in good health and I am now let into the secret that he has had the plague.*
> *There are many that 'scape of it, neither is the air ever infected. I am persuaded it would be as easy to root it out here as out of Italy and France, but it does so little mischief, they are not very solicitous about it and are content to suffer this distemper instead of our variety, which they are utterly unacquainted with.*

But the smallpox—that was a different matter. It was also the heart of her story. She had to think very carefully about how to entice her father onward—the smallpox had remained a forbidden topic ever since Will's death.

Apropos of distempers, I am going to tell you a thing that I am sure will make you wish yourself here. The Small Pox—so fatal and so general amongst us—is here rendered entirely harmless, by the invention of engrafting (which is the term they give it). There is a set of old women who make it their business to perform the operation. Every autumn in the month of September, when the great heat is abated, people send to one another to know if any of their family has a mind to have the smallpox.

The French ambassador had supplied this strange story . . . would her father wish to know that? No. Might toss it down in disgust—French not high in his regard just now.

They make parties for this purpose, and when they are met (commonly fifteen or sixteen together), the old woman comes with a nutshell full of the matter of the best sort of smallpox and asks what veins you please to have opened. She immediately rips open the one that you offer to her with a large needle (which gives you no more pain than a common scratch) and puts into the vein as much venom as can lie upon the head of her needle, and after binds up the little wound with a hollow bit of shell, and in this manner opens four or five veins.

The Grecians have commonly the superstition of opening one in the middle of the forehead, in each arm, and on the breast to mark the sign of the cross, but this has a very ill effect, all those wounds leaving little scars, and is not done by those that are not superstitious—who choose to have them in the legs or that part of the arm that is concealed.

She went on describing the course of the treatment in detail. Waxing into her conclusion, she threw caution to the winds and stuck the French ambassador in after all: *Every year thousands undergo this operation, and the French Ambassador says pleasantly that they take the Small Pox here by way of diversion, as they take the waters in other countries. There is no example of anyone that has died in it.*

To other friends at court, she had written quite similar letters—anything to her father needed about ten drafts, and there was no point in wasting them. But for her intimates, she had added one more tidbit of information: *You may believe I am very well satisfied of the safety of the experiment since I intend to try it on my dear little son.*

For her father, however, she left that red flag out. Time enough for him to discover that another of his descendants would be battling the smallpox—on purpose. Let him mull this much information over for a while first.

She sanded the letter and sealed it, adding it to the tall stack to be dispatched on the next ship for London.

Lady Mary's maid arrived one morning at the head of a double-file troop of slaves invisible beneath armloads of silk, satin, and jewels; the sumptuous Turkish robes she had ordered had arrived. First, the maid sent a filmy smock of white gauze skimming over Lady Mary's head. Then she helped her step into drawers of thin rose damask embroidered with silver flowers, and slipped her arms into a waistcoat fitted to her shape from the same material and fastened with buttons of diamond and pearl. Then came the slender caftan of gold damask, clasped with a broad belt encrusted with cabochon jewels. Over it all—or draped in graceful folds over her arm— went the "curdee," a loose cloak of blue brocade lined with ermine. Bending down, the maid set before her a pair of slippers in white kid leather embroidered in gold. At last, after brushing Lady Mary's hair into a high shine, the maid settled on her head a cap of a light, shimmering cloth-of-silver, fixing it with a plume of heron feathers and a nosegay of jewels carved to resemble flowers in every particular but scent: pearl buds, ruby roses, diamond jasmine, and topaz jonquils.

Except for the face, the figure Lady Mary saw in the looking glass was slender, elegant, and ravishing. Thereafter, she relished playing the Turk with as much ardor as she had disdained to look Viennese, abandoning European dress as much as possible. When Westerners visited her, she received them in the style and appearance of a Turkish princess. When she explored the streets on her own, she went incognito beneath the voluminous outer cloak and veils of a modest Turkish woman. Only when visiting real Turkish princesses did she grudgingly allow herself to be squeezed back into Viennese court dress.

There was a great deal of visiting to be done, and she made use of every minute. She studied Turkish poetry, cookery, music, and dancing—*so soft, and the motions so languishing,* she sighed to her journal, *that the coldest and most rigid prude upon earth could not have looked upon the dancers without thinking of something not to be spoke of.* She studied the language so assiduously that her new friends teased she was in danger of losing her English. She studied their manners and mores, and concluded that beneath their veils and behind their walls, Turkish ladies possessed more liberty than any others on earth. Most of all, she studied Turkish beauty. Men might swoon over it as a glory of nature, but Lady Mary recognized art when she saw it. Turkish ladies, she observed, wore their hair in long tresses braided with pearl and ribbon—she counted 110 on one head alone, and heaven knew how long that took. They plucked their brows and lined their lustrous black eyes with kohl—*at a distance, or by candlelight this adds very much to their blackness*, she judged, *but 'tis too visible by day*. They dyed their nails a rosy pink, but here Lady Mary balked: try as she might, she could not accustom herself to tinted nails.

But their complexions, she sighed, needed no enhancement at all—and was surprised to learn that this, too, was art: one and all, they credited the marvelous powers of the Balm of Mecca. One lady presented her with the princely gift of a pot of it, swathed in thick pity. Lady Mary ignored the pity, and took the pot. That night, she opened the lid and sniffed at it, her eyes watering at its sudden pungent scent. To judge by the lovely bloom of Turkish faces, she told herself, she ought to think well of it. Surely, if they had contrived means to stop the smallpox, they might also be trusted to have found a way to repair its ravages.

She scooped some of the white cream on her finger and spread it onto her face; it burned with cold fire. Staring in the looking glass, she saw the Woman in the pockmarked Moon. The cream that could repair that would truly be a wonder.

The change the next morning was indeed wonderful: her face had gone from ghastly white to glowing crimson, and had swollen to such extraordinary size that she thought it might burst. At breakfast, Mr. Wortley laughed himself into a coughing fit and then dipped into anger. How could she embarrass him so? What if the sultan chose this afternoon to wish to present her to a daughter, or a wife? They would think he had married a giant strawberry. A prize hog's ham, he said the next day, as the red began to fade. Not for three days did Lady Mary's old face return, however. Her Turkish friends insisted that her beauty was much mended, but Lady Mary could see no improvement—and not for lack of looking.

I cannot in good conscience advise you to make use of it, she wrote to the ladies anxiously awaiting news of the legendary stuff in London. *I know not how it comes to have such universal applause. For my part, I never intend to endure the pain of it again. Do as you please, only remember that before you use it that your face will not be such as you'll care to show in the drawing room for some days after*.

It was to be very much hoped, she remarked to Mr. Maitland, that the Turks' method of preventing smallpox worked markedly better than the folly of their favorite restorative.

At last, Mr. Wortley was presented to the sultan. Perhaps the sensuality of Turkey had pierced even Mr. W's armor, or perhaps this brush with power fired his cold, careful soul with a sudden need to exult. In any case, he came to visit Lady Mary among her carpets and cushions, her jasmine and honeysuckle, her songbirds and tinkling fountains. By the time they left Adrianople for Constantinople, Queen of Cities, late in May, Lady Mary was pregnant.

The largest, wealthiest, and most sophisticated metropolis in the world, Constantinople was certainly the most tolerant, and possibly the most ruthless as well. Not that Mr. Wortley could or would grant it such superlatives, of course. The French ambassador found himself freely able to admit that the sultan's capital was larger than Paris, but Mr. Wortley would not own that it was larger than London. It did not seem so crowded, thought Lady Mary; she could at least give him that.

She swept into the city sitting cross-legged on cushions on the shallow floor of a carriage lined with cedar and upholstered in silk, fitfully twitching aside the curtains that kept her decently veiled from the eyes of men. The best way to see the expanse of the Turkish capital, however, was by water. Being rowed hither and yon on the Bosphorus, she wrote home, was much nicer than going in a barge to Chelsea. It offered a beautiful variety of prospects: the Asian side was covered with fruit trees, villages, and delightful swooping landscapes. On the European side, stood the city on its seven hills, with gardens, pine and cypress trees, white stone palaces, mosques, gilded turrets, and spires all rising one above another with as much beauty and symmetry as the treasures in a cabinet, she thought, arranged by the most skillful hands: jars showing themselves above jars, mixed with canisters and candlesticks. *Very odd comparison,* she told herself—and everyone else who would listen, *but it gives me an exact image of the thing.*

Like all other Westerners, the British ambassador and his retinue lived in Pera—no more a suburb, Lady Mary insisted with horror at the very notion, than Westminster was a suburb of London. She was close to the city's teeming wonders, but she was also close to its teeming ills. "The smallpox, my lady, is even more malignant here than in London," reported Mr. Maitland, shaking his head gravely. "As far as I can ascertain, when it flares into epidemics, between one third and one half of everyone who comes down with it dies."

September, she promised herself through clenched teeth, dread once again coiling tightly about her heart. But September and its smallpox inoculation parties seemed to dally in the distant future; they would never come. Her son, whispered her fears, would die before she could save him.

* * *

In the middle of May, the sultan had once again led his army west to defend Belgrade against the emperor and his Austrians, even as his European ambassadors and their families had been sent in the opposite direction. In August, the sultan's troops charged into battle against the Austrians of Prince Eugene of Savoy; a week later, the city surrendered. The prince gave the place over to his troops, and three days later not a house was left standing, not a person alive. Lady Mary presumed her host Achmet Bey dead, and mourned him.

After the siege, Dr. Timonius returned from attending the sultan in the field, and agreed to attend Lady Mary in her pregnancy—for Mr. W most obligingly retained that Italian of inoculation fame as the family physician. Lady Mary's mood soared and then dived. Dr. Timonius was adamant: under no circumstances would he allow her to inoculate her son while she was pregnant, or visit any of the smallpox parties her friends were arranging. Lady Mary might be safe—*might*, he stressed in Italian, French, and Latin—but the danger to her unborn child was immeasurable.

Caught between terrors, she put the operation off.

Mr. Maitland was relieved: it gave him a chance to study the procedure during at least one inoculation season. With her blessing, he visited several of the parties forbidden to her, and she picked his brain upon every return—though it meant an infernal number of visits to the baths, for him. Once he got used to so much steaming, scrubbing, massaging, and oiling, though, he actually came to like it.

"Well?" she asked, pouring him a tiny cup of thick, sweet coffee as he arrived after his first visit to such a party. "What are the symptoms? Are they as salutary as the reports would have them?"

He folded himself onto the sofa. Come to think of it, he quite liked these flowing caftans the Turks wore. Damned sight more comfortable than breeches. "Both before and after the eruption, my lady, the symptoms are so gentle—so very slight—that, in strictness of speech, I cannot really countenance calling the inoculated smallpox a disease."

"Specifics, my dear Scot, specifics, if you please."

In retaliation for that "dear Scot," he sipped at his coffee slowly until she was very near a scream of vexation, when he smiled and relented. "None of the usual complaints of pain in the back," he said. "No vomiting, headaches, thirst, or restlessness." He helped himself to a sweetmeat powdery and sparkling with sugar. "Though the pulse, to be sure, is somewhat fuller and higher than before."

"And the fever?" she asked sharply.

He waved his hand in dismissal. "Scarcely deserves the name of *febricula*."

"I am not sure anything or anyone deserves that," she said dryly. "But is it always so light? Is there never a bad issue?"

"Not one to a thousand, I am repeatedly assured."

"And the pocks?"

"The pustules, madam, commonly number from ten to a hundred, in rare cases more." He leaned forward. "But what I may say I am happiest to report is that they never leave any marks or pits behind—except only around the incisions where they graft the stuff into the blood."

"They are turning you into gardener, too, then?"

He shrugged. "It is a city of gardens, my lady. Why not grow smallpox too? I tell you, if they grow this light kind with any regularity, it will be more valuable than all the pineapples the king can produce in a thousand years."

"How will you ascertain whether it really secures those who risk it against all future danger of catching the smallpox?"

"Ah," he sighed. "That is, of course, the great difficulty." He gave her a sharp look. "And if not fully vindicated, it will render the whole process precarious."

"It will render the whole process trifling," she said. "So let us hope that you will clear it."

"It is not up to me to clear or condemn, my lady. It is my duty to observe the truth."

The next time, he bounded in like a conqueror. "All my inquiries have been fully answered, my lady: I have been assured that there is not one instance known of anyone's being ever infected, who has had any pustules at all, however few have been raised by inoculation."

"Really?"

"Several people have been engrafted a second time—and others have been confined not only in the same room, but in the same bed as the infected. With no effect whatsoever. No one in these trials has ever felt the least twinge of fever or nausea." He was pacing so wildly that he kept sweeping out of the long open doors and into the courtyard, and coming back in, so that she lost some of his ranting.

"I cannot forbear admiring the very great sagacity of the men who first invented this method," he said upon one return.

"What makes you think it was men?" asked Lady Mary, raising an eyebrow.

He stopped in his tracks and stared at her. "I—"

"Men do not practice it. Why should they have invented it?"

In answer, he turned on his heel and swept back out; he did not come back in for some time.

Disaster struck through the mails: Just as Wortley's embassy was building momentum, and the sultan was beginning to take notice of his counsels, a letter came announcing an upheaval in the ministry at home. Walpole was out, and Sunderland was in. As a consequence, Mr. Wortley found that he also was to be out, and another ambassador was to be in. And Lady Mary found that she was to go home, much sooner than was either pleasurable or convenient.

But the departure was not too imminent. She was to have one last winter and spring in paradise.

Lady Mary grew larger and calmer, and then even placid. Her pen stopped its busy scratching, and she sat in her garden on a slope high above the sea, and for hours at a time watched the city undulating away from her perch.

At Christmas, she received a long letter from Alexander Pope; his imaginings grew preposterously extravagant. He had sent her a new poem, titled *Eloisa to Abelard*, "in which you will find," he wrote, "one passage, that I can't tell whether to wish you should understand or not?"

It was a lovely poem, really—unusually passionate for him, she thought. But did he really have to liken his long-distance dreaming of her to poor Eloisa in her nunnery cell, yearning for her long-lost mutilated lover? The man would make a fool of himself one day, surely. But his poetry stirred her. On Boxing Day, she sat in her kiosk and coaxed herself from her contented lethargy into nicely regular verse:

Here from my window I at once survey
The crowded city and resounding sea,
In distant views see Asian mountains rise
And lose their snowy summits in the skies.
New to the sight my ravished eyes admire
Each gilded crescent and each antique spire,
The marble mosques beneath whose ample domes
Fierce warlike sultans sleep in peaceful tombs.

She pressed herself through a classical lament for the ruins of the Byzantine city upon which the Turks had built their present infidel fairyland. But she could not for long maintain a proper sense of doom.

Gardens on gardens, domes on domes arise
And endless beauties tire the wandering eyes.

And endless poetry tires the pregnant mind, she thought with happy sleepiness, letting the quill slip from her hand and watching it float to the ground.

On the nineteenth of January, 1718, Lady Mary gave birth to a daughter, whom she named Mary. Three months later, while Mr. W was off with the sultan's retinue, she dismissed the protesting chaplain, sent her maid on a mission to the Greek quarter, and summoned Mr. Maitland to her rooms.

"I have decided to submit the boy to this inoculation next week. I would be much obliged if you would make it your business to find a fit subject from which to take the necessary matter."

"Yes, my lady."

"Mr. Maitland."

"Yes?"

"I should also be obliged if you would have a word with the girl's nurse. She has not had the smallpox, and she is refusing to undergo the inoculation herself."

"Yes, my lady."

But the nurse was not to be budged, by reward, wheedling, weeping, pleading, or threats.

On the morning of March 18, 1718, Lady Mary had Edward and Mr. Maitland both summoned to her chamber. Soon afterward, the chief inoculatress of Constantinople arrived, veiled from head to toe in black like the Greek widow she was, though she was a Christian, of course, and left her face showing. A kind old face, seamed with countless wrinkles punctuated by faded old eyes and a toothless smile.

The woman was good with children—that much was clear, though she was hindered somewhat by not speaking English, while Edward did not speak Greek. Unfortunately, it did not matter how good she was; the boy did not wish to be scratched, stuck, or otherwise touched by a needle. He dodged away from the woman and made a dash for the door, but two slaves stood there, impassively. He darted away, and began running about the room, overturning what little furniture was available—all of it made light, in the Turkish manner, and easily thrown about by a half-panicked, half-mischievous, and utterly naughty five-year-old.

The slaves made a move to help, but Lady Mary ordered them back to the door; at least, she panted to Mr. Maitland as she sprinted past him at one point, they would keep the chase confined to one room. There was nowhere to hide, but there were a great number of cushions to toss, small tables to throw, and fountainsful of water to splash.

Mr. Maitland had always suspected Lady Mary of being a bit of an athlete beneath the whalebone stays; relieved of them in her Turkish dress, she proved to have a fine gait and a good set of lungs. The old Greek lady, too, showed herself to be surprisingly nimble. But it took all three of them to corner the child, protecting themselves from flailing arms and feet with large silken pillows. One of them burst, filling the air with a snowy feather-fall. And then it was over: Master Edward suddenly went rigid in their arms, shooting them a perfectly wicked smile as they hauled him, stiff as a length of lumber, back into the sunlight in the center of the room.

Lady Mary stood out of her son's reach, holding the jarful of venom so painstakingly provided by Mr. Maitland. The inoculatress pulled out what looked to be the blunt needle she darned her sons' socks with and drew a short line on the boy's left arm, ripping a slight tear in the skin. He wailed and wriggled, but she held him firm. She flicked her needle into the jar once and smeared a tiny dab of stuff into the two or three tiny rubies that had popped out on the boy's arm.

She motioned to Mr. Maitland to trade places with her, but he felt the boy hunch to spring and shook his head. Instead, he drew out the small lancet he always carried with him, pulled off the cover with his teeth, and before anyone could say yea or nay, cut a neat shallow incision on the boy's right arm.

"My lady, if you please, I would take some of that matter."

Lady Mary held out the jar, Mr. Maitland dipped his lancet into the venom, and just as the woman had done, he smeared a bit into the blood—though his cut had produced a thin red line, rather than a row of scarlet beads.

Lady Mary herself tied up the bandages.

The operation over, the boy went rag-doll limp, buried his face in his mother's skirts, and wept. She patted his head.

"That's my boy. Fine spirit and courage," she said.

"Why did you whip out your lancet?" she said testily to Mr. Maitland later, after the nurse had mustered the boy off to bed.

"Because he was ready to spring, the moment we loosened our grips, so we couldn't trade places. I had to operate, my lady. And however highly you may regard this Turkish procedure, you must allow me to regard certain standards of my own profession still more highly." He drew himself up tall. "I do not operate with old rusty needles." The mere thought of it sent him stalking from the room.

* * *

Three days later, bright red spots appeared in Edward's face; a few hours later they disappeared. They bloomed and faded like that for a week.

"When will the illness come on?" Lady Mary asked what seemed like every five minutes.

"Not yet, my lady," was all Mr. Maitland could say.

To His Excellency Wortley Montagu, Ambassador at the Porte
Sunday, March 23, 1718
   The Boy was engrafted last Tuesday and is at this time singing and playing, and very impatient for his supper. I pray God my next may give as good an account of him.
   I cannot engraft the Girl; her Nurse has not had the smallpox.
   LM

The following night, the boy's nurse sent slaves skimming through the palace halls for Lady Mary, and Lady Mary sent them in turn on their way to Mr. Maitland's door. Minutes later, they converged in the boy's nursery—removed to the farthest end of the building from the girl's.

Young Edward was a little hot and thirsty; Lady Mary was a whirlwind of pacing and ordering, checking pulses, stroking his hair and his cheek and pacing again, until Mr. Maitland was sorely tempted to dose her rather than the boy—and with more than a little laudanum. She flat-out refused, however, when he recommended a soothing dose. Unless he wanted to slip something in her wine, she was going to remain awake.

The illness did not last long. A few hours later, the rash began to seed itself across his body, and the fever—*febricula!* exclaimed Lady Mary—went off. Across the next day, he bloomed with about a hundred spots that soon grew round and yellow, like those of the more gentle, distinct kind of smallpox. The red spots that had appeared first grew fullest and largest of all. They began to crust over within the week, and then gently died away without leaving a single mark or pit behind them.

What terrified both Lady Mary and Mr. Maitland—though he tried to maintain the appearance of sure calm—were the incisions. At first, they were barely perceptible—just a bit of red soreness. When the fever came out, though, they bloomed into foulness. Day by day they grew in size, the cuts a green-blue pallor of death, surrounded by pale dripping slime—and that, in turn, surrounded by clusters of tiny yellow pocks. Around the whole was a rosy ring of infection.

By the time the pocks crusted over, the sores encompassed the whole outer side of both Edward's upper arms, and Lady Mary began to fear he might lose them.

On April 1, she wrote once more to Mr. W: *Your son is as well as can be expected, and I hope past all manner of danger.* She did not tell him that the manner of danger she feared was a double amputee for a son.

And then, quite suddenly, the incisions, too, began to scab over. On April 9, she still had received no word from her husband about their son. With relief pouring through her, she lost all patience. She had had a letter from her father, she harped, indicating that the duke was willing to be reconciled to them—if only Mr. Wortley would behave like a civilized man. Mr. W most certainly ought to write her father back: *The birth of your Daughter is a proper occasion, and you may date your Letter as if writ during my lying-in. I know him perfectly well and am very sure such a trifling respect would make a great impression upon him.*

She did not bother treating Mr. W to respect, trifling or otherwise; why should he expect from her what he refused to give?

> *You need not apprehend my expressing any great Joy for our return to England. I hope 'tis less shocking to you than to me, who have really suffered in my health by the uneasiness it has given me, though I take care to conceal it here as much as I can.*
>
> *Your son is very well; I cannot forbear telling you so, though you do not so much as ask after him.*
>
> *LM*

The inoculation behind her, she returned her son to the keeping of his nurse, and set about doing everything else she could not replicate in London.

Unknown beneath her veils, she strolled like a native through the bazaars—noble stone buildings, she thought, full of neatly kept alleys and pillared galleries, with assigned quarters for different luxuries and mundane necessaries: meat, spices, and vegetables, slaves, silk, and leather. The jewelers' quarter glittered so brightly with diamonds, emeralds, sapphires, and rubies that the dazzle made her squint. In their halls, the dervishes whirled. At the baths, the women lingered. Atop the minarets, turbaned muezzins appeared five times a day, as magically as if they had just alighted and folded up wings, and unfurled insistent prayer into the world: *La ilaha illa Allah*: There is no god but God.

In her own guise, Lady Mary rode her favorite white Arabian steed far and fast, admiring the fire with which he pranced beneath her and startling the Turks with her sidesaddle. From a balcony, she observed the sultan riding to worship flanked by a turbaned multitude that made her think of a garden of marching tulips; Achmet III—King of Kings, Emperor of Rome, Refuge of the World, and Shadow of God—was a handsome man, she judged, though his smile was cruel. She met one sultana wearing an emerald as big as a turkey's egg. Another entertained in a chamber wainscoted with mother-of-pearl fastened with emerald studs; in all four corners, fountains poured water in gradual falls, ledge to ledge, from ceiling to floor.

Not everything was admirable. Near her house, the naked, bleeding body of a Turkish woman was found at daybreak one morning. Someone had knifed the lady twice, once in the side and once in the breast. She was not yet quite cold, and so surprisingly beautiful that Lady Mary surmised there were very few men in Pera who did not gather around to look at her. (And very few women, either, she scolded herself.) None of them recognized the body, however, as no Turkish lady's face was known to men outside her own family. They supposed she had been brought there in the dead of night from the Constantinople side, but the government made no inquiries.

She begged official permission to see the Hagia Sophia—built so many years ago by the Christian Romans, kept up by the Byzantine Greeks, and then transformed into a mosque by the Turks. But leave was so long in coming that she schemed to sneak her way in, in the company of a Transylvanian princess almost as adventurous as herself. They dressed each other as Turkish men and walked straight in. The princess, unfortunately, proved a blubberer, and burst into tears at the sight of such a holy place desecrated by infidels. Lady Mary was reduced to hissing at her that they would soon join in the general desecration—probably by being burned at the stake—if Her Royal Highness did not get hold of her tears. The woman obligingly sniffled and stopped.

Lady Mary arrived home to find the official permission awaiting her, so she turned around and went back. This time, she came away with a handful of the mosaic work from the ceiling—it was falling out in a clinking, colored rain, the guides told her. In her hand it looked like small bits of glass, or the paste with which they made counterfeit jewels.

On the nineteenth of May, she seized one final afternoon to sit in her kiosk before the household should dissolve into the chaos of packing, and wrote a last letter—a long, tired sigh for the wonders of Turkey: *I am almost of opinion they have a right notion of Life: they consume it in music, gardens, wine, and delicate eating, while we are tormenting our brains with some scheme of politics or studying some science to which we can never attain or, if we do, cannot persuade people to set that value upon it we do ourselves. I had rather be a rich Effendi with all his ignorance, than Sir Isaac Newton with all his knowledge.*

On the fifth of July, the Wortley Montagus, no longer covered with the glory of ambassadorship, boarded HMS *Preston* along with their children, chaplain, surgeon, servants, and four horses Lady Mary refused to give up, and sailed for home.

❧ 6 ❧

ROSEBUDS IN LILY SKIN

Covent Garden, London
April 1721

L ADY Mary shivered and drew closer to the fire glowering in the library grate.

She was reading John Dryden, as she often did when troubled, or tired, or sad. Since early childhood, his cadences had been as familiar and comforting to her as her own heartbeat. This afternoon, though, even Dryden betrayed her: his rhythms felt disappointingly brittle and his sensibility primly arch. How she longed, some days, for the perfumed sensuality of Turkish poetry, which she had breathed rather than read, it sometimes seemed, in her kiosk by the sea in Pera.

She rubbed her eyes—sore today—and glanced back down at her book, open to a rather bizarre elegy on Lord Hastings, dead many years ago now of smallpox—or the "filthiness of Pandora's box," as Mr. Dryden had put it. Which made the poem really rather relevant, come to think of it, though in fact it had been his first published work.

It was a marvel that it had also not been his last. What was one to make of such passages as this? She read the line again:

Blisters with pride swelled, which through's flesh did sprout
Like rosebuds stuck i' th' lily skin about.

Really, she thought with a rueful laugh, it was all too romantically gruesome. Besides roses strewn upon lilies, Mr. Dryden had turned his patron's pocks into tears, glowing gems, even a constellation of rebellious stars. How had he ever restrained himself from adding in a fiery fall of angels?

A few months ago, she would have clapped her hands in glee at such absurdity and concocted some witty remark to send winging through the more intellectual drawing rooms of Covent Garden, Piccadilly, and St. James's. But then, a few months ago, violets and roses had blossomed in January, and she had thought it a fine omen of unlooked-for loveliness. Now, she deemed it more likely to have been a warning, the last valiant exhalation of beauty they might see for years to come. Perhaps the early bloom had even been a demonic joke: a gorgeous mask that Beelzebub himself had donned just long enough to slip unsuspected into the neverending party of London's western suburbs.

Since then, the demon had tossed off his disguise and pounced. Struggling in his talons, the world had lurched upside down.

But she was being dramatic, she told herself. Mr. Wortley would most certainly say that she was being dramatic.

Surely, though, it would be fair to say that after that early and all-toobrief warm spell, the weather had dipped into unseasonably cold weeping. Worse, the smallpox had begun slashing its way through her friends and family.

In point of fact, her husband had grunted just that morning, the distemper had been trampling through the city almost without pause since they had returned from Constantinople. She had merely ignored it, because it had lingered in the slums and tenements of the East End, St. Giles's, Westminster, and Southwark. Dank and dangerous places, she retorted, where he would have chided her for going. As for smallpox in St. Giles's, it might as well have been fever on the pockmarked moon.

St. Giles's, Wortley had acidly observed, was no more than a few streets away. A few streets, and many worlds, she had said, sailing out of the room.

Soon after their return, Mr. Wortley had gratified her by purchasing a mansion in Covent Garden—Nos. 9–10, the Piazza—quite à la mode, for a woman of artistic bent and intellectual prowess, though the neighborhood was daringly racy by the standards of her more blue-blooded friends. Still, it was genteel, even if its notion of gentility admitted poets, painters, philosophers, and even a few politicians on the basis of merit and manners alone, waiving the need for much of a pedigree. Lady Mary had happily immersed herself in creating a home that was a work of art, and in rekindling old coteries and salons, as well as sparking some anew.

Then Princess Anne, the eldest of the king's granddaughters, had gone down with smallpox last April—could it already be a year ago? Even at that point, Lady Mary had not managed to conjure up much real anxiety, though of course, she had, along with the rest of the kingdom, fretted over the little girl's fate. Anne's illness did not, however, seem a real and personal threat. After all, the palace was a veritable bedlam, people of all sorts endlessly creeping, pushing, battling their way in to see the king, or at any rate, to see whoever happened to be perched on the highest rung they could reach in the cascading hierarchy of royal lackeys.

These days, she had little to do with the palace, though she still often attended the regular weekly suppers put together for the king by the countess of Darlington—the exalted new rank of her fat, witty, half-royal, and wholly loyal friend, Madame de Kielmansegg.

By contrast to the young princess, Lady Mary told herself with satisfaction, her own little Mary was safely cocooned within private walls, surrounded by family and carefully screened servants.

Besides, at the time that the princess fell ill, there had been candidates that seemed much stronger than smallpox, if she really felt the need for a good worry: two and a half years before, the idiotic Prince of Wales, for instance, had turned both the court and the ministry upside down by openly challenging the power of his father in Parliament. In return, of course, the king had determined to crush his son, both politically and socially, once and for all. For starters, he had had him ejected from the palace, and the doors barred behind him.

Far from humbly returning to beg pardon, the prince had flounced off to Leicester Square to scheme against the king from an impertinently short distance. To the king's further dismay, Caroline, Princess of Wales—one of the few persons on earth who could cajole his son into sense—had voluntarily joined her husband in exile. Reluctantly, the king had let her go. He did not, however, allow her to take her children: he kept the three little princesses and their infant brother with him, at St. James's. Hostages for their parents' good behavior, the world had muttered, and for the most part the world had been right. But in some part, Lady Mary surmised, the king's decision had also been purely personal and selfish. Quite simply, he loved his grandchildren. He did not wish to give them up.

For courtiers and ministers alike, this familial war had been a two-year stomach-churning nightmare. In the end, everyone but a few of the prince's most obsequious creatures had adhered to the king—*How could the prince have failed to foresee that?* she clucked to herself for about the millionth time. On the other hand, even the staunchest of the king's men— Lady Mary's own father among them—saw that since George I was not immortal, they could not afford to alienate the prince in any lasting way.

It had been in the midst of this rift, not long after a heart deformity had sent her new little brother, blue lipped, into death, that ten-year-old Anne had fallen ill. Even from this distance, Lady Mary shook her head. Were the doctors not always cautioning their patients to keep their minds and hearts full of good cheer? How could even the most obtuse of ten-year-olds maintains good cheer in such a storm of vicious anger as had ripped Anne's family apart? That poor little princess had surely not been able to count good cheer among her allies as she fought off the smallpox.

She had very nearly lost that fight, rallying back even as the doctors had been preparing her squabbling royal elders for the worst. Remembering, Lady Mary shook her head. The princess had survived, but she was sadly scarred. At least Lady Mary had had a few years to revel in the delights of being young and beautiful in London, before her beauty had been scraped from her. Even so young, this princess was already famously accomplished; she would always be wealthy, always possess the power of her rank and her well-trained mind. Those, as Lady Mary well knew, were delights of their own, in many ways richer, deeper, more lasting. But they were not the same as the bright, fickle flame of beauty. Lady Mary allowed herself a rare sigh of regret. No, they were not at all the same.

As soon as the girl had fallen ill, the king had made quiet arrangements for the Princess of Wales to attend on her sick daughter as much as she liked. This proved to be most of the day and night, except for the hours when the king himself wished to sit and read to his little Annie. He had stood firm, though, on the point of his son's exile from the palace.

Gradually, Caroline had whittled away at his obstinate anger; quite possibly, death's obstinate hover over his grandchildren had also softened him. In any case, it had been in the sitting room just outside Anne's sickroom that delicate negotiations toward a familial peace had been joined. The prince might be too jealous of rank and power to realize that what he really needed was patience, but the princess was a consummate politician. She was quite deft when it came to handling both her husband and her father-in-law, especially when she was allowed to handle them separately, in private.

So she had engineered a tête-à-tête, just the king and herself, in a small chamber next to Anne's, ensuring that no voices would be raised and no tempers lost, if only for the sake of the child only one door away. A few days later, as Anne crept out of danger, the prince himself arrived to make formal submission to the king. All London—indeed, the entire nation—breathed a deep collective sigh of relief.

For courtiers, though, the respite had proved brief. While the king and the prince patched up their differences, the dreaded disease jumped the palace walls. For six months, it tiptoed furtively about the neighborhoods west of the City. Since the New Year, though, it had been cutting swathes of hot agony through the fashionable streets of St. James's and Piccadilly, sending Lady Mary's friends and family blistering and bubbling into heaven or hell.

Lady Mary had been able to ignore it until James Craggs died on the sixteenth of February. Four days later, her sixteen-year-old cousin Lady Hester Feilding succumbed, having shed her precocious beauty almost as fast as she acquired it. Up in Russell Square, the duke of Rutland and two of his daughters had all died within two weeks of each other, leaving Bloomsbury in mourning and mostly empty. All over London, but especially in the west, the whirl of parties and salons had ceased: not knowing who might be exhaling the infection, ladies had grown afraid to face each other across tea tables, and men shunned even old friends at cards. The crowds at the theater had thinned and drooped.

With all amusements off, there was little left to distract her from the smallpox but the crash of South Sea stock. With the help of Mr. Craggs, she had invested heavily. Who could have guessed, she cried at her own walls that such a firm, one of the country's largest trading companies—a financial behemoth big enough to treat with the government in the servicing of the nation's debt—could be a fraud? A collectively dreamed glimmer of soap, bubbling on a breeze? Who was to know that when its fragile film of popularity burst, it would dissolve vast fortunes into thin air?

Her money—a sum sickeningly large, though not bankrupting—had shriveled in a matter of days, but it was not as if she was the only victim. Parliament was sniffing about for a scapegoat; everyone who had made money was suspect. The king himself was looked at askance. Really, it had been just as well that poor beautiful Mr. Craggs had died when he did, for he had been deeply implicated in the scandal. So deeply that his father, unstricken by smallpox, had committed suicide a few days later. Everyone was dying.

A knock at the library door startled her. "What?" demanded Lady Mary, rising.

"It's nurse," stammered the maid.

Lady Mary crossed the room and flung open the door so quickly that she nearly tossed the maid against the wall.

The nurse's room was off the night nursery, two stories up. Just inside, she lay shivering on her bed, flecks falling in an angry red snow down her body.

"Where is my daughter?" demanded Lady Mary, her mind spinning and her heart trying to pound its way out of her stiffly boned bodice.

"I'm sorry, my lady," whispered Nurse. "I've tried to be so careful."

"Where is Mary?"

"Downstairs in your own parlor, my lady. She's fine, not ill at all. I sent her down in Charlotte's care, soon as I realized what was happening. Charlotte's a good girl."

Charlotte, thought Lady Mary, *is a feather-brained fifteen-year-old. But at least she is already pockmarked.*

The nurse began to cry.

"Hush," said Lady Mary, crossing the room and giving the woman her hand. The woman did love young Mary, and had been with her since her birth. But it was hard not to notice that none of this would be happening if she hadn't so adamantly refused to be inoculated while in Constantinople. *Inoculated while in Constantinople.* The full force of those words jolted her through her brain.

The nurse had been saying something in between sobs. Lady Mary couldn't make it out. "It will be all right," she said absently, patting the woman's hand.

Within half an hour, the nurse was bundled up and packed off to a certain house in Swallow Street, down in Piccadilly, where the servants of the aristocracy were sent to suffer through smallpox with kind care, at a safe distance. Footmen had been sent scurrying through the streets with notes inquiring after the availability of suitable short-term nursemaids. And her own carriage had clattered away in search of Mr. Charles Maitland, with orders not to return without him.

Two hours later, Mr. Maitland was shown into a sitting room that resembled a pleasure palace straight out of the *Arabian Nights*.

Sitting cross-legged on an ottoman behind a jewel-encrusted coffee set, Lady Mary was resplendent in her flowing Turkish costume, the thin rose damask embroidered with silver flowers and the jeweled cloth-of-gold rustling and clinking softly as she moved.

He bowed low, in the ostentatious manner of the Turkish court. "You must have a djinn at your mercy, my lady," he said as he straightened. "How else you could have transported such an exquisite corner of Constantinople to Covent Garden, I cannot begin to think."

"I admire the art and the poetry of the Ottomans," said Lady Mary with a smile as she poured out the thick coffee. "And I like to think I can offer some poor shadow of their grace in entertaining," she added, handing him the tiny cup.

He raised the sweet steaming brew to his lips.

"But I fear that in the matter of Turkish medicine I must beg your help," she added.

He froze, and his eyes met her gaze over the rim of the cup.

"I want you to inoculate little Mary," she said.

He set the cup down with a click. "I am honored, Lady Mary, by your trust," he said, stalling.

"Today," she said, leaning forward.

"In such matters, my lady, it does not pay to be hasty."

"In the matter of the smallpox," she countered, "it does not pay to hesitate. In any case, you have had three years to mull over the results of inoculating my son."

"The season is too cold," he objected. "In Constantinople, they operate in a warm season."

"Here, it is a smallpox season," said Lady Mary, never taking her eyes from him. "Mary's nurse erupted this morning."

He had of course, surmised what she wanted. Had surmised several months ago that she might want it. If anything, he was surprised the request had taken this long. He knew her well enough to know that when she set her mind to something, she did not take no for an answer. He knew he was not going to win this contest. Nor did he want to, really. He had seen the experiment work with his own eyes; even a remote possibility that it might work here in Britain made it valuable. But he wished to proceed with caution.

He also wished to make certain demands, though perhaps it would be better to say that he wished to put certain protections into place. For this was not Constantinople, though she seemed to want him to think it was. They were in the heart of London. And she was not asking him just to be a witness, as he had been in Turkey, where he'd merely stepped in to clean up a barbarous operation he had not begun. She was asking him to be the sole operator.

He was less sanguine about the outcome than she was. He had no wish to be charged with the murder of the granddaughter of a duke, and the daughter of an ambassador. It was paramount that he not work in secret. But how was he going to convince Lady Mary?

Let her win a lesser battle, said the voice of instinct. He cleared his throat. "It is not your son I am concerned about, it is your daughter. She must be prepared."

"She's strong as a horse," said Lady Mary, waving that notion off. "Her diet is clean and her exercise regular. I will not have you draining her blood and calling it useful."

He bowed. "Very well," he conceded.

Her eyes narrowed. "You want something else. What is it?"

Really, she was unnervingly perceptive. As smoothly as possible, he came out with it. "For you, my lady, this operation offers great personal benefit, in exchange for grave personal risk, as you well know. I hope, however, that you will consider sharing that benefit. Will you allow me to choose two physicians to witness the operation, in order to contribute to its credit and reputation, as well as to consult on the health and safety of your daughter?"

She sprang to her feet, her eyes flashing. "Certainly not," she exclaimed. "Under no circumstances will my daughter be exhibited to curious crowds like a carnival monkey."

He knew she had no high opinion of physicians, but still, the force of her refusal took him aback. Another, less patient man might have lost his grip on his own patience, and tried to argue with her, but Mr. Maitland knew her better than that. He called her bluff. "Then, my lady," he said, rising after her, "I must regretfully decline your kind offer to make use of my services."

Before she could recover, he had bowed and departed.

Three days later, she summoned him back again. The nurse's case was not going at all well, and fear was thickening her blood by the hour.

This time, he was shown into a proper English room; in the guise of a proper English lady, Lady Mary was standing by a window, with her back to him. "Two," she said imperiously, as he walked into the room.

He bowed. "Three," he countered. There was no need for either of them to specify that it was the number of physician witnesses they were discussing.

"Last time it was two," she said, glancing over her shoulder.

"Now it is three," he said.

She turned away again. "One at a time."

"I agree."

"And I will be present throughout." She whirled around. "I will not have physicians corrupting the operation out of sheer malicious rancor, for fear its success will dry up their revenues, along with the town's pocks."

He let her outburst skid by him. "You will find the city and the nation grateful, my lady. Now if you will excuse me, I will make the necessary preparations."

"No preparations," she snapped. "No prior bloodletting, no purges, no vomits. As I said, she's strong as a young horse."

"Yes, my lady. But that is not the sort of preparation I meant." It had been, of course, but it would not do to let her yet realize it. He liked her on the defensive. "I must acquire some promising matter."

"How hard can it be to scrape pus from a pock in London?" she cried. "Why haven't you already done so?"

"With all due respect, my lady, I was not sure we would come to an agreement. Now that we have, I am sure you do not want me to be quite so cavalier in this matter as you suggest. I must find a suitably clean subject, with no other history of disease, at just the right stage of a light, distinct smallpox. You do not want to shield Miss Wortley from smallpox, only to give her the great pox, or a consumption."

Lady Mary sighed, tapping one foot impatiently. He saw her thinking furiously. "Be quick, then," was all she said in the end.

As it turned out, he had one week's preparation for himself, and his three witnesses, but only after the fact: they were engaged to see Mary as soon as the rash came out, and not a moment before. And he won no preparation for the girl at all, though he kept lobbying for it right up until the last moment.

Lady Mary held her daughter on her lap right through the procedure, kissing the top of her fair downy hair, and singing her favorite songs. The girl wriggled a bit, but not badly: Mr. Maitland was deft and swift, and she had known his voice all her life.

The little girl liked him. To her, he was tall as the clouds and almost as gentle, with a funny way of talking. His *r*'s were furry. Or bumpy. She couldn't decide which. Mamma said he sounded that way because he was from a place called Scotland. Considering this mystery, she sat grave and wide-eyed, only turning away and screwed her eyes shut when he drew out his lancet. She knew he was trying to be kind, so she tried to be brave. But as she felt a prick in each arm, one tear squeezed from each eye and trickled down her cheeks.

The incisions opened and wept early, growing day by day. Two, three, four, five. On the sixth day, Lady Mary was so restless, she snapped at Cook, reduced the new nurse to tears, and sent old Jenkins, the coachman, fleeing for his life, all within five minutes. Directly, she locked herself in her bedchamber lest she transform into a full-blown dragoness. The sixth day spilled into the seventh, and still no fever appeared. Flushes crept across Mary's porcelain skin, sometimes alarmingly bright, but they were accompanied by no hint of heat. The count of days increased to eight and then nine. On the morning of the tenth day, Lady Mary began to fear that she would begin throwing things.

That afternoon, bells pealed all over the city: the Princess of Wales had given birth to a son. Wine flowed in streets crowded with dancing and cheering.

Late that night, the new nurse appeared at Lady Mary's door, frightened out of her wits. The child had grown warm, though still not hot. She was restless and fretful, though, and crying out for her old nurse, or her mamma. Lady Mary, for once, was glad to indulge the child.

The fever was not so high as to be terrifying. Nonetheless, it was a smallpox fever, and rising. She sent for old Mr. Brown, the ancient apothecary who had apparently been serving the neighborhood since the last visit of Caesar.

He was none too pleased to be hauled out of bed at midnight, though his way across the square had been well lit by celebratory bonfires and cheered on by happily drunk crowds. He was horrified to discover that the child had been *given* the smallpox.

He turned reproachful eyes upon Lady Mary. "There is nothing to be done now, my lady, but let Madam Nature take her course. If she behaves, the fever will go off of its own accord by morning."

Somehow, Lady Mary ground out thanks as the man left, and settled down in the nursery rocking chair to wait. To her mind, Madam Nature did not deserve much in the way of trust.

PART TWO

Boston

⧯ 1 ⧮

ZABDIEL AND JERUSHA

Muddy River, west of Boston, in New England
1695

ZABDIEL Boylston flattened himself across his horse's back, sunlight flitting like butterflies, like bright bats through the gloom as his body rolled with the rhythm of the beating hooves. He ducked and bobbed, sweeping aside the claws of trees that tried to rake him from the horse. Was it a book he had been holding only a moment ago in the clearing, when the buck had appeared at the far edge, pale and silent as a curl of the mists that sometimes wound through the forest? No—it was blue steel, the pistol that his father had carried through battles against the Indians. Far ahead, he caught another glimpse of the deer, heard it crashing through the brush—heard, so he thought, the gasp of its breath and the thump of its trumpeting heart.

They burst into a sun-shot clearing, and his quarry crumpled into the grass, though he could not remember having taken a shot. He dismounted at a run and then pulled up short. The body at his feet was not a buck, but his father.

Zabdiel clenched the knife in his hand, turning it over and over. As he stood there, his father's leg began to swell, turned black and green; a sweet stench of rotting slid upward. What was he to do?

In his hand, the blade frizzled and stretched into a saw.

Papa? He heard his voice say. *Papa, I must take it off.* At that, his father quite calmly turned over and sat up. Sadly, he shook his head. *Too late, my boy*, he said, heaving himself to a stand. *Too timid, too slow, too late.* Then he turned and limped into the trees.

* * *

Zabdiel started, felt the ooze of sweat dampening skin on fire, the salt stinging cracked and swollen sores, the wetness failing to touch the thirst lodged like thick, fetid swamp-mud in his throat. His eyes would not open, so he groped blindly for memory. He was not in the woods that pressed around the thinly settled fields of Muddy River, which in any case had thickened, grown orderly, renamed itself Brookline. He had been dreaming, or caught in the net of delirium more likely, judging by the heat pluming within his body. He listened, and heard the ring and clop of streets. A bit farther off, a wet slapping, snap of canvas, creak of wood, and seabirds calling. Wharves.

He remembered: he was in Boston, a north-south strip of town on a peninsula anchored to the mainland by no more than a ribbon of sandy marsh known as the Neck, which disappeared altogether in high seas. A north-south strip of town perched tiptoe between the Atlantic and the high three-peaked hill of the Tremount, like a lady marooned on a stepping-stone in a puddle, holding her skirts out of reach of the wild land behind her and water lapping all around. Having edged as far eastward as she could without getting wet, she peered coyly, anxiously, toward England and home.

He was in Boston, in a year of the smallpox, 1702. Which meant his father was dead. Had been dead a long time. Seven years.

Back in the summer of 1695, Zabdiel had been only fifteen. After shadowing his surgeon father since he could walk, working beside him as an apprentice for a few years, he had been chafing to enter Harvard that autumn when disaster had struck. Had it been the fall of a tree, the poisoned prick of a buzzing snake, the swipe of a scythe? The kick of a horse, crush of an iron-clad wheel, slip of a plow? On a farm, there were a thousand things that could hurl death at even a careful man, even a man as wise in the ways of medicine as Thomas Boylston, gentleman farmer, horse breeder, and surgeon. A thousand things that his son, still a novice, could neither fight nor fix.

Zabdiel's mind had wrapped his father's death in shadow, but could not keep guilt from smoldering through. It had never occurred to anyone else to blame him, but the fifteen-year-old heart still wrapped small and furious somewhere inside his twenty-two-year-old soul would not relinquish that death to the inscrutable decrees of Providence, as the church told him he should. If only he had been faster, better, more daring, the youth grated at his adult self, his father would still be alive. He had worked, ever since, to pluck every splinter of hesitancy from his soul.

After Dr. Boylston's death, Zabdiel's dream of college fast dwindled to dust. His elder brothers Edward and Richard were tradesmen with their own families to worry about—Edward a tailor in Boston and Richard a cordwainer, or shoemaker and leatherworker, across the estuary in Charlestown. Peter, already promised in marriage, had walked into the yoke and the pride of the family farm—or estate, as he insisted on calling it. It was heavy enough for the three adult brothers to shoulder responsibility for their mother, six sisters, and his two little brothers, Dudley, who was eight, and Tommy, only two. The money to send Zabdiel to college suddenly seemed extravagant, impossible.

Still, their father had clearly intended to establish his middle son in the profession of medicine. To honor that intention as well as Zabdiel's obvious aptitude, the family had pooled the money for him to complete his apprenticeship with their father's colleague, Dr. John Cutler, surgeon of Boston.

So Zabdiel had left the fields, woods, and secret glades, the streams and rivers, the horses, his mother, his sisters and little brothers—the hardest good-bye had been Tommy—had traveled north, letting Cambridge and college recede to his left, to arrive among the clamor and crowds of Boston. Under the meticulous Dutch eyes of Dr. Cutler, he had learned anatomy and advanced surgery—which mostly meant cutting things off. He had learned to mix medicines and measure dosages of febrifuges to cool fevers and cordials to heat cold, sluggish blood. He had learned phlebotomy, or bloodletting, had learned how and when to blister, to administer enemas, purges, vomits, and diuretics.

In New England, doctors were expected to master all three branches of the art, to be physician (or diagnostic theorist), surgeon, and apothecary all in one, and he had duly learned all the skills that would make him a real doctor in the eyes of his neighbors. Useful, in their way, he admitted. But to his mind—and the not infrequent exasperation of Dr. Cutler—he had already learned most of what was really useful from his father.

Four short lessons: Do as little as possible. Be clean. When surgery is absolutely necessary—be decisive, precise, and lightning quick. Above all, take knowledge wherever you find it. By which his father had meant *pay attention to the Indians*. Those who are left.

Long before, Thomas Boylston had gone over the sea to England, to be apprenticed in the apothecary shop of a relative in London: where, by law and long tradition, physicians, surgeons, and apothecaries kept rigidly separate. He had learned many things about mixing medicines, but many more about the dangers of blindly accepting the dictums of books—and of tradition. Upon his return, his neighbors had insisted on believing that he carried hidden somewhere about his person the trophy of an M.D. from Oxford. He tried disabusing them of this conviction, but they would not be budged; every cure rooted it more firmly in their minds.

To Zabdiel, though, he acknowledged a rather different source for much of his physic: the Narragansett, the Wampanoag, the last tattered remnants of the Pequod, the Massachusetts, the Cohasset. People his neighbors thought of as savage killers—and God knew, they could be, when pressed to it—but Thomas Boylston, chirurgeon of Muddy River, preferred to know them as skilled healers.

In 1675, the massacres that set off King Philip's War had induced him, briefly, to think otherwise. Heavy of heart, he had ridden to join Captain Thomas Prentice's mounted troopers. A few months later, however, Dr. Boylston had ridden home again from the blood and fire of the Mt. Hope campaign, and had never offered either himself or his horses again; had never suffered his sons to join the fighting. *I can see—just—city fools from Boston mistaking one tribe for another, attacking a peaceful tribe for a warring one,* he would say grimly into a tankard of beer. *But even a fool from Boston should be able to distinguish between battling warriors and barbecuing women and children alive in their homes.*

At the end of the war, there had been a free-for-all, as the settlers rounded up what Indians were left and sold them off to slavery in the West Indies, keeping a few of the likeliest for heavy work at home. To his neighbors' chagrin, Dr. Boylston let a few families live as they chose on his land in return for intermittent tutorials on the medical secrets of the wild plants in the woods and swamp marshes, and a few weeks' heavy work each year during planting and harvest. So, trailing after his father, Zabdiel had learned the secrets of the green life always curling and uncurling in the woods, learned the Indian names and uses for plants that the English blasted as weeds, if they saw them at all.

That knowledge, though uncommonly useful in practice, had proved little or no help in winning him paying patients in Boston. Zabdiel's apprenticeship with Dr. Cutler, on the other hand, gave him cachet. He was just on the verge of setting up a separate practice, when the smallpox had returned, as it did every twelve years, like some vicious clockwork made of hot knives and oiled with pus and with blood.

Dr. Cutler had summoned Zabdiel into his presence. Upon discovering that his assistant had never had the disease, Dr. Cutler had twisted his lips in dismay and looked off into the distance, as if gazing right through the walls and clear across the world to Holland. "You can leave, and hope to outrun it," he said. "Or you can stay, and almost surely contract it."

"What good will I be if I leave?"

"None, to your patients, or to me. But you will be alive, which may be of use to you."

"I want to be of use as a doctor," Zabdiel had said quietly.

So he had trailed Dr. Cutler through his rounds as the epidemic thickened, his stomach rising, his skin prickling, as he bent to cross into every sickroom. It had taken only two weeks until he had shifted places, from assistant to patient.

At first, he had taken notes, right through the first fever and the up-welling of the pocks, comparing what was happening to what various authorities said would happen. It looked, he thought with curious detachment while staring at his forearm, to be confluent. Dr. Cutler, with less equanimity, had agreed.

Within a week, the agony of the still-swelling sores splitting his skin had made further note-taking impossible. The pocks swelled his eyes shut and rattled the air in his throat. He remembered, he thought, chasing his breath, lumbering after it, trying to find it by listening for it. After that, he could remember nothing but agony, all thought compressed into a thin, dark line as he set himself, from minute to minute, to the grim task of surviving. Until now.

"Three days ago, I would not have given you one chance in ten," said Dr. Cutler's voice somewhere above him, the clipped Dutch accent spiking out, as it did whenever the doctor was in the grip of exhaustion or euphoria. "But now I think you will live to be a fine physician. Not a pretty one, maybe. But a fine one."

"Why?" He had not known a word could hurt so badly, cracking the inside of his mouth, scraping it raw. Almost, in the gasp of pain, he missed the answer. Would have, he realized later, had Dr. Cutler not taken time searching about for the right words.

"There is nothing, my boy, to spark compassion like a sojourn in hell."

In autumn 1705, in the heart of Boston, Jerusha Minot ducks inside a shop, and the din and rough smells of Dock Square—the shout and laughter of men, the harsh screams of seagulls, creak of leather and wood, all laced with the rough smells of tar, salt, fish, rum, and tobacco—disappear. The shop, though small, is thankfully open; the last two she tried were shut up. In place of the noise and the smells outside, a thick, twining scent, more luxurious than any silk, envelops her.

Chinese pagodas and island jungles bloom in her mind; she senses red-feathered birds flashing in the sun and tigers stalking through the shadows. It is a green-and-gold vision, hot and insistent with life, woven from bright threads that do not grow in the chill of New England: boxes of lemons and oranges, neatly stacked pyramids of sugar loaves, white and brown, suitable for the finest confectionary or the roughest rum. She senses chocolate, coffee, and green and black Bohea tea. A tease of snuff prickles the air—*to suit any fancy,* a placard proclaims, *whether for Brazil, Barcelona, or Spanish, perfumed or plain.* She catches tangled whiffs of salty anchovies, bitter capers, and sweet oils; plain walnuts and sugared almonds. Pungent jars of pepper, ginger, cinnamon, nutmeg, cloves, and aniseed. Musk, bergamot, and vanilla.

Her uncle and guardian, Stephen Minot, is a prosperous merchant with a large warehouse and his own wharf, so it is not as if she has never sensed such fragrances before. But she has never sensed them with such tactile immediacy, like satins draped over the counter for her own perusal and purchase.

Life does not hold much prospect of luxury for a spinster of twenty-six, a woman of billowing imagination but scarred beauty—and no money to speak of. *Especially,* she tells herself, *one living on the charity of her uncle*—as she has been since the age of eleven, when he found her and her last living brother behind the house, knee deep in earth, trying to scrape out a grave. No one else had dared come near that farm out in Dorchester, on the edge of the wilderness, in the smallpox winter of 1689–90. *Why would they?* When, two days before her eleventh birthday, her beloved father had died, and then the speckled monster had gnashed its teeth and leapt at her and her four brothers in turn. First Israel, then little George, then her favorite, Josiah, had died. And then, last and most terrible, her mother.

The neighbors were either too afraid, or too busy dying themselves, to offer any help. John, just eighteen, had enough to do to struggle suddenly into manhood and look after the farm; he had no patience or skill to look after a young sister as well. Nor was it suitable, in any case. So Uncle Stephen had galloped grimly out of the arch of trees lining the road, had helped to bury the dead, and fetched Jerusha to his home and his overwhelmed wife, the heavily pregnant mother of a two-year-old boy. Jerusha had submerged herself in the squeal and tumble of Uncle Stephen and Aunt Mary's ever-growing brood of children, in their fierce greed for love and their casual generosity in giving it.

For twelve years, she had made herself indispensable, a bulwark against the many woes of childhood—until the next smallpox epidemic. In 1702, she found herself once again helpless against her old foe. First little Peter, not quite eight months old, had died; two weeks later, two-and-a-half-year-old George had followed.

After that, she decided that no one else in her family would die ever again. Standing in this shop she clings to that decision with ferocity, however ridiculous it sounds, however much the Reverend Mr. Colman would chide her for trespassing on the prerogative of Providence. Which is why she is here, she reminds herself. Not that anyone at home is in danger at the moment. But it is never too early to battle headache, stomachache, fever.

She wanders along the shelves. There are the packaged medicines—the latest rage from England: Lockyers Pills, Dr. Salmon's Pills, the Royal Honey Water, Daffy's Elixir. She fingers them idly, curious yet aloof. She would like to know what is in them, though she has no notion of trying them. As for the basics, she herself can do better than that, and if anyone were to fall really ill, beyond her skill, Uncle Stephen would demand the proper services of an apothecary to match the medicine to the particular patient and trouble. He would never allow them to dose themselves with some potion mixed up in an anonymous vat, to be squirted at random at every ill under the sun.

Laid on a shelf she sees a winking of metal: a display of surgical instruments such as those who live out of town might need, or new doctors might care to buy: cupping glasses, urinals, lancets, plaster boxes.

But what catches her attention most is the wall whose shelves are neatly lined with white earthenware jars labeled in blue, full of powders, cordials, spirits, medicinal herbs, and metallic compounds of alum, copper, antimony, mercury, and arsenic; the heavy guns of spirit of vitriol, or sulphuric acid, and laudanum, or opium-infused alcohol. Here she finds rosemary, rue, roses, and lavender. Waters infused with black cherry, peony, or sheep's dung; syrups of violets and marsh mallows. Most intriguing of all are the many jars with no names.

These she picks up, one by one, lifting the lids and scenting the contents. Mostly they are dried herbs, and suddenly her nose fills with the scent of home. Not Uncle Stephen's home. Her home, the farm out in Dorchester: with the sunlit woods, the brown scent of working horses, of turned earth. She closes her eyes, breathes in deeply—and realizes that the scent is coming from behind her, not from the jar under her nose.

"The scent is free," says a man's voice. "I hope you will not be needing the substance."

She turns to see a man behind the counter now: tall, with laughing eyes. She knows Zabdiel Boylston, of course, by sight: they both attend the Brattle Street Church, which her uncle helped to found. But she knows nothing about Dr. Boylston, other than the fact that he is a young doctor with his own new apothecary shop, and that he is proud—justifiably, so far as she can tell—about his horses. Many girls, her young cousin Mehitabel for instance, would call him handsome, if his face weren't so pock pitted.

But then Mehitabel yearns for a dashing young sea captain. Jerusha cannot think why the sound of the blood rushing in her ears suddenly makes it difficult to think.

"What is it?" she asks, holding out the jar in her hand. *Brilliant*, she says to herself.

The name that rumbles out of him is an Indian word.

"In English," she says, a little impatiently.

"It doesn't have one."

"Then you should give it one."

"What matters is what it does. What it's for. Not what it's called. Besides, it has a perfectly good name."

"What is it for, then?"

"Rattlesnake bite."

Unaccountably, the lid leaps from her hands, and shatters on the floor.

"I don't keep a snake in there with the antidote," he says dryly.

She blushes and sinks to the floor, sweeping up the shards with her hands, as if she might fix it.

Then she notices there are other hands on the floor as well: fine ones, long fingered and precise. They seize hers.

"I'm sorry," he says. "My fault. I startled you. Close your eyes, and I'll make it up to you."

She frowns, but he says, "I won't bite. And if I do, you still have the antidote."

She grimaces at him, but closes her eyes, just as he pulls something out of his pocket.

A sweet, earthy scent suffuses through her body. She opens her eyes in surprise. He is holding a small grayish lump of what looks to be wax.

"What is it for?" she asks, giving that last word the faintest flicker of wickedness.

He shrugs. "To smell good. Some say there are medicinal properties, but I don't know what they are."

"What is it, then?"

"Ambergris," he says, a smile hovering at the corners of his mouth.

"You look like a thirteen-year-old boy," she says.

"No one knows where it comes from, but some say it is whale vomit."

Proper ladies, no doubt, would be properly offended, but she is an old aunt loved by many boys who have passed through the age of thirteen. "You *are* a thirteen-year-old boy," she says with a faint tease of amusement.

She tells him what she needs, and he measures it out, wraps it up, and she heads to the door. On the threshold, she turns. "Snakeroot," she says as firmly as any aunt, even as her whole face flashes into a young girl's smile.

"That's your Indian herb's English name. It needs one, you know. Not for its sake: for ours. How will we know it exists, know we need it, without a name?"

Then she disappears, and he watches the place where she was for a long time.

He begins courting her, soon after, with the scents of autumn: apples, pumpkins, running horses, burning leaves, saddle leather.

When scents finally evaporate in the cold, around Christmas, they publish the banns signifying their intention to marry.

That is what makes the official records: *Married, Zabdiel Boylston and Jerusha Minot, by Mr. Benjamin Colman, January 18, 1706.*

❧ 2 ❧

CURIOSITIES OF THE
SMALLPOX

IN a garret at the top of a tall gabled house, a young man shivers alone on a pallet. Around him, the room rocks gently, as if during his months at sea, dry land had taken up rippling in waves, while the water had stilled. Clenching his teeth to stop the chattering, he stares at the shards of light that splinter a small square of night framed in the window. He has not seen the stars since he was forced into the dark belly of that first ship; now he sees that the constellations he once knew as well as the patterns on his own hands have stretched and scattered into chaos.

Everything else is different here, he thinks, *why not the stars too?*

During the day, there is no sky overhead, only a low gray gloom. When this grayness grows thick enough to rain, it does not spit water, but cold, silent salt—enough to blanket the earth in white, but when it touches his tongue, it disappears without a taste, leaving only a cold burning behind. There are no leaves on the gray, jagged trees, and no birds to roost in them: the only birds are the wheeling gray-and-white gulls who cry with the voices of lost souls. This land where he must learn to be a slave is a place of nothingness and absence: no heat, no scent, no taste, no color. Some angry god has devoured them.

Even the people are grayish white, paler than the leathery demon-men who skim the shores of his home, stealing people. Paler than the scalded pink people on the Sugar Islands. Glow-in-the-dark pale, like the nameless things that squirm beneath rotten logs. Some even have eyes drained of color.

He shudders. The stars, the land, the people—everything is different, except one: his determination to find his way home.

In the reek and clank of the ship's bowels, while men stacked around him broke into babble or sank into blank silence, that determination was the rock on which he anchored his sanity. At first, like most of the others chained belly to back, he had dreamed hot red dreams of killing his captors. Then he saw what happened to those who tried. The pale demon-men quickly overpowered the rebels, killing them and hanging their dripping remains on hooks overhead, as a warning.

He heeded that warning by changing his plans, the very drift of his dreams. Not out of fear: out of cold calculation. You cannot take revenge if you're dead, he reasoned. Nor can you go home. First and foremost, he wants to go home. After that, there will be time enough to plan revenge.

To get home, he needs to learn two things. First, where he is now. And second, where, in relation to the first, his home stands. Once he knows both these things, he can draw a line between the two places. Then he will step onto that line and never stop moving until he rounds the last bend and sees home.

His thoughts circle back to the stars. Maybe the whispers he has heard are true: that after swallowing two hundred men, women, and children, the ship—so misleadingly beautiful, even fragile, from a distance—had spread its wings, risen from the sea, and flown through the spaces between the stars to land on the ocean of some other world.

He shifts fitfully on the thin mattress. It does not matter. Such a flight would make his quest harder, but not impossible: as his father, a trader far and wide along the routes that crisscross through their village, likes to say, *All roads except time can be traveled in both directions.*

He is well on his way. Has he not already wriggled into their language? In the auction pens on the bright steaming islands where the ship disgorged them, the others tried desperately to cling to anyone and everyone who shared their words. He, too, had felt that urge. But he squelched it, sidling at every opportunity to the edge of the huddle to grasp at the phrases tossed about by the pale men always watching them.

By the time they were sold, he had deciphered a great many. The two he prizes most are names: "the Gold Coast"—the demon-people's name for his land—and "Coromantee"—their name for his people. He likes the latter word especially: not for its sound, or its nonsense—so far as he can tell, it is confused, lumping together many obviously different groups of the Akan people, some of them long-standing enemies, and naming them all after Cormantine, one of the fearsome island-forts where captives are held until the ships come. No: he likes the word *Coromantee* for the tangled tones with which the pale men say it: a thin layer of contempt failing to mask deep admiration twined with fear. For his people are strong, he thinks proudly. They are warriors. *Untamable*, he heard one of the pink men say. *Bloody trouble*, spat another.

Most of the others from his ship were marched off to the cane fields under the cracking of whips; he was the only man, whole and healthy, to be shunted off into a smaller huddle of women, children, and trembling elders. His curiosity flattened to thin despair as they were herded back to the harbor, pushed aboard another ship.

For nearly the length of a complete cycle of the moon, they sailed ever northward, keeping the rising sun on their right and the setting sun on their left. Day by day, both sky and sea had drained of heat and color, and still they sailed north. He knows this because on this second ship they were not chained below. True, they spent nights locked in a small rolling room, but during the day, they were caged in a pen on deck.

He listened all the while to the boys climbing in the ropes above and the men shouting across the deck. Some of those men were given the job of seasoning the new slaves, teaching them the basic skills necessary to make them salable. In their new lives, most of them would live under one roof with their masters, expected to abide by their customs. So they had all learned the functions of chamber pots and laughable bits of clothing; he alone had learned to pick his way neatly through the dense thickets of his captors' language.

When the sailors figured out he was listening, they began teasing him, tossing out twisted snippets of truth and lies: He had been the prime slave in that first ship, sold for a king's ransom or an amorous queen's bedroom; he was refuse they could not give away to a rat. He would be boiled into stew; he would be made the chief cook of such stews. Their taunts grew so thick that the captain had heard about him, had strolled over to indulge in the curiosity of speaking with a half-wild African.

From the captain, he learned what has proved to be the truth. He was bought as a present for the chief priest of a temple, a man greedy for gifts, who had long made known his desire for a prime slave: adult, male, intelligent.

"He will get a deep well of slow-burning anger into the bargain," the captain had added.

Later, another sailor tossed another snippet his way—the only one that managed to truly alarm him: that this priest whom he must serve battled daily with hosts of demons and witches. This, he hopes fervently, was a lie.

That very morning they had sailed into the harbor that laps at this city.

Two men had walked out to the ship: not on the water, but on the longest of the many wide wooden roads that stretch from the city into the sea like fingers grasping for treasure. The floating road had been crowded, but even from a distance, he saw that these two men were different, swathed in power and respect. They hailed the captain, who herded him off the ship and into their company. Then the two men together with the captain had led him to this house and presented him to his new master, the priest whose title is reverend doctor. Whose name is Cotton Mather.

For all their evident power, the threesome who brought him here not only admire this priest, they fear him: he saw it flare in their eyes.

By his new slave's estimation, the Reverend Dr. Cotton Mather is ferociously intense, his body always pulled taut, fairly humming, like wire pulled almost to the breaking point. As for intelligence and slow-burning anger: the young man has rarely seen their like before. But he refuses to fear him, telling himself that he will fear only the demons and witches this Mather battles, if indeed he battles them.

It did not seem likely, at first. For the reverend doctor is one of those men who must battle to hurl the words from his throat. When this Mather first opened his mouth to speak, it seemed he might be choking. But the priest had closed his eyes, slacked his jaw, and then, as if some floodgate had opened, the words had spilled out in a slow, almost sung cadence of power and beauty. "Henceforth," he had chanted, "your name is Onesimus."

Newly named, Onesimus was so astonished that he barely registered the information that streamed out, though he remembers it well enough now: that the name belonged first to another slave of another chief priest, of the Mather's god: a man named Saint Paul.

Once the reverend doctor had begun, he had no trouble flowing on through words, though they remained curiously distinct and measured, as well as melodic. He began singing out questions. Onesimus's age?

Seventeen or eighteen, near as Onesimus can tell.

His tribe?

Then it was Onesimus who hesitated. Not, as the Reverend Dr. Mather clearly thought, because he did not understand the question, but because he did not trust the consequences of his answer. He feared that these men drawn so close around him might send others to round up everyone from his village, if he betrayed too much.

But he had to say something. "Coromantee," he blurted out.

An inexplicable look of rapture crossed Mather's face. "*Garamante!*" he exclaimed, changing the word a little, hardening it.

"Coromantee," corrected Onesimus, but Mather heard the word he wished to hear: a word, he said, that until now he has heard only in books—the slender boxes filled with layers of leaves that store the voices of far distant and sometimes long-dead men. "Virgil, Lucan, Strabo, Pliny," chanted Mather with reverence. They have all spoken to him of a warrior race in Africa called the Garamantes, a race known by the Pharaohs, the Greeks, the Romans.

At once, Onesimus realized the implications: some of the information in those books concerns the place where he comes from. And if that is so, perhaps somewhere inside one of them lurks the information he needs to get home: where home is; where he is.

Even as he wondered how to make those books speak to him, the Reverend Dr. Mather perceived his interest and promised to teach him: a crucial step, he said, in learning to worship his god.

Up in his garret, Onesimus frowns. He wants no part of a deity who devours color and heat.

But the reverend doctor did not perceive his dilemma: oversensitive to some things, he is strangely blind to others. He sped on to another subject that still, several hours later, startles Onesimus: wanted to know, do his people suffer from the spotted disease? Smallpox, as they call it here, though what about it might be thought of as small, he cannot fathom.

A silly question, he thinks. He frowns again, thinking about it, just as he frowned that afternoon at Mather. "When it gets in among us, people die like rotten sheep," he said.

"Like rotten sheep," the priest repeated happily, scratching black marks on his white sheet. "Have you had it?" he asked, looking up.

"No," said Onesimus. "And yes," he added triumphantly, even as his new master's face began to fall.

And then he held up his arm, showing his scar. "In my country, no person dies of it who has courage." Once bitten, forever after safe. He, Onesimus, this scar proudly proclaims, has dared the hot speckled wrath of the earth god and survived. He is safe.

That is when it happened: across the Reverend Dr. Mather's face flashed a look of confusion that curled through suspicion into respect. It is a look that Onesimus will treasure till he dies: for though Mather did not see his courage, he saw something else.

Up in the dark, Onesimus stretches with the pleasure of it. For the look in the priest's eye told him, for the first time since all his confusion and sorrow began, that the pale demon-men are not, even here in their own land, entirely dominant in the possession of knowledge. He, Onesimus, possesses knowledge that one of them—a chief priest no less—envies.

In his mind, he watches it all over again: sees their eyes meet, sees the flash of incomprehension in the other, and then something still more exquisite: he sees Mather perceive that he, Onesimus, has seen his ignorance.

The priest does not shout, or kick, or beat, like many other men might. Instead, he looks down again and begins making the magic designs that will transfer the voice of his, Onesimus's wisdom, into one of those books.

In the cold, dark room at the top of the stairs, Onesimus curls his body around that memory. In a warm secret flush of satisfaction, he falls fast asleep.

Anno Domini, in the year of our Lord, 1716, on a hot, bright New England morning in July, the Reverend Cotton Mather—Doctor of Divinity (Glasgow), Fellow of the Royal Society of London, and minister of Boston's Old North Church—lies on the floor of his library, weeping.

His fifty-three-year-old figure, stretched, as he likes to say, prostrate in the dust (though the maid, indignantly, disagrees) is gaunt from frequent fasting, punishment for myriad sins not only of the flesh, but also of the spirit. For he has been specially marked out by God to bear a terrible burden of pride, anger, malice, and even hatred; lately, he has been marked out, also, to bear the rare burden of prosperity—*a most wonderful Prosperity! A valuable Consort! A comfortable new Dwelling! A kind Neighborhood! Health and Strength!*—which blessings he must atone for by discovering some certain way to improve himself, his family, and his flock in their piety.

Staggering beneath this load, he rises early each morning and reads a chapter from some pious book to his new wife—*that collection of a thousand lovelinesses, the best of American women*—Lydia Lee George, now Mather, thanks be to God. He lost his first two wives to wracking disease—Abigail to the slow gnawing of breast cancer, Elizabeth to a sudden conflagration of measles. They had been quiet, dutiful doves, but Lydia—*Lydia!*—is a falcon whose wingbeats whip his blood to froth.

Such lust, even in marriage, is not becoming in a minister. So he spends ever longer hours up here in his sun-flooded sanctuary at the top of his spacious new four-story house, as near to heaven as he can get, wrapped in light and submerged in secret prayer.

Prayer is not enough, of course. It must be allied with action. "G.D.," Mather thus begins each day's entry in his diary: "Good Devised." For, as he continually urges his flock, "We all came into the World upon a very important *Errand*, which *Errand* is, To *Do* and to *get* Good!" He knows that some of the young bloods mock his way of making capital letters, italics, and exclamation points audible in his exhortations, though his dramatic emphases spur their better-schooled elders into weeping frenzies of piety.

"In a *Good Man*," he tells his congregation, "the *Grace* of GOD overcomes *Ill Temper;* 'tis a *Burden* to him; and he takes a *Revenge* upon it by multiplying Acts of *Goodness* that shall repair the *Errors* into which Base Passions have betrayed him."

In revenge for evil, he shrills tightly to himself, *Do Good.*

The vengeful good he has devised for this week involves writing. So he rises to his knees, which creak and pop, and pushes himself to his feet, creaking even more. As the tears dry on his cheeks, he settles at his desk, flipping the skirts of his coat on either side of the chair back. Later, at nine o'clock, Lydia, the children, and the servants will knock and enter for an hour of family prayers, after which Onesimus will carry in cups of hot, sweet chocolate, and they will all break the night's fast together, giving thanks to God.

Meanwhile, he has a few precious hours for the private doing of good. He draws out a clean sheet of paper, and dips his pen into the ink.

To the learned Dr. John Woodward
Secretary of the Royal Society

July 12, 1716
Boston, in New England
     Curiosities of the Small-Pox
Sir,
  The history of that grievous and wondrous disease, the Small-Pox, would no doubt be as grateful to the learned as the distemper itself is loathsome. However, I shall presume at this time to entertain you with no more than two or three American curiosities upon it.

He pauses to reflect on the unexpected ways the world unwinds. A few months back, ships from the old country spilled a plague of grumbling Scots onto the wharves of Boston. Grateful for the doctorate of divinity that the University of Glasgow has seen fit to bestow upon him (purely on the merits of his writings, since he has never crossed the sea, much less set foot in Glasgow) and impressed, too, by the severe piety of the Church of Scotland as well as by the visitors' letters of introduction from famed men of learning, Mather welcomed them to town, throwing open the doors of his church, his home, and his library.

The Scots proved a needling blessing, sharp as the teeth of weasels. For debate, it had to be said that they were excellent fellows. But they did not know when to concede. Where reverence was due to superior learning and age, they offered only spleen and spite. One, even, had twisted his words to lies.

Still, on balance, the encounter had been profitable. In exchange for the use of his library—notably large and deep, he thought proudly, even by European standards—he had had free perusal of the books they had brought, some of them new to him, especially those in the collection of young William Douglass, M.D., late of Bristol, but born and bred in the Scottish town of Gifford, tucked between the Firth of Forth and the Lammermuir Hills, just east of Edinburgh.

Small but select, my son, Mather had murmured, thinking briefly that the phrase might as well describe the owner as his library. Douglass's round face belied long years of study at four universities of Edinburgh, Paris, Leiden, and Utrecht. His scowl, Mather had heard his fellow minister Benjamin Colman say, on the other hand, attested to even longer years of dyspepsia, or perhaps ill-fitting shoes. If Douglass had scowled at Mather's assessment, Mather did not see it; he was engrossed in the man's books.

Among them, Mather had come across recent numbers of the *Philosophical Transactions of the Royal Society*—the most learned journal in the world. In its pages were papers garnered from the far corners of the earth, deemed by the Royal Society—the most learned body of men in the world—to be of sufficient importance to broadcast to the reading public.

Several years before, in 1712, Mather had sent to the Society a series of letters he called *Curiosa Americana;* to his lasting delight, these pages, unworthy as they were, had been so well received that the Fellows of the Royal Society, presided over by Sir Isaac Newton, had voted to welcome him into their membership, adding the precious "F.R.S." after his name, following the Glasgow-given "D.D." As was only just, however, the Lord had seen fit to bestow honor only to turn it into a trial: the Society had since then unaccountably omitted his name from their list of members. For several years now, he had failed to receive copies of the *Philosophical Transactions*, though he heard the letters that had so impressed the Fellows had duly been printed.

Bearing up under the cross the Lord had laid down for him, Mather had not informed the Society's secretary of this lapse. Instead, he sent in a second series of curiosities. He was waiting patiently for them to correct the error on their own, or until some angel deemed it time to nudge them toward justice.

Leafing quickly through the pages of Latin, English, mathematical equations, and astronomical charts, in Vol. 29, No. 339, for April–June

1714, Mather at long last found, on page sixty-two, what he had been yearning to see: *An extract of several Letters from Cotton Mather, D.D., to John Woodward, M.D., and Richard Waller, Esq.*

Scanning it, he had felt hot pleasure and pain suffusing across his skin—so sharp that he can feel it again, even in memory. True, they had printed his diligently researched and reported letters, but they had also mutilated them, whittling a hundred pages down to ten: Here, cast up like so much flotsam and jetsam amid the wreckage, were brief, teasing details of giants' bones found buried deep in the earth near Albany, Indian medicinal plants, bird behavior, the force of imagination, monstrous births ("nothing very observable," someone, presumably the publisher, Dr. Edmund Halley, had commented), people cured of wounds that should have been mortal ("In this, little of philosophical information"). Here were his Indian time-keeping, rainbows, mock suns, prophetic dreams, rattlesnakes, thunder and lightning, earthquakes, hail big as hens' eggs, ice storms, exploding trees, and people living to great old age.

Burning and freezing with the honor of it, with the horror of it, he turned the page. And read:

> *An Account or History, of the Procuring of the SMALL POX by incision, or Inoculation; as it has for some time been practiced at Constantinople. Being an extract of a letter from Emanuel Timonius, Oxon. & Patav. M.D., F.R.S. dated at Constantinople, December, 1713.*
>
> *Communicated to the Royal Society by John Woodward, M.D., Professor of Medicine at Gresham College, and F.R.S.*

A twinge of doubt, a flush of fascination. He read on, greedily. Pangs of pride and envy and disappointment swirled through him: his long-researched, carefully written series of thirteen letters had been chopped down to ten pages; Timonius's single offering had been "extracted" to ten and a half. If only he had thought to include that bit of knowledge, which after all, he had been privy to long before Timonius ferreted it out from Greek hags: perhaps he, too, would have been printed at length, without the sniping commentary. But he turned from that thought; he would not rail against Dr. Timonius. He would try harder, labor longer and more clearly, on his own part.

It had taken him a while, but he had an intimation of what he must do: he would write another series of letters.

It could only be seen as a glorious, even wondrous, challenge to his spirit, a blessing indeed, guarding him from becoming too proud.

In revenge for evil, *Do Good*. That was when he knew what he must do.

Not only would he return to writing letters, he would comment as proper upon the other submissions to the *Philosophical Transactions*.

Now he turns to that task:

> *The Small-Pox has usually proven a great plague to us poor Americans, and getting among our Indians hath swept away whole nations of them, and left not enough living to bury the dead.*
>
> *We have been ready to suspect a peculiar agency of the invisible world in the infliction of the Small-Pox upon our city of Boston, when we saw that from the first foundations of it in the year 1630, down to the year 1702, the distemper observed the precise period of twelve years in its mortal visits unto us. Now and then a vessel would, in the intervening space, bring in the distemper among us. However, it would not spread. But on the twelfth year, no precaution would keep it off: it must be epidemical—so raging, so reaching, that it would come at unborn children: They have been born full of it upon them.*
>
> *But at last, two years ago in 1714, when a seventh period for a variolated twelfth year was arrived, our observation has met with an interruption. The compassion of Heaven would not add that calamity unto what we suffered the year before in the measles, which at once arrested almost the whole city, and proved so strangely mortal to a multitude of people that we buried above a hundred in a month, among whom were no less than five in my own family.*

Five gone in two weeks. He cannot help counting them over in his head: his beloved second wife, Elizabeth, her two-week-old twins, Martha and Eleazar, born prematurely in the labor of nursing and the oncoming fever of her own terrible bout with measles, two-and-a-half-year-old Jerusha, and their maidservant. He remembers drawing up a list of his children. A terrible list. Of fifteen, nine dead.

He fears it will get worse, oh yes, he fears it. His favorite, Katharine, his Katy, twenty-five and lovely, a *Lamb* inexpressibly dear, is not only a fine cook, exquisite needleworker, and songbird, but his companion in study. Fluent in Hebrew and Latin, a composer of pious poetry, she is his secretary and scribe. She survived the measles, but for two months now she has been declining daily into a consumption—she is succumbing, in other words, to tuberculosis.

He wrenches his mind back to the smallpox.

The last time it came into the town, in 1702, he writes, he urged the physicians to try Dr. Sydenham's cool regimen, which he had seen discussed in the *Philosophical Transactions of the Royal Society*. He is satisfied, he adds, that through his urgings, many lives were saved.

He flows on with his description of the treatment, forgetting utterly that he got it from the Royal Society in the first place, so the Fellows' need for a rehash is presumably minimal. He has fallen in love, as he so often does, with the very act of writing: with the way that words flow from him in a glory of speed, the thoughts bending, curling, curving at will, stretching to their utmost, but never breaking. So different from the torture of speaking, of smoothing through the stutter that once tempted him, so strongly, to deny the ministry and follow medicine. But he had proved strong enough—with the Lord's help—to deny the lure of ease and pleasure, to take the thorny path of righteousness.

> *All that I shall now add [*he sums up*] will be my thanks to you, for communicating to the public in the* Philosophical Transactions, *the account which you had from Dr. Timonius at Constantinople: the method of obtaining and procuring the Small-Pox by incision, which I perceive also by some in my neighbourhood lately come from thence, has been for some time successfully practiced there. I am willing to confirm you, in a favourable opinion of Dr. Timonius's communication; and therefore, I do assure you, that many months before I met with any intimations of treating the Small-Pox with the method of inoculation, anywhere in Europe; I had from a servant of my own, an account of its being practiced in Africa.*
>
> *Enquiring of my Negro-man Onesimus, who is a pretty intelligent fellow, whether he ever had the Small-Pox; he answered, both Yes and No; and then told me, that he had undergone an operation which had given him something of the Small-Pox and would forever preserve him from it; adding that it was often used among the Guramantese, and whoever had the courage to use it, was forever free from the fear of the contagion. He described the operation to me, and shew'd me in his arm the scar which it had left upon him; and his description of it, made it the same that afterwards I found related unto you by your Timonius.*

Onesimus, Mather sighs to himself, scratching himself with his quill, leaving a faint scribbling of ink on his chin. He will have to do something about Onesimus. He has tried reasoning, cajoling, and beating his servant, and has returned once again to reasoning. But still, the man exhibits some actions of a thievish aspect: he will take small things when he wants them—needs them, as he says. Beads from a broken bracelet. Buttons. A chicken. Herbs from the garden. Bits of bright-colored cloth. This, even though he is allowed to work for himself outside the Mather home, and to keep his earnings, too, so long as some of them are put to pious purposes.

But then, his piety, it must be said, at times appears shockingly—yes, quite shockingly—lax. He still cannot, for instance, be made to see the blessing of losing his small son Onesimulus to the bosom of the Lord last March, before the wicked world had a real chance to corrupt the boy. Furthermore, he is proving a great disappointment as a servant. Growing useless, frorward, disobedient, rebellious. What is the word he seeks? Mather can sense it hiding there, peeping out behind some veil of darkness in his mind. He waits, with the cunning of a cat, and then pounces. *Immorigerous.*

Perhaps he should dispose of Onesimus and supply his family with a better servant. He frowns, bites his lip. Such a grave matter requires *Caution,* he thinks, much *Prayer,* much *Humiliation* before the Lord. Meantime, he has another project to finish.

He turns back to his letter. To the problem of smallpox. The mystery of inoculation. It works, of that he is certain. What he would like to know is, what does the Royal Society intend to do about it?

> *This cannot but expire in a wonder and in a request unto my Dr. Woodward. How does it come to pass that no more is done to bring this operation into experiment and into fashion—in England? When there are so many thousands of people that would give many thousands of pounds to have the danger and horror of this frightful disease well over with them? I beseech you, Sir, to move it and save more lives than Dr. Sydenham. For my own part, if I should live to see the Small-Pox again enter into our city, I would immediately procure a consult of our physicians, to introduce a practice, which may be of so very happy a tendency. But could we hear that you have done it before us, how much would that embolden us!*
>
> *Sir,*
> *Your most sincere servant*
> *Cotton Mather, D.D., F.R.S.*

❧ 3 ❧

THE BEAUTY OF THE SEA

THE ship was sighted homeward bound on October 28, 1720: two snowy pyramids of sail skimming over the cold, gray horizon, threading through the scattered islands of Boston's outer harbor.

Boston watched with mounting excitement. Eight weeks out from London, she was not only expected, but longed for. The North Atlantic would soon shroud itself in winter, making transoceanic voyages all but impossible; she would be one of the last ships in from London until spring.

With a population hovering between eleven and twelve thousand, Boston was not only the largest port but by far the largest town in North America. Philadelphia was behind by several thousand, and New York was just over half her size. She was, in fact, one of the largest towns in the British Empire, home ports included.

It was her ships, her deep-water harbor, and her dour Puritan work ethic that had catapulted Boston to greatness: transformed her, quite suddenly, from a small haven of godliness to a queen of the sea, a trade hub of national if not yet world-class importance. Proud of her success, she draped herself in satin and silk, enjoyed strong Madeira wine and fast horses, and sipped coffee, tea, and chocolate poured from china and silver by black slaves in fancy livery. Deep in her old Puritan soul, she was also dismayed with herself: with her hunger for finery, for rum, for carnal riot. She was falling headlong from grace into giddy luxury, and she knew it. She just didn't know whether to weep or sing.

In the case of a ship from London, she usually chose to sing, and sometimes to dance as well.

This ship, like most in from the capital, would be carrying all the luxuries the town craved. Even better, if more fleeting, she would also be carrying news. In well-thumbed sheets of roughly printed flimsy paper and in stage-whispered gossip, Bostonians would soon learn who was in and out at court and in Parliament. They would trace the downward spiral of the stock market in the wake of the South Sea Company's spectacular, scandalous crash. They would devour news about wars and peace and devious political maneuverings the world over: Paris, Hanover, Vienna, Madrid, Moscow, Constantinople. They would flutter over the latest fashions in dress, hairstyles, and comportment, the very latest in music and books. For it was not just material wealth for which the city yearned: it was sophistication. And ships from London were her chief source.

This ship—properly a merchant brig—was all the more welcome for being commanded with a lively grace by Captain John Gore. Harvard College class of '02, member of the Brattle Street Church, mariner, scientific navigator, collector of fine books, and friend of many, he was only thirty-eight, but already coming to the fore as one of the city's favorite sons.

So Boston fairly craned her collective neck, watching the brig skim in toward shore. *Beautifully made and beautifully sailed*, the citizens congratulated each other—for they all laid claim to the fine ships that called this harbor home. *And beautifully furling her sails*, noted some doubting Thomas, with a frown. The town stood on tiptoe to see.

It was just so. Unaccountably, she was slowing—no, dropping anchor some distance from the wharves. The boat skidding merrily out to greet her veered aside into the wind. Then the town saw what the boat had seen: a flutter of yellow toiling up her mainmast. She was running up the yellow jack, the flag that warned "disease on board."

Pulling oars, the boat drew in close enough to hear the shouted news, far enough off to escape contagion. After a few minutes, the boat drew back toward the town dock; a little while later it returned with one extra passenger, skirts whipping in the wind. Rebecca Gore. After a brief exchange of shouts, she blew her husband a kiss and stepped back, throwing a cloak over her face and turning again toward shore. The boat returned with Madam Gore and a tale to freeze the heart.

Soon after leaving London, Captain Gore had discovered he was in command of a coffin ship: after one sailor erupted into the smallpox, the captain had interviewed every last man and woman on board. He was lucky; they were all lucky. There were no more than seven more people aboard who had not yet had the disease. By the time they reached Boston, six of them had caught it. Again, they were lucky: only one body had slipped, canvas-wrapped, into the sea.

As they glided into the outer harbor, Captain Gore made it clear to his passengers and crew that no one would go ashore anywhere but into quarantine on Spectacle Island until they knew the fate of the eighth man, and beyond that, until the last scab had dropped from the last survivor. He had sailed in so close only to deliver this news and to catch one glimpse of home—not just the town, but the tall brick house high on the slopes of Beacon Hill, where Rebecca awaited him. That Rebecca herself sailed out as near as possible to him had been at once a surprise and a relief: it was just like her.

Soon after, the ship drew away eastward, mooring off the quarantine island named for its resemblance to a pair of spectacles through which the ocean could peer up at the skies. The sick were taken ashore to the Province Hospital, clean and new built for the purpose just three years before, and John Gore settled down in his cabin to wait out the fate of the eighth man: himself.

He did not have to wait long. The following day his temperature soared. Three days later, on All Hallow's Eve, the telltale rash sputtered across his skin, growing thicker by the hour. For a week, he clung to life, to the cool, smooth-skinned dream of his wife, but his luck had run out. On November 7, he died. The following evening he was consigned to a grave scooped from the windswept sand of the quarantine island.

Officially, this was not news. It was a secret, kept out of the papers, whirring in hushed whispers. It spread through town, of course, like fire in a dry midwinter wind. The memorial service, a week later, filled the Brattle Street Church to overflowing—not for the man, though he was widely liked, but for the martyr: the captain with the courage to die in sight of home, yet in exile, for the sake of a city.

"Captain Gore was truly an ornament to his country, to the college, to the town, and to our church," Mr. William Cooper preached at the funeral, his voice ringing out over hushed weeping, his eyes held with kindness on Rebecca. "Very much the honor of his order among us, a glory to his profession, *the beauty of the sea*."

"Ships!" shouted six-year-old Tommy Boylston, dashing into his father's apothecary shop, as Saturday afternoon dipped toward sundown and the Sabbath on the twenty-second of April 1721.

He was Zabdiel Boylston's favorite among his six surviving children, in spite of his effort not to have favorites. At fourteen, Zabby—his namesake—had reached an age when even the best of sons would clash all too easily with his father, and Zabby was wild, though Dr. Boylston hoped not irretrievably spoiled. John, thirteen, was on the other hand alarmingly earnest and good. As for the girls, nine-year-old Jerusha and eight-year-old Mary already twittered like little ladies. Lizzy, the baby at four, was thankfully as fat, firm, and jolly as her elder sister of the same name, lost to death before this Lizzy's birth, had once been frail. But Tommy—he was all imp. Just like his uncle, Zabdiel's brother Tom, after whom young Tommy took his name (or half of it, as Tom said; the boy's grandfather had to be allowed his fair share). Tommy—little thief—had also taken Tom's walk, Tom's talk, and Tom's laugh, as well as the same rock-solid certainty in Zabdiel's invincibility that Tom had possessed as a child. Like his uncle before him, he yearned to grow up to be just like Zabdiel. How could such antics and adoration not fill one with delight?

"*Ships!*" Tommy repeated breathlessly, all other words having evaporated.

There were always ships in Boston Harbor, of course. It would surely take more than a ship or two, thought Dr. Boylston, to produce quite the thrum of excitement streaming through the town's streets. He dropped pestle into mortar and let his son tug him out the door of the shop. The lilacs in his spacious garden would burst any day now, filling the whole street with their sweet lavender foam, but as yet the damp prickle of salt from the harbor still reigned supreme. A few yards down, father and son rounded a corner into the open space of Dock Square at the working heart of the city: and stopped short, eyes and mouths round with awe.

From end to end, the outer harbor was scattered with the plume and puff of sails—twenty, thirty, forty ships—all bearing down on the town like a flock of gigantic white-winged swans chasing day out of the thickening east.

It was the Saltertudas fleet in from the West Indies, ushered home by the sleek power of His Majesty's Ship *Seahorse*. She was a warship, though not one of the behemoth ships-of-the-line meant to spout half a ton of fiery death at France with each thundering breath. In the eternal shifting dance between strength and speed, her makers had turned into the wind, letting it streamline their very dreams, not to mention their plans and their planing tools. She was no lightweight—she carried twenty six-pound guns and so could throw sixty pounds of fire and steel with one roar—but she was built for speed, and speed she had. Zabdiel was no seaman, not by a long shot, but to his eye she was lithe, lissome, and lovely.

The beauty of the sea. How that phrase from John Gore's funeral sermon hung on the mind.

Boston, it had to be said, was overdue for some beauty. Between the ravages of pirates and a scarcity of currency, trade had very nearly ground to a halt. At least the navy was attempting to fix the part of the problem it could reach: assigning ships like *Seahorse* to escort merchant fleets in convoys, sending others in heavily armed squadrons to scour pirate-infested waters from Surinam to Nova Scotia. The provincial government, by contrast, had proved worse than useless in solving the currency crisis.

Within days of arriving, the new governor, Samuel Shute—a bit of a pompous ass, admittedly—had tripped into a petty personal feud with Elisha Cooke, Esq. That gentleman was known as a hard-drinking boor: once, while too drunk to stand, he had been heard to call the governor a blockhead. But he was also the wealthiest and most powerful man in New England, the boss who ran Boston's political machine—and through it, the province's elected house of representatives. These two men, both crucial to the smooth running of any government, had mishandled each other colossally; their mutual contempt had quickly seeped through their circles of friends, which had hardened into factions. By now, the parties were far more interested in thwarting each other than in governing.

Still, Zabdiel reflected, these irritations seemed easy enough to sort into some kind of order—enough to comprehend them, at any rate, if not to fix them. The private troubles that had haunted his family through the autumn and winter were more amorphous, as hard to grasp as sea fog at midnight, impossible to control.

In July, Jerusha—at forty-one, old enough to make pregnancy frighteningly dangerous—had borne their eighth child, a son she named for her brother Josiah. Jerusha, thank the Lord, had survived, but little Jo had not. His first pink bloom gradually, inexorably, faded to blue-gray. All too soon, they had laid him to rest in the churchyard next to their first Elizabeth.

Helpless to cure his wife's hollow-eyed grief, Zabdiel awoke one morning in October to find a professional squabble forced upon him. Not in the open, but in a sly campaign waged in whispers over tea tables and punch bowls, screamed silently in advertisements in the newspapers:

> *Dr. Sharp of London being arrived here at Boston, in his return from Jamaica to England, gives notice that he is to be advised with at the Widow Leblond's in Tremount Street, Boston, he intending to stay but a few weeks in this country. If any are troubled with cancered breasts, or any other cancerous or scrophulous tumours, whether in the throat, or any part of the body, the King's Evil, leprosy, scurvy, rheumatisms, or any sort of stinking rotten ulcers, proceeding from what cause soever: and because he is a stranger, and to prevent the calumny of designing men, the doctor promises where he miscarries of curing (if such a thing should happen) that he will take no money.*

This proclamation was not, for all its air of proud innocence, a lone voice of salvation crying in the wilderness: it was a salvo of heavy artillery.

There were upwards of fifteen doctors practicing in Boston—but this boast was aimed with precision at Dr. Boylston's fame throughout the province as a high-risk surgeon skilled in cutting away cancers as well as excising bladder stones. Almost, it had the flavor of the conniving malice of that young Scottish snake, Dr. William Douglass—except that Douglass would not admit the merits of Dr. Sharp any more than he would admit those of Dr. Boylston.

The part that really grated was the postscript: *N.B. he gives his advice to the poor gratis.* Boylston did not give advice to anyone gratis: which is not to say that he was heartless in the matter of caring for the poor. Jerusha teased that they had traded places: he had become as sentimental as the maiden aunt she used to be. Time and again, he took hopeless cases into their home, nursing them around the clock for months, doing his best to alleviate advanced syphilis, or patch together whatever ribbons and shards were left after knife fights or savage wife-beatings.

He just demanded, as was proper, that someone pay for his services: if not the patients, then the township responsible for their welfare. Some thought his charges high at first glance, but they were scrupulously just. In tricky cases, they included the unusual luxury of room and board in his house, with skilled nursing day and night. Furthermore, his drugs were never substandard, never siphoned off, but delivered at the full dose, in the highest quality he could cull from his garden and orchard, from the woods, from fields and mines as far away as Spain, Turkey, the Spice Islands, China.

He didn't mind if patients who were neither destitute nor flush with cash eked out their payments across years, so long as they made an honest effort meet their debt. He had been poor once himself, on his own in the world after his father died: but had paid off every debt, every bit of charity, to the last penny. It was a matter of respect.

In private, he was hurt by this sly challenge to both his competence and his compassion. In public, he responded with dignified silence.

His admirers had not been so reticent. Eventually, at Jerusha's urging, he had allowed their indignation to bubble over into print. Even so, it had been odd to read this description in the same newspaper:

> *For the public good of any that have or may have cancers: These may certify that my wife had been laboring under the dreadful distemper of a cancer in her left breast for several years; although the cure was attempted by several doctors from time to time, it was without success. When life was almost despaired of by reason of its repeated bleedings, growth, and stench, and she seemed to be in danger of immediate death: We sent for*

Dr. Zabdiel Boylston of Boston, who on July 30, 1718 (in the presence of several ministers and others assembled on that occasion), cut her whole breast off and dressed it in the space of five minutes by the watch of one then present; and by the Blessing of GOD on his endeavors, she has long since obtained a perfect cure.

I deferred the publication of this so long, lest it should have broken out again.

Edward Winslow
Rochester, Oct. 14, 1720

Dr. Boylston had not previously advertised this spectacular case. Partly because he was not sure Sarah Winslow would live: cancers as far gone as hers often came back. Partly because no one in New England had ever dreamed of such an operation, much less performed one. He knew what would happen. Through most people's minds, over and over, would slice the vision of a circle of men holding a woman down on her own kitchen table, while he, Dr. Boylston, stood in the middle, one hand forking the diseased breast, the other scything through it with a ruthless blade. The flesh would fall to floor as he reached for the red-hot cauterizing iron, sealing the wound by searing it, the sizzle and steam pierced by screaming of a kind rarely heard outside childbirth or war.

That was the swift horror of surgery. What the doctor could not make most people understand was that it was also the most compact, condensed part of an operation, lasting mere minutes. The vast bulk of his time was spent cleaning, not cutting. At the Winslows, he had spent hours supervising the scrubbing of that already clean kitchen: the table, the floor, the hearth. He had cleaned his instruments himself, trusting no one else to do it. And he had instructed the maid how to help Mrs. Winslow clean herself just as thoroughly.

Because he arrived with a cask of strong rum, people thought he soused his patients with it, but that was not true. Alcohol only made people bleed faster; he strictly forbade it, at least on the inside. He doused them rather liberally, however, on the outside, all around the area where he was to cut. He allowed opium for the pain, but only after the operation was over.

A smaller but significant bit of time was taken up with study: he had examined Sarah minutely, determining exactly where and how he meant to cut.

Only then had he motioned to the ministers to add physical force to the heavenly might of their praying, and hold the woman down. (That was what they were there for, as far as Dr. Boylston was concerned: there was no way his man Jack, though as fine an assistant as you could wish, could hold her still all by himself.)

The fee of £35, though steep, had been as scrupulously fair as all his others. Mrs. Winslow had been far too ill to come to Boston, so he and Jack, the black slave he had trained as his assistant, had ridden all the way down to her home on Cape Cod. After the operation, they had lingered in Rochester a few more days, until Boylston was sure she was out of danger. He had been anxious about the cautery. Ligatures were much cleaner, and healed prettier: but that wound had been too wide and too bloody for stitching. He had risked an infection-prone burn in exchange for the speed of fire.

When this astonishing report had reached the Boston papers in mid-November 1720, the public, as he expected, paled and went green. *Disgusting*, grunted the men; *horrible*, shuddered the women. But many more of his neighbors than Dr. Boylston would have guessed took deep breaths and firmly settled their stomachs. Captain Winslow and his wife were well liked; their adoration for each other was legendary, and they had three children to think of too. Besides, at the time she had been just thirty-six, not young, perhaps, but too young to die of an old woman's disease. For Sarah Winslow, the operation had meant the chance to watch her children grow up, to scent several more seasons of apple pies baking, to lie in bed next to her sleeping husband and watch the moon wax and wane out the window. On consideration, people nodded to one another, they had to agree: better to have one's breast cut off than to paste the spreading sore with strong (but not strong enough) smelling ointments and drink opium until one died, chased in circles by nightmares and pain.

Daring, said his admirers. *Courageous and kind. The man you'd want by if it was your wife ill. Your husband, or your child.*

Dangerous, hissed his detractors. *A butcherous quack. He calls it a cure, but it might well have killed her. Who was to know?*

Slowly, the jangling had died down. Dr. Boylston's patients had drifted back, while Dr. Sharp shut up shop and slipped out of town—not, as boasted, to London, but to Piscataqua, New Hampshire.

Even as this controversy was coming to a head, John Gore had sailed into the harbor to die in sight of home.

The beauty of the sea: John would have laughed at that phrase applied to himself, but loved it, set to the sight that was stilling traffic in Dock Square. Up and down the Long Wharf, too, and all along the crescent-shaped shore from the hump of the South Battery to the coy curving tip of the North End. *Ships.*

* * *

Zabdiel sent Tommy scooting back to the shop to fetch Jack; they reappeared in a twinkling, Jack with his two-and-a-half-year-old son Jackey perched on his shoulders. The little party threaded its way down to the Town Dock, breathing in the white-winged power of the view, and jostling the others joining the impromptu fair setting up along the shore.

Tommy danced about underfoot all the while, naming as many ships as he could by the shape of hull and sail—*Friends Adventure*, Captain James; *Neptune*, Captain Langsford; and one—no—two *Sarahs*, plus Captain Pitts's *John & Sarah* to boot. And there was Captain Fletcher's *Tryal*—why would you name a ship that? Or *Prudence*? There, see? Still far to the south: Captain Beardmore's *Leopard*, fast and dangerous as her name. Tommy liked her captain's name too: dashingly close to Blackbeard. Best of all, they all agreed, though, was the king's ship: the three cloudbanks of sail—one for each mast—that marked out HMS *Seahorse*.

Tommy Boylston was not the only boy in Boston whose soul was thrilling to ships.

The following morning, Charles Paxton, impatient son of an imperious father, proved so useless in the boat they were bringing alongside the *Seahorse*, that his father felt it necessary to point out that it would do him no good to be seen as an incompetent seaman in full view of the frigate's deck.

The previous December, Charlie had disappeared, leaving his mother in hysterics for three days. It was Scipio, the family's black butler/valet/footman/jack-of-all-trades—specially the heavy or dirty ones, as he put it—who had ferreted out the young master's whereabouts. Ever so carefully, he had coaxed the information from the network of enslaved Africans and indentured Irish who knew everything or nothing about every home, warehouse, shop, and ship in Boston, depending on a mysterious balance of loyalties, bribes, and favors owed. Scipio always made sure that he had many favors owed. Being as least as good a businessman as his master, he had seen immediately that in this instance, he could with a minimum of trouble call in a minor favor or two and transform them into a large debt of gratitude on the part of the young master's parents. Besides, he liked the young spark.

The boy had borrowed his older brother's birth year, declaring himself to be sixteen, almost seventeen, and had volunteered as a sailor on the *Seahorse*. Since he was in truth only twelve, almost thirteen, this news had produced both gratitude and an astonishingly loud wail on the part of his mother, who had screamed *Seahorse! Pirates!* and promptly fainted. In the father it had produced a mottled mix of white-faced anger and flushed pride: No son of Wentworth Paxton's would stoop to the level of a common sailor, especially on a ship Captain Paxton had once commanded. Or just as good as: he had commanded the ship (the *smaller* ship, specified Scipio with malicious glee, though only to himself) that had held the name HMS *Seahorse* twenty years before. But devil take it, the boy had salt in his veins, and daring too: was a Paxton through and through.

Later that day over a bowl of punch in an upper room in the Royal Exchange, Captain Wentworth Paxton, quondam commander of HMS *Seahorse* and now merchant of Boston, and Captain Thomas Durell, current commander of HMS *Seahorse*, came to a compromise. Charles would remain on the ship's books. Furthermore, his rating would remain "ordinary seaman," or mariner-in-training. All the same, behind the words, his status shifted perceptibly, if not yet his duties, or the respect accorded him among the men—which now, more than ever, he would have to earn. Christened in absentia by a toast clinked over rum punch and sealed with a handshake that transferred an untold sum of gold, he became, without knowing it, one of the "young gentlemen," aiming, with help, to reach someday for the rank of an officer.

It would have proved a day of unsullied joy if his mother, too, had not left her mark upon the agreement. Entrusting her son's future to her husband, Faith Gillam Paxton took aim at his present. Charlie would remain on the ship: but only until she shipped out. In light of his age—or rather, since it was not uncommon for eleven- and twelve-year-olds to go to sea, in light of his mother's tender (or *hysterical,* Scipio silently corrected) concern for his age—he would be granted the extremely uncommon luxury of shore leave for the duration of the *Seahorse*'s next voyage to the West Indies and back. Charlie would turn thirteen, Madam Paxton demanded (and it was, after all, her Gillam family fortune upon which their prosperity depended, thought Scipio), before the famous pirate captain Roberts, terror of the Caribbean, would be granted the signal honor of so much as trying to level a blunderbuss at her baby son.

When the ship returned, Charlie would return to the ship. But not until then.

So, when *Seahorse* had pulled out of the harbor on January 6, young Charles Paxton had stood white with rage on the family wharf near the South Battery, his father's hand laid firmly on the scruff of his neck. At least, Charlie thought hotly to himself, they had had to replace him two-for-one, and not with just anybody, no sir. In his rightful place on board were two of the finest sailors in his father's ships: the Indian slave Hector Bruce, thin and strong as a whip, and an indentured man, Richard Kent.

* * *

As soon as the *Seahorse* was sighted inbound, Charles began maneuvering to sail out to meet her. Waiting for her to come in to him might take days, as much as a whole week (maybe two, said Scipio) to reach the town's wharves. It was unbearable.

This time, his father overruled his mother, the danger of pirates being judged minimal within the confines of Boston Harbor. After submitting to a smothering of kisses, Charles stepped into a boat with his father, Scipio, and a few more of his father's men. They scudded across the water, drew alongside *Seahorse*, and soon Charlie and his father were clambering aboard the frigate, Scipio following a bit more clumsily, hoisting up the boy's sea chest, full of greatcoat, warm and cool clothing, Bible, as well as the hamper of fresh food destined for the captain's cabin.

Captains Durell and Paxton exchanged smiles above the boy's head. It was refreshing—was it not?—to see a youngster near to squealing with excitement to be on board, when most of the men around him were panting for release after twenty-six days at sea.

As the captains retreated to the great cabin, Scipio ducked below with his young master's things, down and down again, hatchway after hatchway to the orlop, the lowest deck, suspended in the midst of the hold—no light or air, the bilge water mere feet below; one could hear it sloshing with every roll of the ship. The stagnant air smelled of men's sweat, tobacco juice, swamp, and cistern. Standing at the foot of the ladder, letting his eyes adjust to the dimness, he saw things gone a bit lax, no longer quite shipshape; it was, after all, the end of a cruise. He tried to map out for himself the layout of the low room that yawned into darkness on either side, the width of the ship. Even among the boys and young gentlemen who berthed down here, territory was measured in inches; to encroach in the wrong place, even by so small a bit of turf as the area of a sea chest, would transform young Charlie's initiation from rough jesting to cruelty.

He was threading across the floor, looking for the assigned gap in which to deposit the chest, when he heard a groan. He stopped and looked over his shoulder. The deck had not been left entirely open, as he had at first presumed. At the fore end of the orlop, a thin wall sliced a small space from the rest of the deck, its door propped ajar. The groan came again, from inside.

Scipio had taken no more than three steps forward when the ship rolled and the door swung open, belching forth warm, moist air whose stench made him gag. Just then, a man carrying a steaming, sloshing bowl of water poked his head through the hatchway above as he climbed down the ladder. "You there," he said sharply. "Where do you think you're going?"

"Just delivering my young master's sea chest."

The man laughed, but it was not a sound of pleasure. "Not in there," he said. "Young gentlemen's berth is the palace in the other direction."

"Yes, sir," said Scipio, glad enough to let someone else take care of whatever was amiss in that chamber. The man, wiry and roasted to mahogany by the sun, went by him and kicked the door shut with a practiced thud. Scipio heard a latch slide home from the inside.

On the way south, *Seahorse* had rather ostentatiously draped a suspected pirate in chains and shoved him into the hold, to be transferred to a court in Barbados, which no doubt had raised him up directly to dangle from a yardarm. Perhaps Boston had traded Barbados, one prisoner for another. Poor bugger.

Scipio deposited the young master's things, and hotfooted it back out on deck, where the air was sharp and clean, and one could see the town laid out across the shore like a glistening necklace, the heavy square of the fort rather grandly called Castle William dangling at the bottom like a matron's pendant. It was this fort—or its island, Castle Island—for which the frigate was sailing. He caught the eye of Hector, his fellow among Captain Paxton's slaves, and old Dick Kent, the other sailor who had shipped in Charlie's place, and winked. But they both stared hard ahead, making no reply. Then again, the bosun's mate was watching them most particular, swinging his lash about as if he thought they might make a dash for Paxton's boat, right under his nose. *Maybe they might*, thought Scipio, *if that man keeps lashing the air with such menace*. The young master safely stowed, Captain Paxton and his servant returned to their boat and slipped back over the waves toward home.

The harbor bureaucracy inched its way through the fleet, clearing cargo through customs and passing crews under suspicious medical eyes: there were smallpox epidemics raging in London and Barbados. At five in the evening on April 27, as space opened up at the end of the Long Wharf, HMS *Seahorse* cast off her mooring, weighed anchor, and slipped away from Castle Island, sailing grandly into place just off the end of Boston's longest pier: a road that stretched almost half a mile into the sea, into water deep enough to dock even the largest of ships.

The officers, as usual, were granted shore leave; the men, as usual, were not. For three days, a close watch was kept on them from dawn to dusk as they ground through the heavy work of unbending sails, removing rigging that a New England gale had torn up like so much kindling, and shipping the masts for repairs. As dusk fell, though, the watch turned a blind eye to the bumboats that swarmed the ship, offering their wares for a pretty price: boxes and barrels of fresh meat, butter, cheese, fruits and vegetables, bales of new clothing and bedding, and barrels of rum—all draped with raucous women like a bright, slightly bedraggled flock of parrots.

Meanwhile, the captain concerned himself with more exciting game. Governor Shute had informed him of a pirate ship holed up in Tarpaulin Cove, in the islands southwest of Cape Cod: said to be a rich prize, loaded with a bittersweet cargo of sugar, cocoa, and slaves. The combination of damage and half-done repairs had left the *Seahorse* temporarily unseaworthy, but her commander's eagerness untarnished. After brief consultation with the governor, he hired a sloop, and on May 1 he stocked it with fifty sailors from the *Seahorse* and his equally eager second in command, Lieutenant Andrew Hamilton.

With half the ship's crew gone to seek a fight, the remainder felt justified in equalizing things by seeking action of another sort. That night, as dark fell, the watch looked the other way as shadows scuttled down the ship's cables, stifling laughter, and drifted into the taverns and brothels that crowded the wharves.

On the third day of the riotous celebrations in town—the eleventh since ferrying Charlie to his ship—Scipio at last managed to slip out a back door of the Paxton mansion. A few minutes later, he slid into a crowded room hazy with smoke and filled with fiddling, dancing, brawling, a little too much heat, and a scent of rum so raw it could kick over a mule. In particular, it was full of Seahorses, as that ship's sailors were known according to the navy's proud custom of naming men for their ships. He found Hector and slid in beside him. They were toasting a man's life—a man's death—it was all one—and gathered Scipio right into their fold. Another Seahorse he knew slightly, Jack Dunn by name, had been committed to the ground that morning. They would miss the man's capers in the tops, the rest of the Seahorses declared. They would not miss his loutish ways while his pride was overly damp with grog. A tear or two, long guffaws of laughter, and a jig were in order.

"What happened to ol' Jack?" Scipio asked Hector.

But the Indian was already glassy eyed with rum—had no head for drink—and would only reply with one of his gutteral Indian words, chanted low over and over, before he collapsed face forward on the table.

Two or three taverns later—it was getting hard to keep track—Scipio stumbled into the passage, heading out to relieve himself. He pushed open the door to the garden, and out billowed that rotten-sweet scent he had caught a whiff of before, down in the *Seahorse* hold. The house had convulsed on him, surely, had twisted about, while he wasn't looking. This infernal door did not lead to the garden; it opened on a small chamber where a man lay on the floor. Scipio blinked. A sailor, by his clothes. He knew that coat, that checkered neckcloth. Another black man: Joseph May, the gunner's mate.

Then he saw the man's face—if it could be called a face—and felt the wall on the opposite side of the hall hit him in the back.

He did not remember anything else until the following morning, when the sudden nausea he had suppressed the night before startled him awake up in his own attic chamber. After emptying his stomach, he realized that he had a splitting headache, a throb in his lower back, and that he was not certain, from one minute to the next, whether he was freezing or frying.

It had been one hell of a party, even by sailors' standards: Scipio's feverish nausea didn't break till late on the morning of the third day, when he drifted into a heavy sleep. That evening, as the Sabbath drew to a close, one of the maids, a generous girl, fixed up a tray and carried up a light supper of bread sopped in broth. Opening the door with her hip, she turned into the room, her eyes on the tray, keeping everything in balance. Then she glanced up, and the smile she was unfurling for Scipio—poor man— disintegrated. Her hands dropped the tray into a clatter of breaking dishes, rattling pewter, splintering wood.

Apron to mouth, she was backing out of the room when the captain roared up the stairs and walloped her for carelessness. A little strangled scream escaped her throat, but she still could not form any words, so the captain stepped in to speak with Scipio himself.

Hunched in a corner of his cot, he looked up from his own body and across to the captain in terror. He was covered in a thick rash of bumps, even blacker than the midnight of his skin.

After a hurried interview, the captain retired, ashen faced, to write a short note to the selectmen, regretting to inform them that his servant was ill with what looked to be the smallpox. He had heard, he added, that another black man, a certain Joseph May of HMS *Seahorse*, was also ill in town, but he couldn't be certain where: one of the taverns or inns that clustered around the alleys leading off from the Long Wharf, probably.

This he sealed, and delivered into the hands of a small boy who went speeding off in the direction of the biggest house in town, bar the governor's mansion: the house of Elisha Cooke, Esq., up in School Street.

Paxton watched the boy melt into the night, and then shut the door.

He had not found it necessary to announce that Hector had arrived on the doorstep yesterday with Charlie, the boy shivering with the same kind of high fever that had felled Scipio. Hector had also brought a tale that Captain Paxton had been doing his best to ignore. Was doing his damnedest to go right on doing so too. Charlie, after all, had not erupted in spots.

Yet.

Early Monday morning on the eighth of May, 1721, Boston's six selectmen (Elisha Cooke's finest selection, the joke went) filed grimly into the Council chamber upstairs in the grand new brick Town House at the top of King Street, shutting the door firmly behind them.

Murmuring could be heard outside that thick door, but little else, even by the steward who knew the best ways of listening into any room in the building.

Their meeting was brief and to the point.

Smallpox had been raging in London for a year; only the previous month, it had been killing as many as twenty to thirty people a day in Barbados. But Boston had been vigilant, had carefully designed and manned defenses to keep it out: the town already had laws that all ships with sickness aboard must stop at Spectacle Island or face a steep fine. It already had a fine new hospital there. The trouble was to force everyone to use it: not everyone had the selfless discipline of John Gore.

Boston already possessed a customs bureaucracy that could catch the smallest grain of sugar or gold; rather ingeniously the existing machinery of this bureaucracy had been retooled to catch smallpox, too, pairing every cargo inspector with a medical examiner. No ship could enter the inner harbor without leave from customs, and no ship could get leave from customs unless her crew passed a medical inspection.

No ship, that is, save a king's ship, not subject to customs.

It was a gap that no one had glimpsed. Though naval ships knew damn well they were supposed to pass a quarantine inspection, swore William Clark. Knew even damn better that, rules or no, they ought to submit voluntarily to quarantine when carrying something as dangerous as the smallpox, added William Hutchinson.

Where the smallpox had come from, though, was not their concern at the moment. They much preferred to know where it had got to, and how they could prevent it from going any farther. A full-scale epidemic—or even a small-scale epidemic accompanied by full-scale panic—would wreak havoc with trade, rein the town to a nervous standstill.

Their decisions were practical, made quickly, and set neatly into their minute book:

> *Whereas a certain Negro man is now sick of the Small Pox in the town who came from Tertudos in His Majesty's Ship* Seahorse, *which renders it very likely that that distemper may now be on board that ship, therefore for the preservation of the inhabitants of this town:*
>
> *Voted, that John Clark, Esq., be desired to go on board His Majesty's Ship* Seahorse *and report what state of health or sickness the ship's company are in, especially with respect to the Small Pox or other contagious sickness.*
>
> *Whereas a certain Negro man, servant to Capt. Wentworth Paxton of Boston, is now sick of the Small Pox at his master's house, and it not being known that any other person is infected with that distemper in this town, wherefore for the better preventing the spreading of that distemper,*
>
> *Ordered: That some suitable nurse be provided to attend the said Negro during his present sickness and until she be dismissed by the Select Men, who is to suffer no person to come within the room where the Negro is but such as shall have liberty from the Select Men, and that two prudent persons be appointed to wait at the doors of the house and suffer no one to come in or go out, but such as shall have liberty and allowance as aforesaid.*

These things went into their minutes. What did not go into their minutes was their determination to keep the crisis—*potential* crisis, insisted Mr. Cooke—quiet as long as possible, and *to find the second sick man.*

It was all well and good to run a red landsman's flag of quarantine over Paxton's mansion in the South End, but until they discovered this other sailor and bundled him back aboard, they were sitting atop a powder keg. And he—this missing man—was the fuse.

At the appointed hour the following morning, Dr. Clark met Captain Durell at the Town House. After curt greetings and stiff bows, the two men reentered Dr. Clark's carriage for the short journey down the length of King Street, lined with shops of hushed luxury, to the harbor. There they emerged, tight lipped, the captain turning heads with his silver-laced, cockaded hat gripped firmly in white-gloved hands, his finely tailored blue coat fastened with gilt buttons above the clean lines of white breeches and gray hose, his black wig tied neatly with a bow, the gleam of his sword competing with the flash of immense silver buckles on his shoes.

The doctor's red face, plump outline, and quiet elegance cut no figure next to Captain Durell.

"There is no necessity of an inspection, of course," the captain said smoothly as they stepped onto the planking of the Long Wharf. "However, formalities must be maintained." Except for the hollow clomp of their footsteps and the scent of water wafting up from beneath their feet, they might have been marching along any busy road lined with shops and warehouses, crawling with men loading, unloading, loitering, bargaining.

Minus necessity, thought Dr. Clark, he would not be huffing down the Long Wharf a third of a mile into the sea with this peacock, formalities be damned. The time for formalities—the day the ship arrived—had long since past. Captain Durell, with his love of trumpets (on the Sabbath, no less), of flags, and fifteen-gun salutes, of all ritual pomp, irritated the doctor no end. He was all of a piece with that insufferable snob, Governor Shute—was the governor's good friend and ally, for that matter. Did they not treat each other to elaborate suppers whenever possible, forcing the captive audience of their other guests to suffer through their endless compliments to each other?

Hand in hand with his love of a good show went his rashness. To listen to his tales, the man loved nothing more than to chase pirates, guns blazing, sails nearly popping off the rigging, the ship skimming through warm aquamarine seas. The ferocity of this obsession was the captain's glory. Dr. Clark was hoping that it would also prove to be his Achilles' heel: that the captain would, in short, do anything to sidle out from under a sentence of quarantine.

Engrossed in his irritation, the doctor did not deign to offer his companion a reply until they reached the end of the wharf, where the *Seahorse* rocked gently in the water. Then he let his eyes ostentatiously scan the harbor. A few days earlier, the entire horizon had fluttered with a scattering of immense blossoms from heaven. Now masts shorn of their sails clustered thickly near shore like the trees of a barren and leafless forest in winter. "So many ships," he said, shaking his head. "Difficult, you know, to water and provision them all at once. Beer, biscuit, salt beef—not to mention canvas and line to repair torn rigging"—the *Seahorse* tops, he had seen with a grimace of contempt, were a veritable rat's nest: what foolish seeking after speed had tangled them so? He let his eyes drift back to Durell. "Some ships, I fear, will be obliged to wait as much as a month until the warehouses can replenish their supply."

The man's unctuousness hardened to blank stone. "Difficult, no doubt," said Captain Durell. "But surely if every captain commands no more than his share, there will be plenty for all."

Dr. Clark registered that saucy word *commands* with a slow, smiling lift of one brow and then turned to step up the gangway and onto the ship's deck. The captain could command all he pleased, but if the selectmen willed it, there would be no beer, no biscuit, not a morsel of beef—fresh, salt, or putrid—to be found in all of Boston. The lift of brow had been a warning for the captain; the smile was for himself. He had been right: Durell was susceptible to any threat to tie him to the shore. Thus fortified, he strode into the task at hand.

Unfortunately, the ship's surgeon, Mr. Thomas Gibson, was absent, having been detailed to accompany Lieutenant Hamilton in the chasing of pirates. Even so, working alone on a ship he did not know, Dr. Clark needed no more than fifteen minutes to find what he had no wish to find: the scent of death. Down in a small airless compartment at the far forward end of the lowest deck, two men lay ill with the smallpox. The doctor's nose made the call as soon as his head cleared the hatch through the deck above, as he was still clambering down the ladder. A mere glance into the sickroom, garishly lit by a guttering lantern, confirmed the diagnosis. A third man shivered with fever that might well bubble up into pocks in a day or two.

Dr. Clark hauled his bulk back up several ladders to find the captain at ease with a pipe in his cabin. Durell rose as the doctor entered.

Dr. Clark bowed. "I regret to inform you, sir, that your ship is infected—unequivocally—with the smallpox. Pursuant to the laws governing Boston and her harbor, I am placing the *Seahorse* under quarantine until further notice."

"Surely," said the captain, "two gentlemen such as ourselves can find some way around such an extreme measure." He relaxed back into his chair and offered the doctor his choice of tobacco or snuff.

The doctor declined both pleasures.

"Smallpox," said the captain, swatting lazily at the word as if it were a fly, though the doctor observed that his grip on the pipe had tightened. "You will find, Doctor, it is not of major concern aboard a warship. From time to time it sputters up, but it quickly dies out again." He leaned forward. "Ship fever"—typhus—"or scurvy, now: those are diseases to fear."

Dr. Clark stared at the man in disbelief. "Surely you are not suggesting, sir, that you have been aware for some time that your ship carries this contagion and have disregarded it?"

Captain Durell's eyes flared with anger; the man insisted upon pressing the far edges of gentlemanly behavior. "The health of the men is my surgeon's concern," he snapped. "Mine is to sail this ship."

"And mine is to safeguard the health of this town," growled the doctor. He had not budged an inch since entering: just stood there, his ample girth occupying what seemed like most of the room for air and light that the cabin possessed. "Perhaps," he went on, forcing his voice back to the cadences of pleasantry, as if they were speaking of gardening or husbandry, "you do not realize the gravity of the situation. This town has not seen a case of smallpox in nineteen years, in which time the population has doubled. In regard to that disease, we are a keg of powder. The smallest spark will not sputter, will not smolder: it will ignite a conflagration whose destructive force you cannot begin to imagine. That, sir, is why we have laws governing quarantine."

Laws, hung an unspoken sentence between them, *which you have violated quite flagrantly*. "So perhaps you would be so good as to allow me to examine your logs and paybook, so that I may—in the absence of Mr. Gibson—attempt to piece together the recent history of your crew's health for myself."

It was an irregular, even audacious invasion of the captain's privacy, but Dr. Clark intended to obtain what he wanted. "Meanwhile," he added, "no one will leave this ship without my leave." *Including her captain*, said the ice in his eyes.

The logs were duly produced.

He had, of course, all the evidence he needed to quarantine the ship: sick men in the hold. But Dr. Clark was nothing if not thorough. It was one of the reasons he had become the most prestigious doctor in town. He thought of everything. He explained everything.

For all their neat, spidery writing, their massive officiousness, the logs and books were not easy to decipher. As usual the men were listed by the dates they had volunteered, or been pressed into service. Dr. Clark obtained paper and pen, and in the rock and creak of the ship, he sat at the captain's table, rearranging the information into a list of his own devising, ordering men by their date of death, dismissal, or disappearance, scratching his way through to an understanding of what the captain apparently took pains not to know. Or at least, not to say.

The *Seahorse* had arrived in Boston on October 11, from London via New York, where she had delivered that province's new governor. At the end of November, as she sat in Boston Harbor, three men had died in the space of five days: no reason given.

"What, may I ask," said Dr. Clark, his voice rasping in the silence, "was the trouble in November?"

"You will have to ask Mr. Gibson," Durell answered tightly. "As I said, it is his job to keep the crew healthy. Mine to sail the ship."

It was debatable, thought Dr. Clark, whether his men entirely agreed: certainly they seemed to have concluded that *Seahorse* was not a desirable place to be. By the time she sailed for Barbados with her brood of merchantmen on January 6, 23 men—a fifth of her allowed complement of

115—had jumped ship, though the captain did not mark them down as having run, or deserted, until she sailed out of the harbor without them. Presumably, he had known of this hemorrhage before leaving, even if he refused to know the cause: because he had already replaced quite a few of them.

The problem could have been smallpox, mused the doctor. London—including nearby Deptford, home of the naval dockyards and *Seahorse's* port of origin—had been in the throes of an epidemic for over a year. If the ship had been carrying smallpox, though, surely men would have begun to die during the voyage across the Atlantic. And many more would have jumped ship at first opportunity, in New York: but *Seahorse* had lost only seven men to desertion in that city, plus one more at Staten Island. Furthermore, the disease would not have waited until May to appear in Boston.

More disturbingly, *Seahorse* had been in and around Barbados at the height of the smallpox epidemic there in February and March. Durell had listed eight desertions in Barbados and Tortuga: eight runs, or eight deaths ashore? It was useless to ask. If he could cocoon himself so successfully within the claustrophobic wooden world of his ship, refusing to know what was forcibly held under his nose—well, remaining blissfully ignorant of what happened to his men on shore must be easy.

It was after the first call at Barbados that death began flitting about the ship with the determined abandon of a sailor's whore. One at sea on February 4, just eight days after arriving in Barbados on January 27. Surely, thought Dr. Clark, that could not be smallpox, not yet. No—the logs showed a ship newly burdened with 86 extra armed soldiers, heaving hard on a chase after pirates, until terrible storms had snapped so much of her rigging that they had been in serious danger of the masts tumbling overboard and the ship swamping. Surely that man had died in the mayhem of splintering wood and wet whipping canvas, of waves leaping across the deck: the wild, roaring danger of the sea.

The doctor's finger stopped at a second death, duly noted as drowning, on February 20.

Thereafter, the explanations evaporated. One death, unexplained, on March 30. A second—a Boston man, Samuel Gregory—on April 20, just two days before reaching home. A third on May 4, while the ship lay in the harbor: which made steam rise from the back of the doctor's plump neck.

Again, he asked the captain what had been killing his men. Again, the captain claimed ignorance. Momentarily, the doctor lost his grip on calm. "Damn it all, Durell," he exclaimed, slamming both hands down on the table. "I am not asking for the precision of a medical report. I am asking, did they have pocks, sir? Did you see wens, boils, blisters, so much as a pimple or two?"

But the man clung steadfastly to his ignorance.

Dr. Clark did a few quick calculations. If just the last three deaths had indeed been smallpox, that indicated anywhere from 9 to 18 men ill. Maybe more. Not enough to cripple the ship: as the captain had implied, most of the men had volunteered or been pressed into service in the home ports of London, Deptford, and Portsmouth. Were likely scraped from the floors of jails, from the sewers of the streets: had imbibed that contagion with their gin-soaked mother's milk, and having survived, could now laugh in the face of smallpox and pass the rum.

A fair number of his crew, though, were mariners recruited in Boston since last October: and many more of these would—or should—be quaking in their boots. No matter what kind of strict quarantine Mr. Gibson might have been able to impose when he was present, the doctor thought grimly.

"I should like to see the entire crew, for medical inspection," he said aloud.

Reluctantly, Durell gave the order to muster all hands on deck.

There were 111 men currently on the books. The turnout was just what Clark had feared: pathetic. No more than 15, and a handful of those, by the look of them, too scurvy-weakened to be of any use setting sail. According to the master's log, fifty of the missing were accounted for in the sloop Durell had hired and sent chasing the pirate sheltering in Tarpaulin Cove. That should have left 61 men. Three lay below, ill. Which left the hair-raising number of 43 loose ashore, the devil only knew where, or how many were ill.

Dr. Clark stayed only long enough to demand that the yellow jack be run aloft and to inform Captain Durell that he would have to withdraw to Spectacle Island as soon as a pilot who knew his way through the harbor's shifting confusion of sandbars, currents, and deep sea lanes could be secured.

Fifteen men, Clark reflected, would not be near enough to move her even so far on a fine day. He would have to inform his brother and the rest of the selectmen they needed not only a pilot, but mariners. All pockmarked.

The doctor accompanied the captain all the way back up the Long Wharf in silence: his freedom being the unspoken price of a look at the logs. At the bottom of King Street, where Dr. Clark's carriage stood waiting, they bowed one last time.

"I have every confidence," said the captain, "that it is I who shall prove correct in our differing assessments of the danger at hand." If the doctor had been a sporting man, he would have tossed out a bet; but the Bostonian elders were a singularly unsporting lot, suffering from extravagant over-doses of a noxious, pinched brand of piety.

"You have a taste for trumpets, sir," said Dr. Clark. "Do you recall what will happen after the sounding of the first trumpet?"

"What?" Captain Durell was a Church of England man; it took him a moment to realize that he was being steered, in fine Puritan style, toward the Bible.

The doctor's voice rang out clear and deep. *"There followed hail and fire, mixed with blood, which fell on the earth; and a third of the earth was burnt up."* Around them, men stopped their work, drew in a step closer. "Apocalypse, sir," said the doctor. "Hell on earth. And that is just the beginning." He rapped the driver's box with his stick, and his carriage drove on.

❧ 4 ❧

CAGING THE MONSTER

ON the twelfth of May, a Friday, the freeholders of the town of Boston—the propertied men sworn in to the company of voters— filed upstairs into the great domed representatives' chamber that occupied most of the upper story of the Town House. Slanting through long narrow windows, the morning light skated over polished wooden floors and splashed the yellow walls with sunny foam. Almost, so warm and relentless was its cheer, they might be in Barbados, rather than the center of Boston, convening a town meeting.

As a first order of business, the men elected Elisha Cooke, Esq., as moderator; then they went noisily to work. There were many contentious items on the agenda, from choosing representatives to the General Court to levying the town for the next year's expenses. Just before two o'clock, the men burrowed out from under piles of unfinished business and adjourned for dinner. At three, they reconvened and began tidying up loose ends. Tucked in at the end of the meeting, as if that might somehow make it negligible, Mr. Cooke mentioned the word *smallpox*.

Stillness fell across the room as Dr. Clark rose to detail his inspection of the *Seahorse*. Sitting amid a tight knot of selectmen, Mr. William Hutchinson, the youngest of the town's chief office-holders—and as of that morning, newly elected representative to the General Court as well— watched his fellows listen with quiet gravity to the doctor's formal report, as if they had not already heard it informally. As if, hearing it, they had not already rejected it outright, mulled it over, cursed it, silently shouted it down, leaned their shoulders hard into its obstinacy, striving to shove it aside with strength accustomed to move mountains. The selectmen were, after all, men of a certain stature, men used to command and obedience. They were not used to standing aside helpless or, worse yet, turning their backs to run. Or, worst of all, he thought, scuttling to the governor to ask for help like scared schoolboys.

As Dr. Clark finished, a deep murmur swept through the room and died away like a dark squall scudding across the open sea. A short, sharp debate ensued, presided over by Elisha Cooke's very sour face. And then, respectfully, the men of the town took a vote.

> *Voted: that the Select Men be desired and directed to wait upon His Excellency the Governor and pray him to call a Council in order to advise about the* Seahorse *man-of-war, being sent down to Spectacle Island, Pursuant to a Law of this Province to prevent (God willing) the Spreading of the Small Pox in this Town & Province, two or three men being sick of that Distemper on board the said ship now in the Harbor.*

"If anyone can persuade Captain Durell to just action, it will be his good friend the governor," grumbled Dr. Clark as the company filed out.

If anyone can persuade the governor to any action whatsoever, thought Hutchinson with uncharacteristic gloom, *it'll be the six selectmen arguing the opposite case. And if there is anyone whose advice he will contradict more happily than ours, it's Dr. John Clark.*

In the end, Mr. Cooke and Dr. Clark's younger brother, Selectman William Clark, called on the governor alone, while the rest of the selectmen watched shadows lengthen in the Council chamber. Striding to the central window, his back to the room, hands clasped behind, William Hutchinson looked more ship's captain than fine shore-bound gentleman. Staring eastward down King Street and the Long Wharf, he could see the three masts of the *Seahorse*—the tallest in the harbor—swaying slightly, just beyond the town's grip. They were still brazenly barren, free of the least flutter of a quarantine flag. It put his mind on the ghost of another ship, with a different captain at her helm: John Gore, who had died last year among strangers rather than risk infecting the town with smallpox. Captain Gore had been Mr. Hutchinson's classmate at Harvard. Had been his friend.

Presently, Mr. Cook and Mr. Clark returned with grim faces. The governor had agreed to call the Council, reported Mr. Cook. Meanwhile, he had sent for the insolent puppy of a captain himself. With that, Captain Durell was announced. The blast of air that sprang up as the man strode into the room, thought Hutchinson with a shiver, had been born, surely, in the farthest southern seas, fanged with ice.

Puppy, scoffed Hutchinson to himself. *Here is a puppy who fancies himself a lion.* A vision of the lion—*the King of the Beasts, and the only one of his kind in America!*—on display at Mrs. Martha Adams's place in the South End flitted through his head. That creature lazed all day in the sun, not unlike the captain standing at such arrogant ease before them. Not at all the same sharp attention that Durell granted the governor. Hutchinson shifted his gaze back out the window, lest the captain's report snag on his smile.

The captain regretted, he said, the selectmen's concern that the Salter-tudas fleet might have brought the smallpox into town. *Might?* Hutchinson's attention snapped back, one brow skimming up into the fringe of his wig.

Willing to do his part, of course, continued the captain: he had ordered the commanding officer on board to fall down with the ship to a mooring off Bird Island, so soon as these good gentlemen—small nod, just this side of perfunctory—could provide a suitable pilot.

In spite of himself, Hutchinson snorted. *Suitable, hell,* he thought. *Safely pock pitted is what you mean, and we all know it.* Then he identified the jolt that had bothered him in that sentence. "You mean Spectacle Island," he said aloud.

"I am sure," said Mr. Cooke just a little too smoothly, "that we can trust an officer in His Majesty's Service to keep our few small harbor islands straight in his head."

Hutchinson glanced quickly from Mr. Cooke to Mr. Clark. Their faces should have betrayed surprise—same as his—but all he saw was a studied blandness. *So a deal has been struck,* he thought, *a bargain sealed.* He could smell it: something had been offered and accepted in return for escape from formal quarantine at Spectacle Island. But what? Not money: Mr. Cooke might be grasping, but he was also righteous. He would not sell the town into the smallpox.

Mr. Hutchinson knew as well as anyone that he had been elected so high so young for his staunch support of Mr. Cooke. But if Mr. Cooke's party assumed they had acquired a pliant yes-man, he thought, they might as well be disabused of their error at once. In this case, they would get his support, but for a price; for it galled him to the edge of fury to think of John dying alone in quarantine, while this smug, strutting captain draped in lace got off scot-free. "No doubt," he said with a tight nod to Mr. Cooke, "His Majesty's ship *Seahorse* will be quite as isolated off Bird Island as she would be docked at Spectacle Island. Possibly more so." He unfurled a smile of contempt for the captain. "So long as she flies the yellow jack, of course."

Captain Durell glanced at Cooke, but he offered no help.

"Of course," echoed the captain with a grimace. "We will show the yellow jack."

Hutchinson transferred his smile back out the window, as the man departed.

Another tight-lipped discussion shot here and there between the six men, or between the five men and Mr. Hutchinson's back. There were one or two more decisions at hand.

The outcome went into their minutes, along with several other statements that were not as discreet as the captain might have wished. The selectmen had tacitly agreed, it was true, not to wag any more fingers of blame in public, but they had made no such promise about private conversations:

Whereas His Majesty's Ship Seahorse, Capt. Thomas Durell, Commander, now lyeth in the Harbor of Boston infected with the Small Pox, the greatest part of his company are now a cruise, sundry others sick on shore, so that there is not above ten or fifteen effective men on board, and the said Captain having given orders to the commanding officer on board to fall down to Bird Island with the ship, in order to prevent the infection spreading in the town, upon Captain Timothy Clark's repairing on board to take the charge of piloting her down:

Voted, that Captain Clark be desired forthwith to procure a sufficient number of men to effect that matter.

"Vermin monger!" thundered Dr. John Clark, flinging open the door to the best private room upstairs at the Bunch of Grapes, the plush tavern standing at the head of the Long Wharf and favored by the selectmen. Having worked through the dinner hour, they had at last left the Town House and sauntered the length of King Street to share a late supper of haddock in capers, beef, mutton, salad, and hasty pudding. By the time Dr. Clark found them, the last crumbs had been withdrawn; several half-full bottles of Madeira remained. The six men were gathered around the tavern's newest amusement, a large table covered in green cloth and edged with six holes, or pockets. *"Pox-ridden dog!"* cried Dr. Clark.

All but one of the men seemed to have found something fascinating in the close grouping of three ivory balls, red, white, and blue, in the center of the table. The sixth man, William Clark, turned and leaned on his long mace-ended stick. "Hello, brother," he said. "Perhaps you would care to clarify that you do not intend to indicate any of us?"

"Captain Durell," roared the doctor.

Five backs straightened, and five pairs of eyes swiveled to face him.

"He's discharged them," said Dr. Clark. "The three men sick with the smallpox. Gone. Cast out. Lord only knows where."

William sighed. His brother was trustworthy as well as experienced in both medicine and politics, which was why they had chosen him as their inspector. But in medical matters he was also a perfectionist and a bit of an alarmist as well. Which would make him about as comfortable as a horsefly in the upcoming weeks.

"They're in the Province Hospital on Spectacle Island," said Mr. Cooke, taking careful aim at the white ball with the mace end of his stick. The mace collided with the cue ball, and the cue ball collided with the red ball, which spun silently down the table, banked off the end, and veered back through a hoop called the port. This was followed by a short, sharp silence, like a pop, not entirely due to the marvel of the man's skill at billiards.

Mr. Cooke straightened, though he kept his eyes on the table, assessing the new layout of the balls. "As you say, the captain discharged the three men you told us of. James Mansell of Boston, and the two strangers, John Wilkinson and Gilbert Anthony. Unfortunately, he also offered—as is his right—to go on discharging men, as fast as they should fall ill." He cornered the table and confronted Dr. Clark directly. "What would you have done?"

Most of the time, he and the doctor were wary allies against their mutual foe, the despised governor; occasionally, though, they could be determined, if respectful, opponents.

"That whole damned ship belongs at Spectacle Island," growled the doctor.

"The whole damned ship was not going to go there."

"It's where she belongs," Dr. Clark insisted. *You're a physician by training if not by practice*, he thought. *You know that much*.

Cooke shrugged. "I don't give a ship rat's fart where she is," he said, "so long as she is not here, and Durell is not discharging his sick at will into my streets." With a firm shove of the mace, he sent the white ball spinning toward Mr. Clark's blue ball, which flew into the pocket in the far corner. The point of this delicious new game of billiards was, like its forerunner croquet, as much to wreak havoc on one's opponent as to work one's own ball through the port at one end of the table and back to hit the skittle called the king on the other side. Cooke turned to Dr. Clark and spread a wolfish smile. "I owe you thanks, though, for the tip that he would do anything to remain free to chase pirates. Quite useful information, that. Deal clincher, in fact."

"What deal?" asked the doctor.

"I suggested it might be best if we joined forces to round up all the ramblers and stragglers from the *Seahorse*, sent the sick to the Province Hospital, the healthy back aboard ship, and the ship away from the docks.

After short consideration, and the promise of some likely timber for the repairing of his crosstrees, Durell agreed." Cooke laughed. "Though Mr. Hutchinson quite brilliantly wangled a further promise that they will fly the yellow jack."

"And in return?"

"A promise that the *Seahorse* will not be forced into formal quarantine. And none of her officers or crew threatened with either the fifty-pound fine or the six months' jail time specified by the law. . . . I think it was the threat of time, in jail or in legal haggling, that won him over."

Dr. Clark stalked back to the door. "You have made a deal, sir, with the devil," he said, laying his hand upon the latch.

"No, Doctor," said Cooke with smooth disagreement. "I've made a compromise with reality. Furthermore, the other selectmen have agreed."

"I see that," said Dr. Clark, gazing around the room, his stare coming to rest upon his brother. "Thankfully, this year I am not one of your number." He departed, banging the door behind him.

From dawn till dusk on Saturday the thirteenth there were discreet searches along the docks, the taverns, and brothels frequented by sailors: the Dog and Pot, the Turkey-Cock, three different Castles, Noah's Ark, the Sun, the Swan, the Three (soused) Mariners. Every Seahorse who could be found was whisked away, inspected for fever and spots, and sent one of two directions: the healthy back aboard ship, the sick out to Spectacle Island. A distressing number had melted into the still cold and damp air of spring. One man—Joseph May, the gunner's mate—was discovered dead, curled up in the deserted corner of a warehouse, whispered some, or, muttered others, rolled gently this way and that by the swell beneath a dock. At least, observed one of the gravediggers given the task of consigning him to a pauper's grave, he would not rest in the earth as he had died: alone.

At five in the morning on the fourteenth, forty mariners with pitted faces strode through pearly light down the Long Wharf, grimly ignoring the fourth commandment to do no work on the Sabbath. At seven o'clock, the ship slipped from her moorings, weighed anchor, and glided away with misleading grace. She did not go far: not anywhere near as far as the quarantine dock on Spectacle Island. Her borrowed sailors moored her in five fathoms in the shelter of the tiniest, closest island, named for the birds that incessantly wheeled and called overhead. Castle Island and its fort lay a mere two miles to the southeast, noted the master. He did not bother to note that Boston herself lay at just about the same distance to the west:

where the sailors on board could gaze contemptuously at the town, while the landsmen returned their stares with murderous interest. It was just as well for the Seahorses' safety that they were away from the docks.

As soon as the ship was secure in her new anchorage, the town's mariners shipped back to shore, where they were met with fresh clothing; the old was removed, washed, and fumigated. Dr. Clark would have had it burned, but that was rejected as a needless expense.

In the days that followed, most of the town's elders, those who could remember the epidemic of 1702, hunched down, tense and trembling as a deer that has scented panther. Some of more impressionable among the young thrashed through nightmares, having been haunted since infancy by the ugly face of the speckled demon. Others frolicked in their best scarlet brocade and yellow fringe, fiddling, dancing, and debauching ever harder and faster. Why slow up now, when tomorrow you may be dead?

One day, then two, three, four, crept by. Another and still another. The selectmen waited a week before organizing another search: this time, not to find lagging Seahorses, but anyone whom they might have infected. There were plenty who were anxious to look earlier, but Dr. John Clark held them back. It would do no good to look too soon; might well give false security: this was a disease that bided its time in the dark.

At last, on Saturday the twentieth, the justices of the peace, the selectmen, the overseers of the poor, the constables, even the hogreeves, whose job it was to chase down nuisance pigs and remove them from their happy wallowing in the streets, joined to scour every house, every warehouse, shop, and shed in Boston. They made a strict and thorough inquiry of each and every inhabitant of the town. At the end of the day, a long, hushed roll call turned up nothing.

On the twenty-second, the newspapers blazoned their findings with relief: *They found none sick of that distemper but a Negro man at the House of Capt. Paxton near the South Battery, being the House that was first visited therewith: the Negro is almost recovered, and will be in a day or two removed unto the Province Hospital at Spectacle Island.*

No one mentioned Captain Paxton's son.

On the twenty-fourth, still holding their collective breath, the selectmen authorized Mr. Aeneas Salter to conscript twenty-four of the town's "free male Negroes, mulattoes, etc.," to work six days cleaning the streets and the sewers that ran down their centers: these men might be free— might have worked mightily, for years, to earn the price of their freedom— but the town still considered itself as possessing a right to their time in the matter of doling out the nastiest jobs, namely, the shoveling of shit.

Perhaps by now the sickness had fallen out of the air, out of the infected bodies, had run into the sewers where it belonged. Perhaps now it could be swept away like so much dirt. So twenty-four men of African, Indian, and mixed-race descent—et cetera—fanned out in small groups, plodding through the streets, shoveling the sewers clean, carting the contagion away.

That same day, the sloop hired by Captain Durell returned, along with the pirate ship now manned by Seahorses. They had found her, as promised, at anchor in Tarpaulin Bay. Disappointingly, the pirates had long since fled with most of the slaves and much of the cocoa and sugar to boot. Worse, the ship—a Dutch-built tub, it was true, but one that might be made to blaze with as many as twenty-four guns—was already in the possession of customs officials: there would be a fight in court over the prize money. Nonetheless, Lieutenant Hamilton and his men had, as ordered, assumed control of her and sailed back to Boston to join the *Seahorse*.

The sloop succeeded. The pirate ship, still manned by Seahorses, was sent directly to Spectacle Island, with smallpox aboard.

Two days later, early on the morning of the twenty-sixth, Lizzy Mather, just a few months shy of her seventeenth birthday, slipped through the back door of her father's fast-dilapidating house in the North End, past the parlor where her stepmother sat rocking and muttering, and fled to the top of the stairs, to her father's sacrosanct library. She did not think twice; she yanked open the door and flung herself weeping into her father's arms.

It was some time before he could smooth sense from her, stroking her hair, letting her cry. When at last she managed to spill out a sentence or two, his skin prickled cold, and he found himself fighting the desire to catch the words like so many butterflies and cram them back in her mouth.

She had overheard her uncle returning late the night before; had not slept a wink. Overnight, as it seemed, there were eight more people sick, not just sick, but spotted, spotting, swelling into shapes undreamed of: not in one house or two, but in houses scattered from Bennett Street in the North End, through Dock Square and School Street at the center of town, to Battery March and Winter Street in the South End.

The reverend comforted his daughter as best he could, coaxed her onto her knees, and bent down to pray alongside her: *Our Father which art in Heaven, Hallowed be Thy Name. Thy Kingdom come, Thy will be done, even in earth as it is in Heaven.*

The Lord, Mather thought as his daughter prayed on, had seen fit to bless him with many trials in the past few years. Had he not, for the sake of his Lydia—for the sake of *Doing Good*—agreed to administer the tangled estate of her son-in-law, his stepson-in-law? Whereupon Providence had spirited into the shadows all those in debt to the estate, leaving the creditors howling at Mather's door. From one day to the next, he teetered at the edge of bankruptcy, the gates of debtor's prison mocking him like gnashing teeth.

His small bit of wealth gone, his health deteriorated. Then his eldest son Increase, anointed since birth to replace his father and the grandfather for whom he was named in their famous ministry, humiliated the family name. Creasy had been running up debts for dancing teachers, rioting through the town at night with an infamous gang of rakes, descending at last to father a bastard on a whore.

Worse still, worst of all, thought Mather, his Lydia, once the best of American women, had begun to unravel. In odd moments while he was out, she sneaked through his journals, forcing him to write his many comments on her in a separate, hidden notebook, or in Greek. Passing in and out of fits he had christened "prodigious Paroxysms," she reviled him with screams of fury that both startled and embarrassed him. The congregation, he feared, would surely hear her; she was probably audible over in Charlestown. Possibly as far away as Newport.

Once such a loving mother, her attacks on the girls grew so frequent and violent that he had at last sent them scuttling out of the house. First Hannah, his poor sweet Nancy, who could not hope to defend herself with her withered arm and sightless seared half a face, the permanent marks of a fall in the fire as an infant. But then even his strong, upright Lizzy, now living with her mother's brother, Dr. John Clark: only a few doors away, to be sure, but still, out of the house. For Mather feared that Lydia might be mad, perhaps even possessed.

All these trials, he could welcome with pleasure. But this plague of the smallpox, this was terror beyond bearing—though it did reconfirm his ability to sense the will of heaven: to commune with the angels. Almost twenty-eight years before, as the witch trials in Salem were sputtering out, he had been visited in the midst of prayer and fasting by his first angel, a winged man with a shining young face. Robed in spotless white, crowned and girdled with flashing jewels, the messenger of the Lord had sweetened the world with golden-voiced prophecy. He, Cotton Mather, would be as a tall cedar of Lebanon in the garden of God, sprouting books wreathed in laurels.

In the ensuing years, other angels had flocked to him with their messages, though most were more properly sensations than visions: on some troubling topic Mather would suddenly be filled with a pure ringing clarity. Everything had come to pass, just as they let him know it would, which had lulled him into a dangerous trust closely resembling pride. The Lord had been merciful, had allowed Mather to puff up with spiritual reassurance that his first wife Abigail would recover from her cancer. When she had not, Mather had taken the point, of course: it was a lesson that demons took pleasure in leading the godly astray with pleasant voices. He had been wary of such visitations ever since.

But this latest presence had not been pleasant, did not require such suspicion. A destroying angel was looming over Boston, talons ready to swipe, verminous, scaly wings poised for a thunderous downstroke, hot breath ready to engulf them all in a poisonous wind. In recent months, had Mather not lectured, had his father not preached doom like the prophets of old? Had they not called the wicked to repentance, warning that the smallpox would soon descend upon them like one of the seven plagues of Egypt?

Creasy, Nibby, and Nancy, at least, were safe: had suffered through the distemper the last time, when his library had become the family hospital—so many small bodies lying all in a row, burning up. But Lizzy and Sammy had not yet been born.

He squeezed Lizzy's hand.

The one scrap of glory in this welter of fear was knowing once again that the Lord favored him, had chosen him as a vessel fit to sense the presence of angels. Instantly, he regretted this brief flash of triumph: he would have to humble himself exceedingly and lie in the dust, lest his vanity provoke the Holy One into doing some grievous harm to him or his family, by way of just retribution. In his mind, he saw his two youngest children cowering in the shadow of terrible dark wings, and he gasped aloud.

He prayed for a long time with Lizzy, crying to heaven for direction, for the strength to submit to the sacrifices no doubt fast approaching. When their prayers had ebbed into calm, he rose and escorted his daughter down to the front door. Lydia flew shrieking out of the parlor like a harpy, but he shut Lizzy safely out in the street, and then turned and marched silently past his screaming wife. She followed him up the stairs, but he locked her out of his library, still screeching in the passage. Then he sat down, flipped his coattails on either side of the chair, smoothed open his diary, and dipped pen into ink.

The grievous calamity of the smallpox has now entered the town, he scrawled. He looked up, his eyes scanning the shelves until they came to rest on not one but two volumes of the Royal Society's *Philosophical Transactions*. For there had been a second report on inoculation since the first by Timonius, this one by a certain Pylarinus; it, too, he had borrowed from that surly Dr. Douglass. He nodded to himself, and began again. *The Practice of conveying and suffering the Small-Pox by Inoculation, has never been used in America, nor indeed in our Nation*—here he paused with a sigh—*but how many Lives might be saved by it, if it were practiced,* he added longingly. How to urge it into practice? When the Royal Society itself balked? Surely, now if ever, was the time to try. He bit his lower lip and wrote on: *I will procure a Consult of our Physicians and lay the matter before them.*

The news that Lizzy had delivered to her father hit newsprint three days later, on the twenty-ninth—though by then it was doubtful whether there was a soul north of the Neck who could still call it news. As before, guards were placed at the doors of the infected houses and red flags run up to flutter over their gables with perverse gaiety.

The papers also reported that at six o'clock the morning before, Thomas Newton, Esq., aged sixty-one, had passed from this long travail his life. As controller of customs, he had been the man in charge of the bureaucracy that inspected all incoming shipping. *What had killed him? Was it the smallpox?* One could fairly hear the question skittering up and down the streets. *From the Paxtons, from the pirates, from the multiple ships in from Barbados? Was it?* The Newton family remained staunchly silent: there were many things that could spirit away a sixty-one-year-old at dawn's turning of the tide.

Still—barely—the selectmen managed to keep order. Only eight houses, they said. Only eight ill. And all these might have been infected before they had learned of the first incursion; this was as far as it might spread, now they knew to take precautions.

Might, others moaned darkly, hollow and filling fast with doubt.

Still, they waited. Only a month would tell. A whole month, free of pocks.

On one of these tense days, Cotton Mather saw four black men go by with shovels, brooms, and a cartload of dirt, singing as they cleaned the street. Musing upon free black men put him in mind of Onesimus, who had long since purchased his freedom, or most of it—Mather had carefully retained rights to his occasional help in such heavy work as carrying corn to the mill and fetching water on washing days. The sum he had required Onesimus to pay was the purchase price of his younger, less immorigerous replacement: once again, a prime, healthy, intelligent black lad, this one quickly christened Obadiah. This musing upon Onesimus, in turn, led Mather to another memory.

Obadiah in tow, he stepped out to speak with the men sweeping the street. Onesimus was not among them, but Mather was not looking for Onesimus, in any case. Not yet. The four men stopped singing; two of them chattered away in some language Mather could not follow. They laughed, and one of them rolled up his sleeve to show a round scar, grayish-pink and puckered in skin otherwise smooth as polished ebony. Very like the one Mather had seen on Onesimus, so many years ago.

"In my country, grandy-many die of the smallpox," said the man with the scar, his Creole lilt dipping into exaggerated gravity. He tapped his arm. "But now they learn this way: people take juice of smallpox; and cutty skin, and put in a drop; then by'nd by a little sicky-sicky." He flicked his skin lightly in several places, and broke into a wide smile. "Then very few little things like smallpox; and no body die of it; and no body have smallpox any more."

Entranced, Mather listened with a strange mix of envy and greedy delight. He, too, half sang when he talked, but he could never have managed the easy freedom with which these men bandied words about, mixing West African tongues with English, French, and the Spanish of the Caribbean. What he could do was trap every word, just so, in the vise of his memory, holding them firm until he could pin them onto paper with a quill.

It would be a while, yet, for he loped off toward the house of Onesimus, and soon, with his old servant's guidance, he was making his way, street by street, through the homes of other men and women born in Africa and now free. Neat homes, he saw to his surprise. Pious and scrupulously clean, many quite prosperous, more than a few of them nearer neighbors than he had supposed.

One after another, the people who lived in them told virtually the same story.

For a week and a half, Mather dithered, dancing forward, dancing back. He sat down at his desk, meaning to write, but got distracted by reading the *Philosophical Transactions* again. He caught up Obadiah—again—and went out to yet another house: as if out there, somewhere, down the next street, through the next door, would be lurking the information that would make him certain. A rock, an anchor, a smiling Fellow of the Royal Society staying for the length of an experiment in the home of one of their free blacks: *Why, Dr. Woodward, Dr. Newton, Dr. Halley, so honored to meet you,* he would say, *so unexpected yet so timely. Do tell me what you have discovered, if you please: does it work?*

He hinted, rather broadly, to his medical friends and acquaintances, but they returned his inquiries, the most delicate of hints as to a useful experiment, with blank stares. He fretted about his own safety, that of his children, his neighbors, all hunched down beneath the angry angelic shadow spreading over the town.

He was not alone. On June 1, still squabbling with Governor Shute, the

House of Representatives demanded to be adjourned from Boston to Cambridge: the men staring at one another, wondering who might be breathing death upon the company. While they waited, the moon rounded through full and began to wane. Squally rains, haze, and lightning fluttered nervously through the air. At last, summer muscled spring aside, clearing the skies to a brilliant blue. The land below began to smolder. Still, all around town, people peered at each other, brooding.

On the fifth of June, the selectmen ordered the grammar school moved from the schoolhouse to the representatives' room upstairs in the Town House. Three different people were sick of the smallpox in three different houses in School Street, far too close to the school itself for the comfort of parents.

On the sixth of June, Mather's servant Obadiah finally and absolutely refused to go out of the house and into the cloud of contagion he was certain lay just outside the door.

Mather sighed and retreated upstairs to his library. He would write that letter to the physicians, at last. The Royal Society, he wrote, had not so long ago described a sure preventative for the smallpox. It was untried, untested by the Society: but they had among them an army of Africans who had tried it in their own country, and who could swear to its efficacy. Carefully, with unusual brevity, he outlined the general notion of inoculation, and urged the doctors to meet, read the reports, and discuss their merits:

I will only say, he summed up in his pinched handwriting, further cramped with underlines, capitals, and exclamation points, *that inasmuch as the Practice of suffering and preventing the Small-Pox, in the way of Inocula-tion has never yet, (as far as I have heard) been introduced into our Nation; where there are so many that would give great Sums, to have their Lives insured from the dangers of this dreadful Distemper, nor has ever any one in all America ever yet, made the trial of it (though we have several Africans among us as I now find who tried it in their own Country) I cannot but move it be WARILY proceeded in. I durst not yet engage, that the Success of the trial here will be the same, as has hitherto been in the other Hemisphere. But I am very confident no person would miscarry in it but what must most certainly have miscarried upon taking it the Common way. And I would humbly advise that it be never made but under the management of a Skilful Physician who will wisely prepare the Body for it before he performs the Operation. Gentlemen, My request is that you would meet for a Consultation upon this Occasion and to deliberate upon it that whoever first begins this practice (if you approve that it should be begun at all) may have the concurrence of his worthy Brethren to fortify him in it.*

That was it: if they would not gather themselves, he would herd them together, urge them on like recalcitrant children. No time to be lost. After some careful thought, he addressed the letter to Dr. Nathanael Williams, at the eye of the storm in School Street. At the bottom, he added a particular request that it might be forwarded to Drs. Douglass and Clark, along with all the others Dr. Williams saw fit. Then he blotted it, sanded it, sent it away.

Even as the letter sped across town, the *Seahorse* sailed back into shore. The governor had declined to countermand the captain's decision regarding the location of the ship's anchorage. Out there in the shadow of Bird Island, she seemed to have been far luckier than the town. The heavy work of bringing three immense pyramids of rigging down, repairing them, hauling them back up, had been completed, all hands healthy and helping. Or at least most hands: one more man was discharged June 1, branded "unserviceable." On June 7, the *Seahorse* was grudgingly allowed to return to Long Wharf. With the strict provision, of course, that no one was to have liberty ashore without leave from both a selectman and the captain. Demurely, she began taking on biscuit and beer: not so demurely, Captain Durell made it clear to everyone that he was more than ready to pound a pirate or two, so soon as the rest of his company should be released from Spectacle Island.

So the days crept by, everyone on shore and ship watching one another for the least sign of fever: a bright eye, a flush, a shiver that might not be fear, or anxiety, or merely the memory of the cold, wet, disastrous month of May.

⚛ 5 ⚛

DEMONIC WINGS

TO and fro through the second week of June, Dr. William Douglass paced the length of his rooms upstairs at the sign of the Green Dragon, at the southwestern end of the North End, between Hanover Street and the reedy shore of the Mill Pond. Admirably plush rooms, he thought—yes, quite admirably so—yet not satisfactory, not really, because only rooms, even though rooms in the most elegant bachelors' quarters in town. Still, not as yet the grand achievement of a private house. But soon, soon, no doubt, that would come.

For—not quite thirty—he was about to make his mark on the world. He was certain of it.

He was anxious for it, too, which was why he was wearing a groove into the floorboards, listening intently for the clatter of a carriage, of horse hooves, of the service bell below. Listening for desperate pounding at the door.

Having passed safely through two weeks with no further cases of smallpox, the selectmen were already breathing sighs of relief. *Daft pack of ninnies*, snarled Dr. Douglass.

Only that morning his friends had teased that he was reckoning the city's chances with a particularly Scottish sense of gloom. He had responded as a true son of Scotland, with argument: "The span of time between the first patient's eruption into the telltale rash on May 7, and the eruptions of the second parcel of eight patients on May 25, amounts to eighteen days," he had said. "It stands to reason, doesn't it, then, that we ought to get through eighteen rashless days before congratulating ourselves with having escaped? For even in disease nature is a precisely tooled machine, mind you, aye running in regular rhythms, down smooth paths.

In short, if the smallpox took eighteen days to spread itself the first time, might it not be expected to take eighteen the second time around?"

So irascible was his temper that his companions had tiptoed away, leaving him to glower and pace, pace and glower, alone.

Tomorrow would be June 12, by God, the day Dr. Douglass had set his sights upon as the very day, give or take one or two, when Boston would either pull back from the edge, or leap headlong into epidemic. To say "Boston," though, he objected to himself, conjured up a lone figure hesitating at some brink. By his calculation, checked and rechecked, seven or eight thousand people huddled in the disease's direct line of fire: totally vulnerable. And though Boston abounded with upwards of fourteen medical practitioners, there was only one legitimate physician among them. Himself.

He spun on one heel, heading back the other direction.

Not that the town had, in the past two years and odd months in which he had made his home here, recognized his worth. Quite the reverse: his practice still consisted mostly of strangers rather than local citizens. Which is not to say that he didna have a right comfortable practice: there were many long-term and well-to-do "strangers" here, mostly Englishmen from London and Bristol, kept company by not a few of his own countrymen. A fair smattering of French Huguenots, Germans, Dutch, Danes, Russians, even a Spaniard or two. Enough for him to live handsomely on the income of his practice, with a black servant in livery and a coach and four.

His fellow foreigners, at least, knew how to pay him: kept him on a retainer of five pounds per annum for advice, sick or well, and then paid fees by the case when they needed more serious attendance, as was proper. The New Englanders, on the other hand, would only pay by the visit, requiring him to tot up every charge to the last groat in endless itemized lists that made him feel more like a shopkeeper than a physician.

Still, he wished to crack the smooth, taunting egg of Boston's ruling caste, the Cookes and Clarks, Bromfields and Bronsdons, the Foxcrofts, Olivers, Sewalls, and Hutchinsons. He envied John Clark's position, in other words, as the most prestigious medical man in town. Was owed that position, was he not? After years of medical study at the universities of Edinburgh, Leiden, and Paris, culminating in an M.D. from Utrecht? After slaving to learn the latest advances under the mentorship of such men as Dr. Hermann Boerhaave in Holland and Dr. Archibald Pitcairne in Scotland? Whereas Mr. Clark—he would *not* grant him the title of doctor— had a paltry few years reading out-of-date theory at no better place than the small local college Bostonians were all so unaccountably impressed with. *Harvard!* He stopped in his tracks and snorted.

At least Clark could claim study of some kind, Dr. Douglass told himself, leaning into his pacing once more. Most of the others were quacks— Zabdiel Boylston, for instance—no better than surgeons, mere barbers, or worse, apothecaries, pretending to the profession of physician and the title of doctor on no foundations whatsoever. Not that any of them had the least notion of what that august title indicated. Not a single proper dose of decorum among them. Even Clark operated as his own apothecary. *Shopkeepers, the lot of them.*

And provincial, myopic Boston could not, would not, be made to see the difference between the mountebanks and the real article, a genuine M.D., dedicated, talented, living right here under their uppity noses. They called everyone who had once tripped into a cure "doctor."

All this was about to change. In the upcoming epidemic, they would need him: they would need him, all right. Eight thousand divided by fourteen does not yield a pleasing number, in terms of proportioning patients to doctors in time of crisis. Five hundred seventy-one and almost one half to one, to be exact. Not pleasing, no, and certainly not comfortable, yet Dr. Douglass happily acknowledged, at least to himself, that it would be useful, fair useful indeed. Had to clasp his hands behind his back at times, to keep from rubbing them together with glee, which of course would not be seemly, even when alone.

That self-satisfied, inward-looking egg of Boston society was about to feel a tap that would send a thousand cracks spidering through its walls. The hammer of smallpox would make him—he would make himself— both desirable and necessary. In the panic and the chaos, Bostonians would take what help they could get, and he would see that as many as possible, especially among the quality, got him. He was not afraid of hard work, nasty work. He welcomed it. They would see his skill, and having seen it, they would develop a taste—no—a need for it.

But it was not just Boston's attention he wanted. This coming epidemic, he had decided, would make his name in the medical community, perhaps the entire learned community throughout the civilized world. For he would conduct three studies, which he had been planning nonstop now for two weeks: a bit of an Atlas-proud undertaking, no doubt, but he knew he could shoulder it.

First, he would observe the course of the epidemic in detail: had indeed already begun, by noting the exact span of time it took for decumbents, as he called the rash-ridden patients, to cross into different stages of the disease. It might reveal much about how it spread. He would face little threat of competition: it was a study that couldna be done in the more cosmopolitan cities of London or Paris, where the distemper was always skulking about, so that the source of infection was never clearly demarcated. Boston's isolation—the very isolation that he had for so long heartily despised—made it a near-perfect laboratory, a whole city kept separate by the sea, scoured clean by salt air.

"Pox in a box," one of his rummier companions had chortled the previous evening at a meeting of the Scots Charitable Society. In regards to one of his experiments, Dr. Douglass had not found such half-drunken flippancy funny.

Second, he would insist that his patients rigorously follow Sydenham's cold regimen, so that he might determine, definitively, its strengths and weaknesses. It was the best available treatment, sure, but he was not entirely satisfied that it was incapable of being made substantially better. He meant to find out how.

Third and most important was the study that was to be his triumph: he would investigate the cases the common people called the purples, the black pox, the flat pox. Ignorant housewives and apothecaries still often confused the bleeding smallpox with scarlet fever or measles. But he, Dr. Douglass, knew otherwise. After this epidemic—which would surely be large enough to offer enough of these admittedly rare cases for study—he hoped to be able to give a more precise description of hemorrhagic smallpox than had previously been offered to the world. He would explain how and why it developed, advise how to avoid it, and how best to treat it. Perhaps, just perhaps, future physicians might look at once hopeless cases and confidently prescribe the Douglass regimen.

His reverie was cut short by the beat of a horse approaching at speed. Was that a clatter of dismounting in the yard below? Footsteps, the bell— *yes*. It was so hard not to run to the window that he white-knuckled a chairback to anchor himself into dignified place.

There was a knock on his door, and his servant, a grizzled black man in blue livery, entered bearing a letter on a salver. Dr. Douglass did not like possessing a servant taller than himself, but he had not been able to purchase one of suitable shortness who matched his other requirements for well-spoken English and an unflappable adherence to correct manners.

"Dr. Nathanael Williams's compliments, sir, and your pardon is to be begged for tardy forwarding of this letter from Dr. Cotton Mather, Dr. Williams having been so busy with the smallpox outbreak in School Street." Dr. Douglass snatched the missive up from the tray, as Pompey's voice rolled on in the monotone that was both impeccably polite and irritatingly patronizing. "He trusts that you, being a fellow physician, will understand, no doubt being equally occupied with a sudden flurry of business. And he begs that you will take upon you the responsibility to forward the whole as you see fit."

"Out," snapped Dr. Douglass, shoving Pompey from the room with his foot. "Tell *Mr*. Williams's man to wait on answer," he added as the door swept shut. Williams was another popular Harvard man who fancied himself a polymath. It was not enough that he was a schoolteacher and a preacher, but he must claim the triple role of physician, surgeon, and apothecary as well. And Boston happily granted it. No doubt he had enjoyed that snide comment about business, thought Dr. Douglass as he crossed to the long rectangle of light streaming in the window. And Pompey, knowing the lack of business as yet, had enjoyed delivering it. He would beat him later, for insolence.

He tore open the seal. As he read, the hand holding the letter began to quiver. His cheeks, then his temples, then the back of his neck flushed, mottled beet-red. *"Meddling muck-brained minister!"* he roared, tossing the letter down. Cotton Mather had not only stolen the contents from the books he had lent him, he had gone and publicized them without so much as a by-your-leave or a thank-you. No public attribution of his source whatsoever. It was an outrage.

To make matters worse, the topic he had chosen to gabble on about was that Turkish flumgummerie about inoculation that the Royal Society had tossed around a few years ago. Mather had actually called upon Boston's physicians to convene, in order to read and discuss the two articles in question. He, Dr. Douglass, was not only supposed to read this drivel, he was supposed to pass it on, as if he condoned it. *Ha!*

Did every American who had learned his letters think he could waltz into the practice of medicine as he chose?

Suddenly, he felt a centipede of suspicion crawling up through his insides. Perhaps Mather, so jealous of his place as the most learned man in the province, was now pushing for honors in medicine. Perhaps he meant to be the first to try some newfangled notion in medicine, and had lit upon this one. Dr. Pitcairne himself, after all, had been rather fond of the idea of inoculation. Dr. Pitcairne, however, had never been able to bring himself to attempt it, because Dr. Pitcairne was neither a fool nor crazy.

Mather, in Douglass's opinion, could be both. Besides, what other possible reason could the man have for stirring things up just now?

Standing in full sun, Dr. Douglass went cold and began to splutter. Mather had influence. If he yapped long and loud enough, he might well sweep aside all the interest that ought to be focused on Dr. Douglass's carefully planned studies. Worse, he might muddy the waters, so to speak, if he actually got people to try it. Might dirty the clean, closed arena that Boston now presented to the natural spread of the smallpox. Might ruin, in short, Dr. Douglass's experiments.

That was unthinkable.

But having thought it, Dr. Douglass found he could not unthink it.

Mather had to be stopped.

Two minutes later he shouted for Pompey, hurling a slipper at the lazy gomeril when he finally appeared—no doubt he had been smoking and probably tippling, too, downstairs with Williams's servant. Dr. Douglass demanded his coach, demanded to be dressed, demanded clean paper, a new quill, and sealing wax, all at once.

With infuriating calm, Pompey said he would call for the coach and be back with the second-best suit, the yellow camlet. Dr. Douglass threw the other slipper at him, too, but it bounced off the door that Pompey had already closed.

At Mather's house, he did not wait to be announced, but followed the servant up three flights of stairs—*must the man store himself in his own attic?*

He had been in the reverend's library before, of course, but he always forgot just how many books lined the walls—nigh on three thousand. As much as Dr. Douglass loathed to admit it, Mather's library was fine or finer than many universities possessed. Even if one discounted the several hundred volumes authored by Mather himself, it was a collection that would have made most provosts salivate in their sleep. He was pleased to note, therefore, that the curtains were patched and the carpet moth-eaten. The legs of the chairs looked like they had been gnawed by mice who had long since given up hope of cheese.

Mather looked up sharply from his writing, but his annoyance rather oddly melted away as he recognized his guest. To Dr. Douglass's surprise, a sudden burst of pleasure spread over the reverend's face. "Delighted to see you, Doctor," he said, sweeping a pile of books from a nearby chair. "By all means sit down."

Dr. Douglass bowed and declined. "Regrettably, sir, I must request the return of the two volumes of the *Philosophical Transactions* which you have borrowed from me." He had practiced his smile in the looking glass before leaving: stiffly polite, noncommittal.

Mather failed to notice. He leapt up, crossed to the exact spot three quarters of the way down a shelf next to the far left window, and drew them out.

Of course he would know where they were—he had just used them, and rather thoroughly, hadn't he? Dr. Douglass took a step forward. "I must further request, sir, in light of the extraordinarily free manner in which you have publicized the contents of my possessions, that in future you will not ask to borrow my books." *There, that silly smile was withdrawn—snapped—from the man's face.*

Mather paused ever so briefly, then continued on his way, not directly, but tracing a finger along a shelf about shoulder high, all the way around the perimeter of the room, so that Dr. Douglass found his eyes traversing the whole of the collection. Having wrapped the room around him like a cloak of books, of deep-voiced knowledge, debate, and intelligence, of the scents of paper and leather, Mather stepped forward and laid the two volumes on a table that now lay between them. "I cannot, sir, conceive of any future necessity to rely upon your library," he said. He was the master, Dr. Douglass saw, of a smile that has just enough hint of a sneer to make the viewer uncertain of its presence or absence. "As a Fellow of the Royal Society, however, I thank you for the opportunity to peruse information that my Fellows in London have seen fit to publish to the world at large."

Dr. Douglass tried to display polite indifference to such brazen effrontery. The man was not only refusing to apologize or to recognize Dr. Douglass's proprietary rights to the information in the books he possessed, but was waving his F.R.S. about as if it gave him some prior claim to it. Having almost succeeded in swallowing his own sneer, Dr. Douglass bowed once again and departed.

Back at the Green Dragon, Dr. Douglass marched upstairs and flung his stocky frame into a chair. He skimmed the two articles in question, and then clapped the books closed, stood up, and crossed the room. Drawing his watch chain from his waistcoat pocket, he disentangled a key and unlocked the lowest drawer of his desk. Withdrawing the letter that Williams had forwarded earlier that morning, he thrust the books inside, shoved the drawer closed, and locked it once more.

He could honestly say that he had convened the blasted physicians' meeting that Mather had asked for. Every last medical doctor in Boston— namely himself—had attended, had read the articles in question. He let out a single snort of laughter. The consensus, by God, was unanimous: inoculation was a dangerous bit of quackery. An old wives' tale—and an Oriental old wives' tale at that. A conversational curiosity, not medicine. Furthermore, that vain, credulous preacher named Mather should not— *would not*—be allowed to spoil Dr. Douglass's imminent glory.

Despite the fact that it was bright afternoon in the middle of June, he lit a candle. Holding Mather's open letter above the flame, he watched the pages brown and blacken around the cramped writing, until in a whoosh of orange, the letter disappeared into nothingness and gray ash.

Late on the twelfth of June, right through the thirteenth and fourteenth, and into the early hours of the fifteenth, demonic wings swept down across the town in a silent arc of terror, sowing the fecund red seeds of the rash through upwards of fifty houses. Within days, the seeds were blossoming foul yellow and white.

This time, no attempt was made to put guards on the newly infected houses; there were too many. Those posted at the first eight houses melted away or were swept away by a fast-rising tide of panic. People began to flee, first in furtive trickles, then in a steady stream. By week's end, wagons, coaches, light two-wheeled chariots, even wheelbarrows clogged the streets in an endless jostling flood heaving its way out of the city.

"Eighteen days," said Dr. Douglass with satisfaction to his brethren among the Scots Charitable Society, assembled as his guests at the Green Dragon. "Did I not predict eighteen days?"

They had to agree, he had said eighteen days. Often. They raised their glasses to toast the scientific, the orderly, the neat and predictable number of eighteen.

Not that he *wanted* the smallpox to come, Dr. Douglass reassured himself. Only, that if it were to come, as it indeed had, he wanted to understand it.

What shall I do? Cotton Mather wrung his hands as he walked, as he talked, as he prayed, as he scribbled in his diary. *G.D. What shall I do? Oh, What shall I do, that my Family may be prepared, for the Visitation that is now every day to be expected!* His silent wails harmonized with the quavery terror of his two youngest children. Just as smallpox began to spread, Sammy came home from college in Cambridge and refused to go back again. It was spreading there too; he felt safer—or at least more comfortable—at home.

Caught between the Charybdis of Dr. Clark—quite possibly trailing poison from one house to another, she cried to her brother—and the Scylla of her stepmother—barking mad—Lizzy was even more terrified. For her, nowhere seemed either safe or comfortable.

Dr. Mather looked to heaven for direction, but heaven was strangely silent. Meanwhile, he determined to improve, with all the contrivance he could, his children's interests in Piety. To impress upon them the need for subservience to the will of the Lord. To prepare for whatever sacrifices He might demand.

* * *

On the night of the thirteenth of June, with the second wave of rashes blooming around them in the warm, moonless dark, Jerusha Boylston waited up late for her husband. He found her standing barefoot in her shift by the window in their bedroom, the casement open wide to the garden in hopes that a breeze might ruffle the close, damp heat of June. She was forty-two; she had borne eight children and buried two, one within the year. She was tired, not as slender as she once had been. Not yet matronly, but she knew with a sigh of amusement that her thickening waist and hips were headed that direction. She still held herself straight and strong, though, like a dare. He thought her more beautiful than ever.

She held out her arms, and he went to her, enfolding her; the top of her head fit right up under his chin. When she drew back a little and looked up, he could see the wisps of crow's feet that edged her eyes and the laugh lines lacing her mouth. She was not laughing tonight. He ran a finger delicately about her face. For a long time, they stood there breathing in each other's musky scent, curled about with the rich sweetness of roses.

They had never discussed what they would do if and when it came to this, for it had been clear to them both: She would leave with the children, and he would stay with the sick.

The question that circled unspoken around them was not what to do, but how to do it, as quickly as possible.

"How long?" she asked after a while.

"A few days yet," he answered. "Tom rides south beyond the Neck tomorrow, to find a suitable house. We must also hire a coach: Sarah is too far gone with child for a rough ride. It will be better, too, for you and the girls. Pack the—"

"No." She bit her lip and turned her head to the side, pressing into his shoulder and looking determinedly into the starlight until she trusted her voice not to waver. Then she drew back and looked up into his face. "How long before I will see you again?"

He ran a finger down her cheek and gave her a smile, but his eyes were dark seas of sadness and trouble. "I don't know, sweetheart. If we're lucky, the distemper could burn itself out in a few weeks. But it may be many months."

"Many months," she whispered, burying her face once again in the cambric that covered his chest.

He stroked her fine hair, once so blond, now the pale brown of late autumn leaves, of young fawns or panthers. "The children are in more danger from me every day I walk back into this house."

She shook her head. "Not from you. From the smallpox."

"It will amount to the same thing soon enough," he said. "I will be no better than poison to my own children."

"Never say that," she whispered.

"Would you have me lie?"

"No," she said, flinging her head back to answer the glitter in his eyes. For a moment it was hard to say whether they were clinging to each other or pushing each other away. Then a wild, wicked smile no one but Zabdiel had ever seen broke across her face. "I would have you lie with me, though."

He swept her up and carried her to the bed, where they curved and arched over each other, swimming fiercely toward union and the troubled sleep that lay beyond.

The following day, Zabdiel's brother Tom stopped by the house briefly at dawn and then rode away south toward Roxbury. He did not return until late into the night.

Thirteen-year-old John was supposed to be sleeping: his brother Tommy had dropped off hours ago, breathing slow and even beside him. But John could not sleep. He was too aware of the humming tension on the floor below. He knew, without seeing, that his father was pacing in circles around the parlor, while his mother sat rigidly still at its heart, gripping her needle with such ferocity that the square of linen she was skewering might as well be the devil himself. So he heard his uncle ride up, coming straight around to the kitchen door and handing the reins to Jack. He heard their voices, low and indistinct, three stories below. Heard Jack stomp off to the barn, and then silence, as his uncle paused on the doorstep. After a long while, he heard his uncle sniff, and then the door creak open.

He crept out to the landing, to the place where the shadows always lay thick enough to hide in, and peered downstairs. Uncle Tom took the stairs up to the second floor three at a time, as usual, but not with his usual bound: each step was a leaden, deliberate threat. In the parlor, his mother laid her needlework neatly aside and stood up, reaching out for his father, who took her hand in a hard grip.

Tom stopped just inside the doorway, partially blocking John's view.

"Good or bad?" he asked quietly. "Which first?"

"The bad," said his mother.

Tom shook his head. "Nothing," he said. "Nothing we can afford." The words peppered out like angry shot. "Hovels with no drains and a two-mile walk to water are going for rates that would give Mr. Cooke pause."

"And the good?" asked his father.

Uncle Tom set his shoulders. "Rebecca and William have agreed to take Sarah, my girls, Jerusha and your girls as well as Mary and young Mary."

Whatever was wrong, thought John, it must have something to do with girls. For his uncle had just named most of the girls in the family. Aunt Rebecca, one of his father's sisters, lived down in Roxbury with his uncle William and all his Abbot cousins; that was who Uncle Tom must have been visiting. Aunt Sarah, Uncle Tom's wife, and their two baby girls. His own mother and sisters, and his father's other sister in town, Aunt Mary and her daughter, cousin Mary Lane. To find any more girls, you'd have to get on the ferry for Charlestown, or ride all the way out to Brookline.

"*The boys*," whispered his mother in a strange harsh voice.

Tom shook his head. "William was quite firm. The women and the girls are all they can manage. More than they can manage in comfort."

His mother did not weep or wail, or even gasp; she made no sound at all. But a dark wind of despair seemed to pour from her eyes, blowing out all light and warmth, wrenching open a pit at the bottom of John's belly. He had never seen her like this, except once, when they had nailed the lid on his baby brother's coffin. She had not known he was looking then either. As had happened then, her whole body disappeared, wrapped in the strong arms of his father.

Then, the way that his father had held her had reassured John: encased in that grip, the seams of the world would not come apart. This time, the hole in his stomach split wider. For he saw the look that shot from his father to his uncle, over her head.

Rage, frustration, and something he had never seen on his father's face before.

Fear.

The whole of the next day and well into the night, Jerusha packed. She found jobs for the girls all over the house; Tommy she somehow needed nearby, almost underfoot. It was times like this that he envied John his shiny new apprenticeship, a present for his thirteenth birthday; he would not be thirteen for seven long years, thought Tommy darkly. Meanwhile, John was learning to be a merchant—or a merchant prince, as he put it. Usually, Tommy rolled his eyes just thinking about it. His brother stuffed his head with numbers from morning to night; he would eagerly trace not just sums but full-blooded trigonometry problems on the wall with a finger in his sleep. Tommy wanted to be a doctor, or maybe a ship's captain, not a merchant. This morning, though, he had to admit it would have been useful to have John's irreproachable reason to be somewhere else.

All day, Tommy helped his mother pack clothing, bedding, and food for what seemed like a year. Warming pans, pots, utensils. Pickles, preserves, cheeses, dried fruit, and meat. A precious chest full of books and writing paper. Another, even more dear, of medicinal supplies—all that their father would spare and some he was hard pressed to give up. "You must leave some for me and the boys, Jer," he heard him chide, though gently. His mother nodded and ruffled his hair so fiercely that he had to swallow a yelp.

The next day, Uncle Tom arrived, riding alongside his coach. The men stowed the baggage up top, while the women nearly suffocated everybody else with farewells. Finally, his mother and the girls stepped into the carriage to join Aunt Sarah, looking faintly green, and his cousins Sarah and Annie who stuck out tiny pink tongues. Tommy crossed his eyes and waggled his own tongue back, until they squealed with laughter. Moll, Jack's wife and Jerusha's godsend, as his father said, gave Jackey one kiss and a pat on the rear, and climbed up to sit ramrod straight next to the driver.

And then with a groaning heave, they were gone, swallowed by the shout and chaos of the streets.

John bustled off in Uncle Tom's wake. Tommy's father and Jack, too, rode away soon after that, his father on a fine gelding, and Jack on the long-eared, strong-hearted mule he loved—because it was his, and because they had a sort of running tussle over which of them was boss. They would be gone all day, his father had said; it would take that long to visit all the sick people.

There was sure a lot of leaving going on, thought Tommy as he stood with Jackey and waved at everyone else. No doubt, he would miss his mother. On the brighter side, he had just been freed from the girls' endless demands to play the Indian game, reenacting over and over the attack on their mother's girlhood home, such ages and ages ago that his mother hadn't been born yet. The three girls traded off the roles of the heroic maid and the two babies whom she had saved by popping them under overturned kettles. Tommy always played the lone Indian warrior, which would have been brilliant if it hadn't meant that he not only always had to lose, but to crawl off and invent some new spectacular way to die as well. True, he got to take a few pretend pot-shots (he was very proud of the pun) through a window at the kettles. But then whoever was playing the maid got to bean him with yet another pot. And if that weren't bad enough, she then tossed coals in his face. Mary tended to get carried away with the beaning, even though they used a pillow; his sister Jerusha had a wicked arm with the leaves they used for coals. Sometimes he thought the taste of leaves was the last thing he remembered at night, and the first thing he thought of in the morning.

But he would not have to play the Indian game for a while. For a whole glorious week or maybe even two, he was a man in a man's world. Tommy decided to celebrate. Jackey might be only two and a half, but he already knew how to roar like a lion. Also, he worshiped Tommy, which Tommy reckoned was an excellent character trait. "Pirates," decreed Tommy. "We'll play pirates."

At crucial moments, though, just as the Dread Pirate Roberts (Tommy) threatened with magnificent rage to send the scurvy, thieving lubbers among his crew down the plank, directly into a frenzy of sharks, Jackey (the crew, good, bad, and middling) would wander off after a squirrel, or a bee, or the place where he remembered he had left some raisins two days ago. Or he would ask, *What do sharks sound like?* And keep asking, until Tommy came up with a good answer.

Tommy decided that being the man of the house, as his father put it, from dawn until dusk was not going to be easy.

Dr. Cotton Mather had the privilege of being attended in medical matters by his brother-in-law, Dr. John Clark. Nonetheless, on the twenty-first of June, one of the goods he devised was to encourage others in the neighborhood—those who could not, perhaps, be expected to bear the expense of Dr. Clark's services—to rely upon Dr. John Perkins in the matter of the smallpox. His skill and piety made the doctor eminently worthy, Mather judged; his need was self-evident. Newly released from debtor's prison, Dr. Perkins quivered at the threat of return. It was a fate for which Mather had developed a certain sympathy.

While canvassing the neighborhood, urging the services of Dr. Perkins upon his flock, however, Dr. Mather became aware of a certain reticence.

"If you please, sir," one maid squeaked at last, "My father says to say he don't want none of your advice in matters medical or physical, sir, though he would be pleased to retain your services in a more ministerial line. Prayers and sermons and whatnot."

It did not take him long to plumb the source of both her terrified embarrassment—she was bobbing through curtsies like a jack-in-the-box—and her father's obstinate reluctance. Though she was the bearer of bad news quite against her will, she was voicing an alarmingly general murmuration against him. The Lord, it seemed, was blessing him with a new set of trials. For it appeared that Dr. Douglass had not only squelched his plea for a physicians' meeting, but had proceeded to spread lies of a most abominable sort.

In return for evil, his inner voice bristled, *Do Good.*

In this case, there was a particularly satisfactory good within his reach.

The next morning, Dr. Mather shut himself up in his library and drew from a cupboard a sheaf of papers carefully wrapped up in ribbon and labeled. These he carried to his desk and settled down to write a Treatise on the Small Pox, in three parts: first, a section awakening the sentiments of Piety necessary in order to face death in a godly manner. Second, a section delineating the best medicines and methods the world had yet seen for managing the disease. And third, the new discovery of Inoculation.

For he had, of course, copied out both Timonius and Pylarinus word for word—as close as would signify, at any rate—upon first reading them. Long before the miserly Dr. Douglass had locked them away in some secret treasure hoard of knowledge.

Day brightened, and then faded again, and still his pen scrabbled on. Dusk had crept through most of its long summer-blue hour when he at last laid down his quill and wrung the cramps from his hands. He stood up and considered what to do with his treatise, a fine piece of work if he said so himself. In the right hands, he flattered himself—hands that would not burn it—these few humble pages might save many lives.

Shall I give it to the Booksellers? he asked his diary. *I am waiting for Direction.*

Direction came in the night. He would not spread it abroad indiscriminately, pearls before swine. He would see, however, that everyone fit to comprehend it, to judge its worth, should receive a copy. The next day, he noted in his diary, *I write a Letter unto the Physicians, entreating them, to take into consideration the important Affair of preventing the Small Pox.*

Actually, he had written the brief letter out once. It was Sammy and Lizzy who were copying it, along with the treatise, many times over, one of each for every doctor in town. It was a task that had the double good of easing his worries about Sammy's hours of idleness.

The last letter he wrote out himself, signing and addressing it with a grand flourish. Cotton Mather, D.D., F.R.S.

To William Douglass, M.D.

❧ 6 ❧

FATHERS AND SONS

O N the twenty-fourth of June, Zabdiel Boylston arrived home exhausted, long after dark. He had sent Jack home earlier, to get dinner for the boys, so Zabdiel unsaddled, watered, and fed his horse himself. He stopped, too, at the stall of his bay stallion, Prince, who snorted and stamped softly. As he did every evening, Zabdiel fed him some raisins. "Tomorrow," he promised, stroking the horse's nose. "We'll ride tomorrow."

Then he stepped into the far stall, empty save for a bucket of water, soap, and towel. Kicking off his shoes, he stripped, working upward to the day cap that covered his close-shaven head. He had given up wearing a wig at the first cry of smallpox. In his estimation, the thing trapped contagion like a net; in Jerusha's estimation, it would be impossible to comb out the smell. For a few days, he had felt naked and light headed, but now he liked riding out with nothing but a velvet cap between his skull and the sky. The cap, too, soon went flying across the stall, and then he washed himself from head to toe. It felt good to bare his skin to the summer night. To pretend, at least, that water faintly astringent with rue and rosemary could rinse the day's filth from his memory, as well as from his skin. Still mother naked, he walked the length of the barn and ducked into the stall at the opposite end, also near empty, in this case save for a clean set of clothes.

He had decreed this measure for both himself and Jack, to safeguard the boys. Extreme, to be sure, and quite possibly absurd, especially if the contagion turned out to be climactic, settling on the whole region like some foul mist. He could not tell about that yet, though, while he knew for certain that garments could carry the infection. Bedding, too. That infernal practice of auctioning off a dead sailor's clothing at the mainmast within an hour of the unfortunate's expiry might well be what had spread it with such deadly and particular deliberation around the *Seahorse*, for instance. He had heard about that from Dr. Clark: how the worst cases on that ship had seemed to follow one another in single-file procession.

The boys were ready for bed. He said prayers with them, and then told a story about the Dread Pirate Roberts and a Pearl of Great Price. Tommy let himself be swept away quickly on the tides of sleep. From the look on John's face, though, Zabdiel guessed he had sadly fallen off his best story-telling, though John was not going to say so. *Papa needs rest*, said the worried expression on his face.

He was right.

He descended from the boys' eyrie on the third floor to the parlor that stretched the full length of the house on the floor below. It was his favorite room, with his and Jerusha's armchairs drawn close to the cozy fireplace in winter, turned to face the windows and the open sky in the summer. Jerusha had left—on purpose, he guessed—a bit of half-finished cross-stitch on hers, so that he might pretend that she was just across the hall, upstairs with the children, down in the kitchen with Moll. Somewhere, anywhere nearby, rather than five miles off, where she might be fighting fever in one of the girls without him knowing, much less helping. Where she would sit ignorant herself when Tommy and John fell ill.

For they would fall ill. Unless Zabdiel could spirit them out of town soon, they would fall ill. And it would be Zabdiel who infected them, no matter what precautions he thought up. Something would slip by, and he would carry the infection home from some sickroom and feed it straight to the boys. Might as well get over it now, said the crisp voice of reason. But the father in him balked, choked at the thought of his sons swollen and covered in an ash-gray crust of scabs, or scattered with flat black sores seeping into one another. Already, the flat pox was sowing its seed among Boston's children with deadly abandon.

Zabdiel shook the vision off. A letter lay on the table between the chairs; a big, bulky letter. He picked it up. From Cotton Mather, fire-breather. He opened it.

June 24, 1721

Sir,

You are many ways endeared unto me, but by nothing more than the very much good which a gracious God employs you and honors you to do to a miserable world.

I design it as a testimony of my respect and esteem that I now lay before you the most that I know (and all that was ever published in the world) concerning a matter which I have been an occasion of its being pretty much talked about. If upon mature deliberation, you should think it advisable to be proceeded in, it may save many lives that we set a great value on. But, if it be not approved of, still you have the pleasure of knowing exactly what is done in other places.

The gentlemen, my two authors, are not yet informed, that among the Guramantees 'tis no rare thing for a whole company, of a dozen together, to go to a person sick of the small pox, and prick his pustules, and inoculate the humour, even no more than the back of one hand, and go home, and be a little ill, and have a few, and be safe all the rest of their days. Of this I have in my neighbourhood a competent number of living witnesses.

But see, think, judge; do as the Lord our healer shall direct you, and pardon this freedom of, Sir,

Your hearty friend and servant,
Cotton Mather

At the very bottom was his name, Dr. Boylstone, as Mather spelled it, with that old-fashioned curl of an *e* at the end, the only personal word on the page. Otherwise, the missive had the distinct distance of a form letter. As if ten, fifteen, identical letters had been written, then each marked out for a different doctor, ticked off some list.

Zabdiel frowned. He had heard the skirling gossip that Mather was championing some new bird-brained notion of a cure for smallpox. He had also heard that it was the dour Scots plumage of Dr. Douglass that was most ruffled. But Mather was a meddler, and Douglass a complete snarler. Zabdiel had had no time for their nattering.

He glanced at the first page of the enclosed treatise:

There is a Great Plague which we call the SMALL POX, wherein the Misery of man is great upon him: A Distemper so well known and so much Felt that there needs no Description to be given of it.

If only Dr. Mather could obey his own calls for brevity. Zabdiel riffled through the treatise, ream thick. Here and there, a phrase or two leapt off a page: "a *New Distemper* . . . *the Ancients* unacquainted with it." The reverend began, it seemed, with history. Next, theology, or the "Sentiments of PIETY to be raised in and from this *Grievous Disease*." No surprise there. Smallpox, like every other ill, cried Mather, was the hot lash of a wrathful God. "*Ah, Sinful Generation, a People Laden with Iniquity, a Seed of Evil-*

doers, Children that are Corrupters." Zabdiel could hear Mather's voice ringing from the pulpit, deep and doom laden with the cadences of Jeremiah, of Isaiah, of Ezekiel—surely this had been delivered in a sermon?

He shivered. The reverend had the poetry, the bright burning visions of a prophet too. *"Behold an Angel with a flaming Sword over thee giving of it; Prepare to meet thy God,* O thou Traveller thro' a Land where *Fiery Flying Serpents* are hovering Everywhere about thee!"

Zabdiel sensed no shadow of God in the merciful person of Jesus anywhere in the treatise; Dr. Mather seemed concerned solely with God in the wrathful person of Jehovah. To those fallen ill, he recommended self-abhorrence and self-abasement, directing them to cry out, *"Unclean! Unclean!"* and confess, *"Lord, I am a Filthy Creature!"* On and on he fulminated. "All the nasty *Pustules* which now fill thy *Skin,"* he thundered, bringing down his arm to point with terrible sure directness, "are but Little Emblems of the *Errors* which thy *Life* has been filled Withal. Make thy Lamentation: *Lord, from the Sole of the Foot, even to the Head, there is no Soundness in me; nothing but putrifying Sores."*

Zabdiel did not know whether to laugh or cry. Such self-loathing was hard to avoid at certain stages of the distemper, but in his experience, breast beating and panic contributed little to nothing toward curing the body; he had his doubts about their usefulness for the soul. Did he not spend all day from dawn to full night urging his patients and their families that the best restorative for those fallen ill—the best preventative for those still healthy—was cheerful calm?

He was tossing the papers aside when another phrase caught his eye: "Yet let us be of *Good Courage;* yea, be *Very courageous."* For there is, wrote Mather, a way to manage the beast. Zabdiel's arm stopped of its own accord and drew the treatise back under his eyes.

It was a false alarm: Mather launched into detail on Sydenham's cold treatment. Useful, well done, but not news. Zabdiel had learned a modified—moderated—version of Sydenham's regimen long ago, from his master and mentor, Dr. Cutler. He skimmed on. The minister had certainly done a fair amount of medical reading: everything in print concerning the smallpox, it seemed, had been digested and discussed here. Quite impressive, really. A fair amount of sound advice. Authorities like Archibald Pitcairne and John Woodward, in addition to Thomas Sydenham. But, as yet, nothing new.

Zabdiel rubbed his eyes, let the papers fall to his lap. Again, an image of the boys sick rose into his mind. He sighed and picked up the dissertation once more. There was supposed to be something new here; he would find it no matter how deeply Dr. Mather had buried it.

Ah. An appendix.

"There has been a *Wonderful Practice* lately used in several Parts of the World, which indeed is not yet become common in our Nation."

Yes, this was it.

"I was first instructed in it," wrote Dr. Mather, "by a *Guramantee* Servant of my own, long before I knew that any *Europeans* or *Asiaticks* had the least Acquaintance with it; and some years before I was Enriched with the Communications of the Learned Foreigners, whose Accounts I found agreeing with what I received of my Servant, when he showed me the Scar of the Wound made for the Operation; and said, That no Person ever died of the *Small-Pox*, in their Country, that had the Courage to use it.

"I have since met with a Considerable Number of these *Africans*, who all agree in one Story . . ."

Zabdiel stood up, hardly knowing he did so. He took a step forward in his excitement, and another. Soon he was striding around the room as he tore through the remaining pages, devouring every word through to the end. Africans along the Gold Coast, old women among the Greeks, the Turks in Constantinople, all of these people knew this practice of inoculation. Said it was not just workable, but damned near infallible. Into this appendix, Mather had transcribed reports made to the Royal Society several years earlier by two Italian doctors in the Levant, Timonius and Pylarinus. According to them, all one needed for delivery from Mather's destroying angel was a needle, a clean glass vial, a lancet, a bandage, and a small curved bit of shell from a walnut.

That, and the poisonous white paste from the ripe pock of a healthy young person—as healthy, at any rate, as it was possible to be while stricken with the smallpox.

Zabdiel made one more circuit around the room, thinking furiously. Then he yelled for Jack, who appeared in the doorway a moment later. "Listen," he said hoarsely, without interrupting his stride. He read the appendix all the way through again, this time aloud, gripping the pages so tightly the paper came near to ripping.

"Have you heard of this?" he cried, wild eyed, waving the papers before him.

Jack gripped both sides of the doorway, on the theory that somebody needed to keep the house still, or it would fair begin to spin from the force of the doctor's crazed circling. "Yes, sir," he said. "Never seen it—born in Barbados, not the Gold Coast. But I heard of it. Everyone's heard of it—everyone of us, Doctor, begging your pardon."

The last sentence brought Zabdiel up short; he had never given much thought to that black, recently African *us*. But of course, there was one, with its own remedies, traditions, knowledge. A great deal of it discreetly shielded from English view, no doubt, if that *us* was anything like the Indian *us*. He licked his lips, which suddenly felt dry. "What do you think?" he asked, his sudden stillness even more urgent than his circling had been.

Jack watched him unblinking for a moment, then cocked his head, and said, "Takes a brave man to try it, Doctor. So they say."

Zabdiel nodded. "Thank you," he said, and Jack withdrew. He ran his hand across his head, rubbed his eyes. He paced across the passage and dropped to a seat on the edge of the bed. He was tired. So tired already, and it had just begun. He knew what was coming, though: in the worst cases, purple spots and convulsions, bloody urine or no urine, or involuntary, unstoppable urine; sweats and salivations, grossly inflamed eyes, throats, and groins. Scarred faces. Many people would lose one eye; some would lose both. Women big, but not big enough, with child would abort before their time, swimming through their own blood to follow their too-young babies into death. Parents left childless, and children left orphans; parents and children carried off in one fell, family-shattering swoop. And everywhere, the thick, choking smell. Blisters and pustules. Pus, pus, and more pus.

Death was terrible in all its shapes, but this was one of its worst. Mather's newfangled notion was no cure. It was deliberate infection, its only merit an unfounded claim to offer future protection. Surely it was a demonic joke, a bit of laughter fallen from the destroying angel's throat.

Takes a brave man to try it, Jack had said.

What kind of a man did it take to try it on his sons?

The following morning, Tommy was up and into the shop early, helping his father fill the cordial bottles and powder papers he would take with him that day; it was a new job, one that made Tommy stand as tall as he could. Still not tall enough to reach the higher shelves, though. He was on the footstool, reaching for the black cherry water, when the front door banged open, though it was not yet time for breakfast. He glanced over his shoulder and saw a woman slump to the floor; a funny sound came from her throat.

"Tommy," said his father, "step down, please, and fetch some salt from the kitchen."

It was an odd request, but his father's tone of voice was the one that meant *Act now, ask later*. He stepped down at once, though in such a way as to get one good look at their visitor. The woman—was it a woman?—in the midst of that heap of widow-black skirts had sores over every visible inch of skin, flat round sores the size of coins, deep crimson and purple.

Her swollen nose was bleeding, and blood seeped from her mouth. Just as he rounded the corner of the door that joined the shop to the rest of the house, he caught a queer impression that she was crying tears of blood.

His father patted him as he went by, then gave him a quick shove through the door, shutting it between them; Tommy heard the latch drop home from the other side. It was a sound that seemed to cancel the strange request for salt, and in any case, he had reached the outer limits of his capacity for obedience. He did not go on to the kitchen, but stood listening to his father's voice, kind and calm, on the other side of that door: the woman was to go home, he would send a nurse around, he would come himself directly, but she was not to stir out again, not to put others at risk, not to waste her precious store of energy that must be put to use fighting the distemper.

Tommy heard a scraping that must be his father pulling her back to her feet; heard the front door open, a whistle, muffled voices of men, a clatter of wagon and hooves. Heard the front door close again, and then stood to attention, waiting for his father to come back, unlatch the door, and explain everything. But his father did not come; no footsteps crossed the shop. After a moment's careful thought, Tommy scuttled through the passage to the kitchen, just in time to catch a glimpse of his father's back disappearing into the barn, forbidden territory since the smallpox had descended on the town.

Jack called him to the breakfast table, but Tommy shook his head impatiently. He stood lookout at the window until he saw his father emerge in his work clothes and ride away.

It was a consequence of dispensing with guards on the infected houses, thought Zabdiel angrily. Well-meaning friends and family visited the sick and then each other; the solitary sick wandered out into the streets, half delirious, to find help. It left one in the untenable position of ordering a dying woman from the house, for the sake of one's children.

He set his shoulders, put his head down, and went to work; to his visitor, first of all, though all that remained to do for her was to make her as comfortable as possible and send for the minister she trusted most.

Then all day long, in and out of bedrooms sumptuous or spare, of garrets, cellars, sheds, and ships, Zabdiel dutifully tended the sick and comforted the still healthy. It was not where either his mind or his heart lay, though. Some odd detached part of him watched from above as eagerly, even greedily, he asked in each household to speak to every person there, slave or free, who had been born in Africa.

Evening stretched into night, and this time Jack stayed with him.

"Boys'll be all right," he said when Zabdiel tried to dismiss him. "Left 'em some venison pie and salad." Then he took the lead, guiding Zabdiel to several households of free blacks who had stories to tell. Scars to show. In one of those houses, they heard the very tale that Cotton Mather had transcribed word for Creole word.

To a man, to a woman, every person Zabdiel spoke to all day long upheld that story. Not exactly: not as if they had been discussing it among themselves. Some displayed scars on the fleshy parts of an upper arm or leg; some showed the back of the hand, or the thin web of skin between thumb and forefinger. Sometimes they spoke of an old woman who pricked people with a thorn. Others had put themselves in the hands of tribal elders, sometimes even priests, bearing ceremonial instruments. But the central part of every story was the same: they had been infected with a small bit of pock matter. They had sickened briefly. And they had survived to face down the speckled demon, unscathed and unafraid.

Zabdiel rode home deep in thought. Once again, he stripped, washed himself, and walked naked to the other end of the barn, to dress in clean clothes. Jack did the same, if rather less absently.

As they stepped out into the yard, Zabdiel stopped. "What do you think?" he asked Jack, once again.

Behind them, Prince snorted softly and stamped.

"I think you better ride that horse," said Jack. "He's tired of standing in a stall day in and day out."

Zabdiel nodded. In the moonlight, the shadows under his eyes looked like bottomless gulfs of exhaustion, but at the thought of a ride, his whole body perked up.

"I'll see the boys to bed," said Jack.

Still, Zabdiel hesitated.

"I tell a fine bedtime story," said Jack. "You go on."

"Thank you," said Zabdiel. He watched Jack walk off toward the house. He was thirty-six, only a few years younger than Zabdiel; he, too, had a son at risk.

"Jack," he called, just as his servant reached the back stoop. "What do you think?"

He heard a catch of breath, a sigh; saw a gleam of eyes looking about for an answer. It was not common for a white man to ask a black man his opinion. Not unheard of, but uncommon. On such a dangerous subject as this, Zabdiel realized, Jack'd have to pick his way into speech with extreme care.

"Same as I thought last night."

"Right," said Zabdiel wearily.

"Wait there a minute," said Jack. Zabdiel heard the faint whoosh of the door opening, a creak of floorboards, a footstep or two. Then Jack said, "Catch." A tiny stone of darkness arced toward Zabdiel through the night; without thinking, he put up his hand and caught it.

"Good night, Doctor," said Jack. "I got to go see to those rascals upstairs." Then he was gone.

Zabdiel opened his hand. In his palm, silver in the moonlight, lay the old-man wrinkles and folds, the doubled ship's-hull curve of a walnut.

A few minutes later, he was astride Prince, trotting west up Queen Street, the stallion's hooves ringing over paving stones. A few more minutes, and that clatter melted into a muffled thud as the ground relaxed into deep turf. Both horse and man breathed deep sighs upon outrunning the town's plucking panic, escaping into the windswept freedom of the fields that sloped away up the Tremount. Zabdiel had no particular destination in mind; he gave the horse his head, and soon they were cantering along a bridle path, a narrow ribbon of silver that seemed to lead straight into the stars.

Near the top of the tallest of the mountain's three peaks, the Beacon Hill that rose three hundred feet above Boston, Prince slowed to a satisfied walk, the lights of the sleeping town now twinkling far below. Beyond lay the infinite darkness of the sea murmuring to itself in sleep. With a satisfied whinny and a thorough shake of his mane, Prince stopped to graze in the summer-sweet grass.

Zabdiel leaned across his back. The horse smelled of fresh brown earth, newly turned and clean; all around them, June had draped the earth in green growth, the scents of wild roses, hawthorn, and budding apples. The air was warm and moist, rippling with mischievous winds from the sea.

He closed his eyes. There were only two paths off this mountain. One led to a familiar hell. He saw a small girl with Jerusha's eyes, digging a grave. He felt the heat and stretch of his own skin on fire. The other was a road that stretched into an unknown distance. Flickering through his mind he saw an august body of learned men in London, sensed the undulating beauty of Turkish harems. Heard the lilt of African voices, high and low, telling, again and again, the same story.

Heard again the suspicions that had wafted across his path in low whispers all day long: *It may be a plot. Why not? They are not so numerous as to be able to rise against us, as they do in Barbados, in Jamaica, aboard slave ships. But they are cunning. They will tempt us into killing ourselves. Our own children.*

He did not think there was a conspiracy. Too many upright, God-fearing people had told stories that were similar, yet not the same, not spread out regularly, easily, like bait. But brought out hodgepodge, jumbled. Some were the worn flotsam and jetsam of men and women stretching back to long-ago memories of a far-distant land. Some were newly broken shards, scooped up and waved with fierce pride, images of a home still clear in mind and desire, described in voices not yet accustomed to English or refusing ever to become accustomed to English.

In the west, the moon was setting, swollen and white like some vast celestial pock. Far in the east, a thin spear of gold lanced between sea and sky. Prince had been grazing steadily downward; Zabdiel now gathered the reins, spurring him on faster, down and south across the Common, skirting the town to their left, taking a hedge or two for the sheer pleasure of flight. The stallion was more than willing, his black mane and tail streaming behind the rich reddish brown of his body as he roused the winged creatures from their roosts, earth against air. Southward they sped, in among the sparse houses at the bottom of the South End. Then the houses drew apart again, and fields ran up to the road, their heels nipped by water on either side as the solid land funneled itself into the Neck. At its narrowest point, just forty yards wide, a high wall guarded all entry and exit to Boston. One gate for pedestrians, one tall enough for riders and wide enough for carriages. The porter had seen Dr. Boylston coming and had already opened the big gate, waving him through with a call for good luck. Assuming, no doubt, that he was off to some emergency.

Just beyond, as he passed the gibbet, Zabdiel wrinkled his nose at what was left of Joseph Hanno, the black man hanged a month earlier for murdering his wife. A few more minutes of cantering, though, and salt marshes stretched away on either side. Out here at dawn, the world was made mostly of lavender sky and towering castles of pink, orange, and gold. Out here, it did not seem possible that the world could hold such filth as smallpox.

The marshes were crisscrossed with a web of trails more or less solid at ebb tide. Zabdiel set Prince on a course for a sliver of beach beyond; as they raced still southward, hundreds upon thousands of ducks, geese, herons, and cranes filled the sky with wings, wheeling white, blue, dun, tan, emerald-green.

These birds migrated every spring, thousands of miles, from the steaming wetlands of the south toward the blue glowing icebergs of the north, and back in the fall. No one knew how. But human ignorance had never stopped it from happening.

At the sea's edge Zabdiel reined Prince in and faced east as the world caught fire. *Take knowledge where you find it,* he heard his father's voice say, though perhaps it was his own murmur. He tried to shake the thought off, but it grew wider and warmer, along with the day.

He could not try it on both of his boys. He would have to choose. John, highly intelligent and just as highly strung, already agitated to sleeplessness by tales of sick friends. Or Tommy, who certainly knew about the epidemic—he had seen a dying woman just yesterday—but who seemed not to know fear. Tommy, who wanted to be a doctor and would therefore have to get through the distemper someday, just as he once had. Tommy, who was, a very small voice whispered, his favorite, the one he would least like to risk.

The sun rose burning from the sea. He watched it for what might have been seconds, or might have been centuries. Then he turned Prince's head for home. They ran all the way, galloping through dawn, not bothering to slow up even for the clutter of town, scattering pigs from their wallows, irritating the roosters, unsettling the hens.

When Zabdiel walked into the kitchen, Jack was stirring porridge; he turned and stood there, just holding up a ladle like a steaming question mark.

"I can't try it on myself," said Zabdiel.

"No, sir," said Jack, understanding the apology offered in the doctor's voice.

"I'm going to try it on Tommy."

Jack nodded. "I hope you'll try it on me, too, then. And Jackey."

Zabdiel said nothing, but he felt a surge of relief, maybe even triumph: he had been right. There was no conspiracy.

Jack turned back to the pot hung over the fire. "Guess I can be as brave as you, Doctor." He began spooning breakfast into wooden bowls. "Just hope you'll be quick about it, before my mind has much of a chance to change." He set the bowls on the table, and wiped his hands on his apron. "Shop was locked up from the inside last night. I went around and opened it from the front while you was out. Now excuse me, while I go rouse those three slug-a-beds."

Zabdiel ducked down the passage and into the shop. The counter was spread with a clean white cloth; neatly lined up across it lay a small glass vial and stopper, a quill newly sharpened into a toothpick, and a lancet. Off to the right, by itself, lay a nutcracker.

There was a walnut in Zabdiel's right hand, a walnut that he had rolled this way and that all night like a Mohammedan worry bead.

*   *   *

John, Tommy, and Jackey pelted down the stairs to find Zabdiel already gone, which was disappointing. On the other hand, for no apparent reason their porridge was not only sweetened with sugar and thickened with new milk, but also studded with raisins and freshly cracked walnuts.

"Is it someone's birthday?" asked Tommy, plowing into it as soon as grace had been said.

"Always," said Jack. To John, he added, "You finish up, now, and head on back upstairs and pack a few things. Your uncle Tom'll be needing you to stay at his place for a few days."

Zabdiel rode off at a trot to a certain house that held everything he wanted: a young man progressing nicely through smallpox of the most distinct kind, the pocks having scattered themselves sparsely across him nine days since. This morning, they were plump and white.

The boy's mother was surprised at seeing Dr. Boylston so early: her boy was doing well, and she knew for a fact that others nearby needed him to ward off dying. However, no doubt the poor man wished to start the day with something easy and cheerful; her boy was just the thing. That thought made her cheerful herself, though she was a bit pressed for time, it being baking day and the oven not heating quite as evenly or quickly as one would wish. She sent the doctor up alone.

Zabdiel examined the boy's legs and chose a fine large pock. Explaining what he wanted, he pricked it near the base and gently pressed the matter out into his vial. It was fetid, but not rancid. The boy watched the whole operation with keen fascination.

When he was finished, Zabdiel stoppered the bottle and shoved it into a leather pouch that hung on a thong around his neck, tucking the whole inside his shirt to keep it warm.

Back at home, he forced himself through the ritual of changing clothes in the barn; he could not tell whether he was hurrying or moving in slow motion. Inside, Jack had explained to the boys that they were to have a small operation, like big boys. It would not hurt so much as bloodletting, but blood would come. It was practice for being a man.

Zabdiel did Tommy first; Tommy insisted. A little scoring of the skin on the outer arm, just above the elbow, a glossy red bead of blood welling up. A tiny bit of white matter drawn from the vial on the point of a quill. Only a little shaking of his hands, almost imperceptible. The two drops, red and white, swirled around till they were one. A curved bit of walnut laid over the scratch, bound up with clean white linen: keeping anything else from touching it, wiping it off, spreading it. But letting air circulate.

Zabdiel had Tommy lie down on his stomach a bench, and he did the same to the inside of one leg, up near the buttocks.

Next he operated on Jack. As he finished his arm, Jack scratched his head and said, "I been thinking. How'm I supposed to sit that cantankerous old mule if I got a rear full of smallpox?"

Zabdiel looked up from the lancet he was wiping clean and shook his head. "Maybe that mule's out in the barn thinking, *How'm I supposed to walk pretty under a cantankerous old man with a rear full of smallpox?*"

Jack blew a sigh of relief. "Suppose any other part will work?"

After a short consultation, they agreed upon the muscle that swept from his neck, across the shoulder blade, and into the back.

At last, it was Jackey's turn. He had screamed at the first scratch of Tommy's skin. By the time his father was done, though, he was so eager to be one of the big boys that the hard part was to get him to stop squirming with excitement.

It was all so prodigiously, preposterously easy.

"Now what?" asked Tommy, as if a few words of hocus pocus would suddenly produce a painless crop of spots.

"Now we wait," said Zabdiel.

Later that morning the light breeze off the water died away, leaving heat to settle heavily on the streets. Out in the harbor, the great guns of the *Seahorse* began to roar in slow, pompous succession.

Well into his rounds despite his late start, Zabdiel reined his horse, the big patient gelding called Exeter, to a stand and turned to face the sea. Everyone else in the street was doing the same. Earlier, the *Seahorse* had hauled herself up to the end of the Long Wharf to load her refurbished guns back on board; Captain Durell was wasting no time in testing them. No doubt he would justify the noise and the expense in powder by claiming to be celebrating some royal birthday or other. To Zabdiel and many of the Bostonians around him, though, it sounded like a preemptive funeral salute for a city, the reverberating footfalls of fast-approaching doom.

Behind Zabdiel, a ways up the hill, someone began shouting. He glanced over his shoulder and saw that the commotion centered on the gilt frippery of Dr. Douglass's carriage. It was an absurd vehicle that might have been at home in the boulevards of Paris or possibly the more palatial districts of London, but was sorely out of place in Boston, whose streets were as narrow and crooked as cow paths. The doctor had thrust half his body out the window and was griping at a couple of teamsters who had halted an ox-drawn dray in the road. Having pried open a trap door in the ground just outside a shop, they were stolidly proceeding to transfer their load of barrels and boxes from cart to cellar.

Unfortunately, the dray occupied half the street—at a squeeze—just at the point where someone had dug up the other half to lay a drain. Not knowing of the blockage ahead, traffic had gone on pouring into the street behind. The gunfire had then induced many to turn back halfway for a good look, so that in no time at all the road had become a thick jumble of carts and carriages facing every which way. For Dr. Douglass, there was now no going back, while there would be no going forward until the dray popped itself like a stopper from the bottleneck. For the foreseeable future, however, it appeared to be settled as firmly as a lump of solid cement.

"Make way," shouted Dr. Douglass. "Make way for a doctor!"

The teamsters, both the size of trolls, paid him as much mind as they might have given a gnat.

"Are you men or mutton?" shouted Dr. Douglass, waving his walking stick about in a fury. "Make way for a doctor!"

Zabdiel sighed. He did not care for the man, but he pitied his patients. No doubt someone had sent for him in a panic and was now anxiously awaiting his arrival. At this rate, though, they would not catch a glimpse of the doctor before dinner. Reluctantly, Zabdiel turned Exeter about and picked his way to the carriage. "I would be happy, sir," he said with a nod of greeting, "to give you a lift to your destination, if it would be of help."

A look of horror rippled across Dr. Douglass's face as he registered Boylston astride a tall horse. "Thank you," he said, bristling with all the hauteur he could muster. "But I must refuse. I do not mind telling you, sir, that my patient is a lady of some consequence." He returned Zabdiel's nod. "I make no doubt that she expects me to arrive in a style befitting her station. I cannot think that arriving pillion, like some flibbertigibbet maid out for a country ride with her beau, will quite answer."

A smile twitched at the corners of Zabdiel's mouth. "If she's as ill as you suggest," he said, "she'll surely find the speed of your arrival more to the point than the style of it."

Withdrawing into the coach and motioning Dr. Boylston to lean in, Dr. Douglass lowered his voice to a conspiratorial whisper. "I wouldna have yon oafs know it, sir, but her condition is not yet so acute as to justify dispensing with form. Nevertheless, she may present an intricate case," he added with pride, pulling out a handkerchief and mopping sweat from his face. "I make no doubt of being recommended most warmly to her acquaintance if I should satisfy: so you see, I must endeavor to satisfy in all particulars. Including appearance, which, as you know, is of great importance to the ladies." He shot out of the window to shout once again at the men ahead, and then he turned back to Zabdiel. "Have you had the good fortune to be called to a case of smallpox yet?"

"No—" began Zabdiel, intending to add that he had been called to something closer to twenty, but Dr. Douglass cut him off.

"Not a one, sir?" he cried with something like triumph. "I wish you may have better luck in upcoming days. A most fascinating distemper, sir. Most fascinating. And one must make hay while the sun shines, no?"

Down in the harbor, the last of the shots—fifteen, all told—faded away. "I have never thought to equate smallpox with sunshine," said Zabdiel quietly.

Far from registering his companion's distaste, Dr. Douglass positively gloated. *"Carpe diem,"* he cried, waving his walking stick about with excitement once again. *"Seize the day,* you know. It's no different for men with fortunes to make than for young maids with beauty to bargain, *n'est-ce pas?"* He cast a quick, sharp glance up at his companion. Craning forward conspiratorially, he said, "As long as we are thrown together in this morass, sir, may I take the opportunity to ask whether Dr. Mather has sent you one of his letters?"

"Yes—" began Zabdiel.

"Ah! Then may I count on you, sir, to join me and the other practitioners in this town in—shall we just say *quarantining?*—this bit of foolery to the oblivion it deserves?" His rumble of mirth at his clever choice of words faded as he registered the gravity on Boylston's face.

"No," said Zabdiel, shaking his head. "No, I am afraid you may not."

"Surely, sir," said Dr. Douglass, quite aghast, "you cannot be considering undertaking the practice?"

"No," answered Zabdiel. "I have already performed it."

An odd noise escaped Dr. Douglass's throat as mirth, triumph, and relief were all knocked to the ground in a hard little rain of surprise. *"Already—"* he croaked. *"When—?"*

"This morning," said Zabdiel. "On my youngest son and two slaves."

Dr. Douglass swept the pieces of his dignity into a glowering mass of disapproval. "You are aware, sir," he said darkly, "that as a medical doctor I cannot recommend or support this practice?"

"I am now," said Zabdiel. "Luckily, I was not counting on either." He did not want to hear doubt, not now, not even from such a predictably sourpuss source as Dr. Douglass.

But Dr. Douglass was beyond voicing doubt, or anything else. His mouth was opening and closing in silence. *Curious,* thought Zabdiel, *how periwigs make some men's faces expand toward greatness, while others seem to shrivel until they resemble nothing so much as a South Sea Islander's shrunken fetish*. Beneath his borrowed mane, Dr. Douglass began to shake with what was presumably rage. If he were an Islander, wondered Zabdiel, would he feel obliged to dance about in some kind of savage idolatry, to appease him?

Zabdiel pulled himself out of his reverie. He must get away, he realized, before either of them said something they would both regret. "You are sure, sir, I may not give you a lift?"

Douglass was still too shocked to provide any answer beyond a vigorously negative shake of the head.

"Then I must bid you good day and good luck, sir, and head off to my own patients." Zabdiel set his horse into motion, threading through the tangle of carriages and carts. The dray, he saw, had not moved an inch. As they reached the ditch, Exeter took it in stride, leaping it with ease. After winding through the equally dense thicket of vehicles on the opposite side, they were soon trotting away through streets that were clear, save for a thick shimmer of heat.

By nightfall, the entire town knew that Dr. Boylston had given smallpox to his own flesh and blood—*on purpose*—and as if that weren't enough, to two black slaves as well. The boy whose pock Zabdiel had pressed talked to his mother; she talked to everyone she could find. Dr. Douglass also let the news slip once or twice, in well chosen houses. *No better than murder,* sniffed one of his more excitable old gossips; she had ample opportunity that day to practice her tone of outrage and offended motherliness, tweaking it to perfection.

The next day, Zabdiel began to sense whispers, silences, averted eyes, but he told himself he was imagining things. He managed to believe it, too, until the first door shut in his face. At the next house, though, he got a hearty slap on the back, and a request to try it on a child or two there. If it should succeed on Tommy, that is.

The word went on sputtering, flickering, flaring through town, sometimes burrowing to hushed bass depths, sometimes accompanied by gale-force gasps and shrieks that would do banshees proud. Nervous giggles. Blanched horror. For four days, the glares thickened around him as he rode about his business; Jack, who felt entirely well, still rode out with Zabdiel, but he began drawing his mule as close as possible behind. At home, Zabdiel changed all their dressings, two each, morning and evening: they had flamed red by the end of the first day; after that they looked as if they might go on holding that same angry shape until the Day of Judgment.

On the fifth day, another wave of eruptions began to appear around town; this time the sick numbered in the hundreds. Castle William, too, was infected. Men had been deserting in hordes, it seemed, for a week. In the streets, the glares following Zabdiel thickened to hatred. The whispers hardened to muttering, exploding here and there into jeers, as if he might be to blame for the spread of the disease.

G.D., wrote Cotton Mather in his diary, *the Affair of preventing the Small-Pox, in the way of Inoculation, is begun, and has raised an horrid Clamour, which Occasions new Cares upon me.*

On the sixth day from inoculation, the first of July, Tommy, Jack, and Jackey all grew feverish, their skin a little warm to the touch. Zabdiel insisted that Jack stay home with the boys. That evening, a jeer broke loose from a huddle of men, and then another, and then a stone skimmed across the street, not quite at him, but too close for comfort. Zabdiel's horse shied. He said nothing, however, just rode on as if nothing more untoward than the sudden flap of a bird had startled his mount.

All three of his patients at home were a little restive and feverish that night, on into the next morning. That day, more doors shut in his face. Early on, one or two women begged him, quietly, to return later, after their husbands were out. In broad daylight, one or two more whispered for him to come back after dark, when the neighbors would not see. As he rode home that evening, someone spat, hitting him square on the cheek. Zabdiel shook out a handkerchief and wiped the spittle away, looking straight ahead.

At home, he found that Jack's fever had dissolved, and the sores on his neck and arm were drying up. "Are you sure you haven't had the small-pox?" asked Zabdiel.

"Don't remember," said Jack.

"You've had it," said Zabdiel.

Jackey and Tommy, though, remained feverish; their incisions had blossomed, so that each showed a red halo burning around a single large pock.

The next morning—the eighth day, July 3—Jackey's fever limped on as before. Tommy, however, began twitching and tossing in his sleep, his skin papery and burning to the touch, the fever creeping ever higher. With a heavy heart, Zabdiel left the house on his rounds. The air, too, was feverish, hot and moist, pressing like a headache against his temples.

Jack rode out with him again; this time, Zabdiel did not complain. When Jack drew up alongside on his mule, unbidden, neither man remarked upon it, but they both felt safer that way. That afternoon, crowds began to jostle around their mounts; Prince reared and flailed out with his hooves, scattering the crowd. Zabdiel stared the crowd down, and then said one word under his breath to Jack: *"Home."*

It was just as well. No, it was a godsend. For Tommy lay in a wet heap on the kitchen floor, his fever so high Zabdiel thought he could fairly see steam rise from his son's skin. Jackey was sitting next to him, petting him and singing a wandering little lullaby.

"What happened?" Jack asked his son.

"He was hot," whispered Jackey. "He went out and stood under the pump. Then he came back in and went to sleep."

Jack built up the fire, while Zabdiel stripped his son and toweled him dry. Tommy muttered and twitched, but did not wake, even when Zabdiel lifted him in his arms and carried him upstairs. He was already soaked with sweat by the time Zabdiel could lay him on the big bed. His and Jerusha's bed. He tried not to think of Jerusha. Of the face she would turn to him if she were to walk in this instant. Jack brought up a bucket of cool water and some cloths.

Zabdiel sat up late into the night, laying cool cloths on Tommy's head and feet, while the boy shivered and mumbled, struggling against the darkness. On his arm, the large pock in the middle of the incision had exploded into an open sore two and a half inches across. Green and yellow rottenness dripped at its heart, while the red ring had stretched huge, its perimeter thick with tiny pocks.

Faint and far away, he thought he heard a commotion. "Doctor," said Jack from the passage, "I think you had better come into the parlor."

He had made up a cot there for Jackey, within calling distance from Zabdiel. Jackey was fitful and hot, too, but not dangerously so. His arm looked just like Tommy's.

It was not Jackey or his arm that Jack had called him to see, however. The light in the parlor was a strange glowering orange, and the noise seemed louder here. Was louder—was a roar of voices shouting. A bang rattled the window glass, and Zabdiel instinctively stepped back. A splatter of filth dripped down the glass. Then came another and another, until the front walls and windows reverberated as if under siege.

In the back room, Tommy moaned; just behind them, Jackey cried out.

Zabdiel strode across the room in three steps and threw open the window. A shriek rose, hung before him, and died away. Zabdiel stood gazing at the mob below. A crowd of men unsteady on their feet. Others still solid in their rage, but flickering like ghouls beneath their torches. A few women; one of them screamed, *"Murderer."* "House of filth," shouted a lower voice. And in the front, in the middle, stood a large man he did not recognize, silent, square on bowed sailor's legs, swinging a rope. *"Negro lover,"* he said in a voice that needed no shout to carry.

Zabdiel let his eyes roam the entire crowd, till he held every last ounce of attention. "There are sick children up here," he said in the voice that could seize women out of hysterics, pull men back from the brink of panic, send children and animals hurtling safely out of harm's way.

"*Murderer!*" the woman screamed again.

He found her face, her jaw still hanging open from the cry, and pinned her beneath his gaze until she closed her mouth. "Sleeping," he said firmly. "Not dead." *If they die*, he thought, *you can have me. But not until then.* "They need quiet."

The mob shifted sullenly, muttering. Under his stare, they went silent, though they did not go away, standing like sentries of wrath in the street. "Thank you," he said. "And good night to you all." He shut the window and turned back into the room.

To be two and a half thought Zabdiel glancing at Jackey, *and sleep through a riot.*

Jack, for his part, was watching the doctor. "Come on," he said, heading back into the bedroom and stepping up to the bed, taking Zabdiel's place wetting cloths and laying them across Tommy. The boy was sweating, shivering, and muttering on the bed, stripped save for the bottom sheet.

"Sit," said Jack. Zabdiel dropped into the chair by the bed and took hold of the tankard filled with a cool draft of small beer, which Jack had set on the nightstand.

"Yesterday," said Jack, wringing out a towel, "Lieutenant Hamilton of the *Seahorse* bought himself a new servant and named him Cotton Mather: in honor, he said, of Dr. Mather's fine trust in men with black skins, black hearts, and blacker magic."

"Christ Almighty," said Zabdiel into his tankard.

"They're scared," said Jack, turning back to Tommy.

"Everyone with an ounce of sense in this whole damned town is scared," said Zabdiel. "Strange excuse for a killing spree."

"Oldest excuse in the world," shrugged Jack. "Oldest and strongest. What do you reckon we do now?"

Zabdiel shook his head, and looked up at Jack. "Now we wait," he said blankly. After a while, Jack tiptoed back out of the room.

The pages of Dr. Mather's treatise lay, already dog eared, on the table by the bed; Zabdiel had long since committed it to memory, the writing burned into his brains with letters of fire. There was no hidden word of comfort to be unearthed there. He picked up the Bible that lay next to the treatise. The cadences of this book were as deeply rooted in his soul as the voice of his mother singing, or the gaits of the horses he had ridden with his father long before he could walk. His fingers drew the book open to a chapter in Genesis.

Take thy son, thine only son Isaac, whom thou lovest, God had once tempted Abraham, *and offer him for a burnt offering.* So his son and two servants went up to the mountain with him. At its feet, the two servants halted, while Abraham and Isaac toiled into the heights. Side by side, father and son built an altar and collected wood. Then, without warning, Abraham bound Isaac and laid him on the altar as the sacrifice.

Zabdiel did not need to read on to know what came next, but he ran his eyes over the words anyway. *And Abraham stretched forth his hand, and took the knife to slay his son. And the angel of the Lord called unto him out of heaven, and said, Abraham, Abraham: and he said, Here am I. And the angel said, Lay not thine hand upon the lad.*

No voice, thought Zabdiel wearily, had called out to him. Mather sensed angels everywhere, incessantly. Zabdiel had scoffed at him for it, in his heart. Perhaps he should have been listening instead. Perhaps he should have shouted at the heavens, *Here I am.*

But he had said nothing, had heard nothing. His knife had come down.

Another sentence, about another father and son, drifted up from far later pages, twisting slowly through his mind: *Father, if thou be willing, take this cup away from me.*

He slid onto his knees by the bed.

Please, Lord, be willing.

PART THREE

Hell Upon Earth

⇥ 1 ⇤

SALUTATION ALLEY

ZABDIEL startled awake. In the dull gray heat of dawn he lay curled on the edge of his bed, one arm flung over his son. Tommy was shivering and muttering incoherently in his sleep, still dangerously hot.

Zabdiel leapt from the bed; in two bounds he landed in the stair passage and called to Jack, who was there in half an instant.

"Jackey?" he said hoarsely.

"Fever broke in the night," said Jack. "He's fine."

"Good," nodded Zabdiel, though his heart squeezed into an even smaller ball and plummeted toward the center of the earth. "Watch Tommy," he said, and ran barefoot down the stairs, skidding through into the shop. At the shelves holding his drugs, he paused a little wild eyed, scanning the long ranks of jars and canisters. *What was good for the boy?* He needed something to drive out the poison, to send it flowing out into his skin, where it might escape; as it was, it was festering within, feeding on his vital spirits.

A vomit. He needed a vomit. There wasn't anything worth worrying about left in his stomach: but the emetic action would work on the boy's pores too. Nothing too strong—not now. Usually Zabdiel preferred antimonial vomits, but after three days of broiling in his own juices Tommy was far too weak. He'd have to make do with a gentler vegetable concoction. *Ipecacuanha.* He pulled down the jar and mixed up a light dose in some oil. He also concocted a cooling draft to fight the fever: two ounces of sweet almond oil and two ounces of the syrup of marsh mallows, shaken together.

With a vial in each hand, he raced back up the stairs. Jack offered to dose the boy, but Zabdiel shook his head and Jack tiptoed away again. Zabdiel sat down on the side of the bed and with infinite gentleness began spooning the vomit into his son's mouth. Then he held Tommy over a bowl as he retched. When he stopped, Zabdiel wiped the spittle away and fed him a few spoonfuls of the cooling oil, but Tommy shuddered, puckering his face and turning away. Surely that was a good sign that he had not drifted too far away from consciousness or life?

Zabdiel sat on the edge of the bed, holding his son's small hand. Twenty minutes later, he thought Tommy might be shivering less. Maybe, just maybe, he wasn't as hot. He would not believe it yet, though, not until he was sure. He sat rigid, counting his own heartbeats, wishing them to go by faster. An hour later, he called softly to Jack.

Jack laid a big calloused hand on Tommy's forehead, and then he broke into a wide grin. "Fever's passing," he said. "He's going to pull through." He turned his eyes on Zabdiel. "But I ain't so sure about you, Doctor. You go on and get some sleep now. Let me watch the boys."

"Jackey?" asked Zabdiel once again. His tongue felt thick.

"Jackey'll be right as rain, soon as those spots come out, and so will Mr. Tommy here. Cot's right over there." He nodded.

Zabdiel stood up unsteadily and crossed to the window, laying his cheek against its coolness. In the paddock below, two foals frisked about, watched by their dams. *Thank you*, he whispered. Jack collared him where he stood, propelling him to the cot, or he might have fallen asleep standing up. *Fallen right out the window, if it'd been open*, thought Jack.

Later—much later, to judge by the light and the heat that had filled the room—Zabdiel woke to a shout of triumph; he blinked and sat up with a start. "Spots!" shouted Tommy, waving one arm about. "Papa, I have spots!"

Zabdiel strode to the bed. Tommy did indeed have small red speckles, about five that he could see and ten or fifteen more he could not. Zabdiel plucked his son out of the bed, whirling and stamping, whooping and hollering, with glee.

Tossing Tommy on his shoulder, he ducked across the hall. Jackey, too, was sprouting bumps, only on Jackey they were not bright red, they were an even deeper black than his dark skin. Zabdiel and Tommy whooped and whirled away again. After a split second, Jack caught up to Jackey and joined in the dance.

A few minutes later, the Reverend Benjamin Colman walked out of his house with a heavy heart, ready to keep vigil at a child's deathbed; the news had slithered into his study at first light, in the whispering of servants. Not that it was anything like a secret. As he emerged from his own door, he saw a knot of people gathered around Boylston's house, gesticulating and pointing. He quickened his step, and the crowd parted silently to let him through.

It sounded as if Indians were celebrating a massacre upstairs. He was obliged, in the end, to loose the clarion call of his pulpit voice to rouse a servant through the commotion. Neither the wild-Indian dancing nor the laughter faltered as he mounted the stairs behind Jack. Of course, it was proper to coax even the smallest child into calm prayer just before the end. But in Reverend Colman's experience, if a dying child asked for it, the most sober man in the world would turn somersaults and quack like a duck. So it was not the father who made the minister's brows float upward in surprise. It was the boy himself.

Perched on his father's shoulders and hollering, Tommy looked tired, a little washed out and peaky, but not remotely in danger of dying. "I've got spots," he shrieked as he caught sight of the minister's head rising through the gloom that pooled in the hollows of the still-shuttered ground floor.

"So you do," said his father, glancing back to see whom his son was shouting at. Seeing the minister, Zabdiel stilled his feet a little sheepishly, but he made no move to put Tommy down. "So you do. But you must also have some manners. Give Reverend Colman a proper greeting now." He tried to look stern, but the twinkle in his eyes refused to cooperate.

"How d'ye do, Reverend," said Tommy, slightly lowering his voice. "If you please, sir, I have spots." He thrust out an arm for inspection. "So does Jackey." Jackey's arm shot out too.

The Reverend Mr. Colman duly peered at the proffered arms. "Hurray!" he cried. "Hurray for a fine crop of spots!"

Tommy's laughter rose to gale force, and the dance took hold of them all—this time including the minister—once more.

Hurray for a little boy's life, thought the Reverend Mr. Colman in midspin. Tall and fine boned, with fair hair and blue eyes, he was something of a renegade among Puritan ministers: the very soul of moderation, a champion of tolerance, he was so elegant as to be swooningly popular with the ladies. He was also endowed with almost unnatural powers of sympathy. Swept up in the unseemly dance, he was still aware of the crowd gathered in silence outside, aware that Tommy's survival had repercussions far beyond the scope of his doting family. Furthermore, he was aware of Dr. Boylston keeping the same knowledge at bay; right now, the man wanted to think only of his son.

Let him, thought Mr. Colman. *There's time enough for the troubles ahead.*

Almost as one, they slowed and stopped, for they were all exhausted. The two boys were deposited on the big bed, the men standing before them with bowed heads, still breathing hard as Mr. Colman led them all in a psalm: *O Give thanks unto the Lord, for he is good: for his mercy endureth forever.*

Zabdiel tried to focus; Jerusha would want this prayer said well, from the heart, but he wasn't ready for the certainty that thanksgiving implied. With his body at rest, his mind wandered. They had reached an oasis where they would be granted a three-day rest, that was all. They were not yet out of danger, much less home. If Tommy's rash grew as thick as his fever had been high, he would die, and the dying would be terrible. *The Lord is my shepherd* . . . he whispered, clinging to hope.

That evening, after Tommy, still blessedly cool, dropped into a profound, healing sleep, Zabdiel took himself off to the Salutation Inn for a pint. It was a squally evening, splattered with fat drops of rain that many a night would have convinced him to stay home, epidemic or not. But tonight he needed quiet celebration in the company of friends. So he set off north toward the tavern, hoping that his friend Joshua Cheever would be there.

His gelding's hooves clopped over the drawbridge across the creek that sheered the North End from the rest of Boston. From there, Ship Street wound northeast in tight little curves, clinging to the wharves bristling along the eastern shore. Across the street from the sea clustered the taverns that balanced the city's Puritan zeal with more worldly cheer. At Cross Street he passed under the dripping sign of the Red Cross, and then past the Three Crowns, the Turkey-Cock, and the Red Lion. The steeple of the Old North Church loomed into sight a little off to the left and lumbered on by. To the right, Clark's wharf, the grandest of Boston's private wharves, jutted out of sight into the sea. The Mitre, the King's Arms, the Castle, and then the Ship, better known as Noah's Ark, lumbered by in the dark, and then just beyond Scarlett's Wharf, up on the left, the long, low two-story expanse of the Salutation Inn slid into view, its thirty-five windows gleaming in welcome. The familiar sign creaked and swayed in the wind: two men bowing low to each other in ostentatious greeting, sweeping their cocked hats before them. The Two Palaverers, its patrons affectionately called the place.

Zabdiel handed his horse to the stable boy and stomped up onto the porch, shaking off some of the rain, hoping Cheever was there to palaver with.

He was. Tall and fair as a Viking, Mr. Cheever was stretching his long legs before a summer-bare grate and chatting with John Langdon, the butcher and victualler who'd bought the inn fifteen years before as an outlet for his cooking and had since made it famous for solid, homely fare—

New England boiled dinners, juicy roasts served with bright peas and nicely brown Yorkshire pudding to sop up the drippings, chicken pot pies. Langdon was almost as tall as Cheever, and almost as wide as he was tall. The jolly giant, they called him.

As Zabdiel walked in, Cheever looked up, and the question flashed wordlessly in his eyes. *Is he alive?* Zabdiel's whole body must have answered for him, for Cheever leapt to his feet and gave him a slap on the back that nearly knocked Zabdiel's lungs back into the street.

Langdon called for beer all around, and soon a knot of Salutation regulars had gathered to hear the news: Langdon sons and sons-in-law, their neighbors Bill Larrabee and John Helyer from down the street, various Thorntons and Greenwoods, and several Webbs, the clan of brewers and distillers who filled the inn's barrels and kegs. Even Joseph Dodge, the sour little publican who'd recently bought the inn's liquor license, lingered to listen after handing out the last tankard.

Zabdiel had married into the Minot clan of Dock Square, fast rising into the mincing ways of the gentry; for Jerusha's sake, and for the sake of his business, he kept his shop and his home at the center of town. But it was here, at the far northern end of the North End, where he made his friends. These were men who built ships and houses, who manhandled hundredweight bags of flour into bread, or hops into beer. Men who beat iron into anchors, crafted hides into shoes and slats into barrels, men who fired sand into glass windows and wax into candles. They were close knit, proud, and deeply devout, but they were also, at times, deeply devoted to downing their fair share of pints among friends. *Hard work and hard praying merits hard playing*, they joked among themselves. Zabdiel didn't pray as hard as most of them, but he figured he made up for it in working. Especially lately.

Recounting the battle for his son's life made the events of the last week begin to seem real. As Zabdiel finished, his companions touched off a burst of congratulations and questions, shot through with praise, both of Boylston and the Lord, and quick prayers for continued success. Sensing his exhaustion, though, the men soon trickled off, leaving Boylston and Cheever to work their way through tankards of ale and pipes full of tobacco in comfortable silence.

It was then that George Stewart ducked in to escape the rain, calling for a private room upstairs. He passed them by with no more than a quick nod, but a few steps on he slowed and stopped. He turned back, a quick flash of surprise replaced with oily solemnity, and then he swept off his hat and bowed to Zabdiel. "May I offer my condolences?"

Zabdiel's eyes widened and his face grew flat as it always did when he tried to squelch laughter. "Very kind"—he nodded—"but I'd rather you kept them till I have something to condole about."

Cheever groaned inwardly. Dr. Stewart was a Scot, another surgeon who'd arrived in town a few years back and in very short order had married the daughter of Zabdiel's old mentor, Dr. John Cutler. When Dr. Cutler had died four years ago, Stewart had been none too pleased to find that most of the man's rather considerable regular practice had drifted to his eldest son, John junior, or to Zabdiel. Since Stewart had to maintain familial bonhomie with John junior, he'd channeled his growling disappointment toward Zabdiel—who made it all the worse by regarding the whole matter with detached amusement. Especially the Scottish growling. Zabdiel could rarely restrain himself from baiting the man. *He's like a snapping turtle*, he'd once said to Cheever. *He and Dr. Douglass. Endlessly fascinating to see what they'll snap at next.* So long as it ain't the nose on your face, Cheever had observed.

"I heard your laddie was at death's door," Dr. Stewart was saying with a frown.

"Try not to look disappointed, man," roared Cheever, coming out of his reverie. "It's a boy's life you're moping about."

Zabdiel waved him off. "His fever was high, far higher than I expected," he said to Stewart. "I'll admit that. But it's gone off, and he looks to do very well now."

"From what I hear," said Stewart, "you stirred up a right bourach such as set your street all tapsal-teerie into the wee hours last night." He sniffed. "A brave experiment, no doubt, if a bit hasty. Glad to hear it's not been a total hash."

"Far from it," said Zabdiel gravely. "I'm still hoping it will prove a total success."

There was a brief silence. Stewart did, in fact, have a long, leathery turtle's neck and a mouth that sloped down in a point like a beak. He blinked. "You can't mean you're thinking of proceeding?"

Zabdiel tossed his arms wide. "Why not? We might save hundreds, even thousands, of lives." He said it to annoy Stewart, but suddenly all three of them sensed a strange future glimmering there between them.

Stewart shook the vision off first, drawing himself into a prim punctuation mark of disapproval. "Let me be the first to wish you equal luck with regard to the secondary fever," he said with a curt nod, and stalked away.

"Ghoul," said Cheever. "You'd think he wished Tommy dead."

"I think he wishes me—the whole inoculation experiment—to fail," said Zabdiel, looking thoughtfully in the direction he had gone. "And he isn't alone."

Cheever gave him a sharp look. "Has it been bad?"

Zabdiel pulled the pipe from his mouth, and shot his friend a wry grin. "You heard the man: a right tapsal-teerie bourach." He blew a smoke ring toward the ceiling. "Which translates, close as I can tell, to nearly having the house burned down around me."

"Rough night, eh?"

Zabdiel stared into the depths of the fireplace, feeling the warmth drain away. "I almost lost him, Joshua." He turned a haggard face his friend. "You should take Sarah and get out of town."

But Cheever shook his head. "She won't go without me, and I can't leave the shop. Don't have anyone to leave it to. Besides, we don't have children to worry about."

Zabdiel nodded. It must make a difference. It must make all the difference.

"You really mean to try it on others?"

"I don't know," said Zabdiel. "Mostly I just wanted to irritate George." Cheever caught his eye, and he grew serious. "I'm waiting to see how Tommy and Jackey do, before I even think about anything else. Stewart's a gloomy old tortoise, but he's right about the secondary fever. It's the one that kills."

Cheever shifted in his chair. "Tommy's tough," he said.

"He is," nodded Zabdiel. They returned to their beer and smoking in silence.

Across the next three days, the rash sowed itself quickly and lightly across both boys: they had about a hundred bumps each, not counting the tiny pocks that clustered around their incisions. To be sure, it was far more than the ten or twenty pocks that Timonius estimated, but still exponentially fewer than what he and Jack saw day by day in sickrooms all over town: a thousand or even fifteen hundred pocks crowding onto one small body were not uncommon. And those were the patients whose pocks remained distinct enough to count.

Within the first twenty-four hours, the boys' bumps had ballooned into blisters filled with a clear, viscous liquid that clouded to a dull, turgid gray across the next two days. Both their fevers disappeared. The blisters didn't hurt, but they were growing a little itchy. Zabdiel put Tommy in charge of keeping Jackey from scratching himself, arming them with a little calamine lotion and the advice to keep each other busy. Then he and Jack returned to spending all day, dawn to dusk, away from home, running between houses where death was pounding at the door. They returned that first night to find their own transformed into a ship. Briefly, Zabdiel wondered what Jerusha would make of her best sheets rigged as sails, but then he fig-ured that if it would make Tommy scud through the smallpox with ease, she'd rig them herself.

He told himself that he should write to her, but decided against it: not yet. He could not bring himself to put paper to pen until he should know what he would have to tell her.

Meanwhile, a few irregular blocks to the north, Dr. Mather went on weep-ing and prostrating himself in the dust, begging the Lord to spare the lives of his two children. Out in the streets, the clamor receded; the crowds withdrew to a watchful, muttering distance.

For the most part, the doors that were going to close against Zabdiel had already closed. Oddly enough, others began to open. People he had never spoken to before began hailing him in the street, curious for minute-by-minute appraisals of the boys' progress.

For a while, he was happy to give it. Few in number and strangely small, the pocks sat lightly on the top of the skin—more like chicken pox than the deep-set pustules of smallpox. Also, they went on ripening at double speed. As the boys rounded into only the fourth day of the rash, the blisters were already beginning the critical process of congealing into pustules. Zabdiel subsided into tense, prickling quiet. It was toward the end of this third stage, as the pustules matured, that the secondary fever would blow its hot breath through Tommy and Jackey, if it were going to come.

Day crept by day with agonizing slowness but no hint of a fever, though Zabdiel sensed it hovering like a hurricane just beyond the horizon. Scat-tered like seed pearls across the boys' skin, the pocks grew plump. They were perfect, thought Zabdiel: robust enough to hold the poison at the outer rim of their bodies, but not so big that they'd pop like hot corn, leav-ing patches of ragged skin and oozing filth behind.

The next morning, just five days since the first appearance of the rash, the boys' pocks began to crust over, transforming from pustules to brown scabs without ever bursting. Gingerly, Zabdiel began exhaling the fear he had stored up inside him.

His attention began returning to other matters. As countless people in-formed him in urgent undertones, the *Boston News-Letter* had devoted al-most the entire issue of July 10 to "pestilential contagion" and the correct methods of preventing it. Anxiety eddied in the streets all day long, but Zabdiel could not pause to read it until he rode home for dinner. In the kitchen with Jack, he took it up, and very nearly tossed it down again in dis-gust. For the paper failed to point out that the pestilence discussed by Dr. Mead in the treatise it reprinted with such dire flourish was not smallpox.

It was plague of the blackest bubonic sort, then ravaging Marseilles and the whole southern coast of France, and it had ignited panic—and a fair amount of latent Francophobia—all across Europe and England. Apparently Mr. John Campbell was keen to strike similar sparks in New England.

"Keen to sell his paper's more like it," said Jack, stomping here and there around the room, swatting at specks of dust with a towel. "Put fear of plague in, get twopence out. I bet he's sold two, three times the number of papers he usually sells."

Zabdiel's mind was headed in other directions. *Who had given Mr. Campbell this treatise in the first place?* he mused as he mounted the stairs toward bed. It was too detailed to have come from a dispatch. And far too technically medical in parts to have come from Campbell's own library. Zabdiel wondered briefly, and then he lay back and fell deep asleep.

Early the next morning, as Captain Durell paraded down the Long Wharf toward his ship, he was hailed—most irregularly—by one of the Seahorses. Captain Paxton's Indian man. At least he bowed and scraped obsequiously, acknowledging his temerity. Unfortunately, he was also holding out a paper. Two papers.

Two very disagreeable papers, the captain saw as he took them. One was a note from that coxcomb of an ex-captain Paxton, requesting—though the tone was insufferably more like demanding—the release of his slave. The other was a discharge, complete but for Durell's signature.

"So you're begging off, are you, Hector?" he said.

"The captain's request, sir," said Hector in his soft, vaguely singsong voice. "I just saw Master Charles off at the ship, though," he added. "Captain says, I was taking his place and now I'm to go back and serve at the house."

The way the man referred to Paxton as "the" captain irritated Durell. In any case, he did not recall that those were the terms of the agreement; he did recall—it hung on his mind from sunup to sundown—that his ship appeared once again to be hemorrhaging men. He sniffed. Hector was a crack seaman, while young Paxton was no more than a raw boy. It did not even approach a fair exchange. As Captain Paxton had no doubt counted on, however, there was no time now to wrangle. Durell could force the man back aboard, clapping him in irons until they were safely far enough at sea that there was no hope of escape. But Boston was HMS *Seahorse's* home port, and it had been brought home to Captain Durell quite firmly in recent weeks that he needed the town's goodwill. He signed the man's discharge, shoved it at him, and stomped on his way.

He would never have signed it, had he reached the ship first. Another man had died the night before, which Lieutenant Hamilton had wisely kept as quiet as the fact that he had been sick in the first place; Captain Durell agreed that they should go on keeping it quiet until they had reached a proper deep to which they might commit him. That was only a minor irritation, though; the major problem was that the desertion rate was far worse than even his worst projections. Another twenty men had failed to show up this morning. Neither the press crew nor volunteers— few and far between, and heavily pockmarked—had even begun to make up the losses. Word must have oozed out that she was a coffin ship with a demon perched on her prow, digging cruel claws into the neck of the figurehead mare—*You can see the marks for yourself, mate*—his tail flicking spotted death behind him.

Durell swatted a sailor out of his way. "Take that man's name," he barked to Lieutenant Hamilton, who'd see that the bosun meted out some fit punishment for disturbing the captain. *Disturbed* was an understatement of ludicrous proportion, thought Durell. After deaths, discharges, and previously acknowledged runs, his ship was left a crew of only ninety-three, and that was counting himself. Barely enough men to sail the ship, much less fight her. For a while, he had the ship linger, but when the tide would wait no longer, HMS *Seahorse* slipped her moorings and set sail twenty-odd men too light.

Captain Durell sighed as she tacked clumsily out of the harbor. If it weren't for the matter of his wife, whom he was leaving behind eight months pregnant, he'd have been relieved to be free, for a while, of blasted Boston: her intrigue, her finger pointing, her groveling weakness in the face of the smallpox. He had no respect for weakness.

In the Boylston household, the dreaded fever played coy. The boys' incisions, however, were another story. They grew, even as the pocks shriveled into hard little brown discs imbedded in the skin.

"Good thing I took it in the neck," said Jack, looking at the green-and-yellow dripping sore, clustered with small pocks, that now covered his son's upper leg. Not that it would have mattered, on himself. His own incisions had dried up and healed over a week ago, leaving nothing but guilt behind. "That'd make for one sore seat in the saddle, Jackey boy." He whistled, squelching the question he really wanted to ask—*They going to spread till the whole arm and leg rot off?*

"It must be where the body is venting the poison," reasoned Zabdiel. "At least, I hope that's the case."

That was good enough for Jack. It had to be.

On the twelfth, Zabdiel and Jack came home to dinner to find both boys shedding their scabs like pennies tossed at a wedding. Zabdiel thought he had never seen such a beautiful sight in his life. The fever still had not showed; now it likely never would. One more time, they sank to their knees, but this time Zabdiel had no trouble with his prayers. He would not declare victory, he told himself, for another two or three days: the incisions were still bubbling with fresh pocks.

Hope was becoming harder to hold down, though. So hard that right after the last amen, he let out a mighty yell. Instead of a bedtime story that night, a full-blown game of pirates raged through the house, with Zabdiel leading the way as a wily captain sailing through seas boiling with leviathans and giant squid that hoarded treasure like deep-sea dragons. Armed with a pot and tongs, Jack was brewing up a magnificent storm just reaching gale force when they became aware of a thunderous noise not of their own making. Someone was pounding on the front door.

The game dissolved into silence.

Zabdiel slipped downstairs into the front hall, where he picked up a cudgel, hefting it twice, and stepped toward the trembling door.

"Who is it?" he called, but whoever it was had no chance to hear over his own rhythmic pounding. Dogs were barking all over the neighborhood, and a rooster or two had begun to crow.

Zabdiel raised his cudgel overhead and slowly unhitched the latch.

Torchlight flickered on the stoop just outside, but he could see only one figure in its angry glow, so methodically hammering away that he did not realize the door had opened until the next thump sent it crashing into the wall.

It was Joshua Cheever. "It's Sarah," he said hoarsely.

Zabdiel took the torch from his hand and doused it, seizing his friend by one sleeve and dragging him inside, pulling the door shut behind him. "What's wrong?" he asked quietly.

Cheever slumped into a chair. "Fever. Vomiting. Jabbing headache and backache. . . ."

The smallpox, shrilled a mean little voice in both their minds.

"I should've taken her away," said Cheever dully.

"Let me get my things."

"Things," repeated Cheever, as if it was a new word he had to think about. He nodded, but as Zabdiel turned away, he leaned forward and snatched at his coat. "For the love of God, make it quick."

They rode hard up to Cheever's home off Salutation Alley, the narrow lane trailing west from the inn, where many of their friends had built snug homes set in neat gardens. After a brief examination, Zabdiel stepped out of the sickroom. Cheever leapt to his feet. "How is she?"

Zabdiel shook his head. "I won't feed you false hope, Joshua. The fever is a bad one: not the purples, but I can't guarantee it won't go that way. I don't like her flush."

Cheever turned abruptly to look out the window at a tall row of hollyhocks edged with Queen Anne's lace. Not easy to grow so close to the salt winds off the sea, but Sarah could coax anything into bloom. "When will you know?"

"Not for a day or two. Even then," Zabdiel went on as gently as possible, "we won't really know what we're dealing with until the rash comes out." He cleared his throat and said the hardest thing of all. "You should leave, Joshua. Tonight. Jack and I'll move her to my house and care for her."

Cheever stared out the window in silence. "What are my chances, if I stay with her?"

Zabdiel just shook his head.

Cheever caught his reflection in the glass. "Inoculate me," he said quietly.

Zabdiel frowned. He must be hearing things.

Cheever turned. "Inoculate me," he said again, more forcefully.

"No."

Cheever crossed his arms. "You said yourself that it could save hundreds or even thousands of lives."

"It could kill that many too," retorted Zabdiel. He took a step back. "It came a lot closer to killing Tommy than I like to think about. I'm not trying it again until I'm sure it works. Or at least, until I'm damned sure it isn't going to kill."

"When will that be?"

Zabdiel had no idea, but he did know that at the moment Cheever could not stomach such hazy truth. "Three more days," he said.

"I don't have three days." Cheever slid off his coat and began rolling up a sleeve. "I'm not leaving her, Zabdiel. Not even to you. So either you inoculate me, or I'll inoculate myself."

"You won't."

"Like hell I won't."

"*No.*"

Cheever turned dark eyes on him. "My wife is fighting for her life, Zabdiel. I can't afford to be any sicker than I have to be. Not now. And from everything you've said, inoculation is the easiest way out of this mess. If you won't do it for me, do it for her."

The old vision of a little girl with Jerusha's eyes, digging a grave, swam

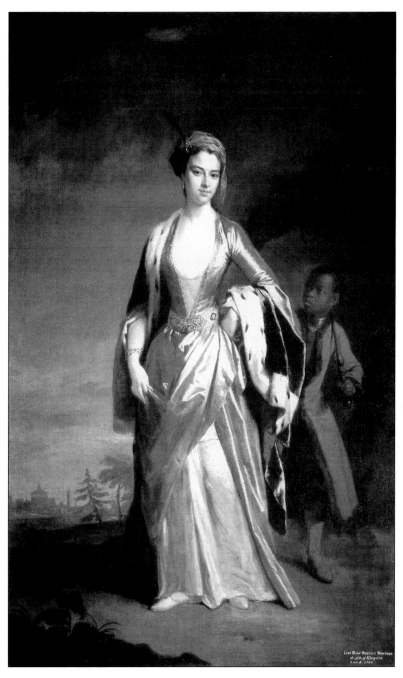

Lady Mary Wortley Montagu in her Turkish robes, by Jonathan Richardson, circa 1725. Society portraitists regularly brushed delicate roses-and-cream complexions over smallpox scars. (Courtesy of a Private Collection/Bridgeman Art Library.)

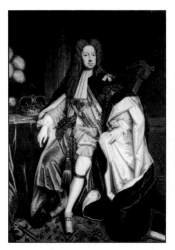

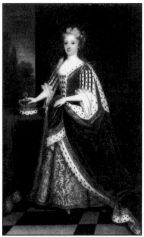

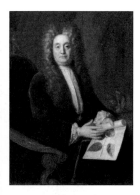

Sir Hans Sloane, by
Stephen Slaughter,
1736. (Courtesy of
the National Portrait
Gallery, London.)

King George I of Great
Britain, 1714, from the studio
of Sir Godfrey Kneller.
(Courtesy of the National Portrait
Gallery, London.)

Caroline of Brandenburg-
Ansbach, Princess of Wales,
1716 (later Queen Caroline),
after Sir Godfrey Kneller.
(Courtesy of the National Portrait
Gallery, London.)

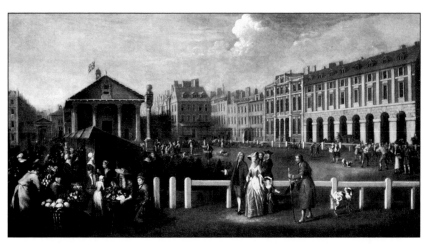

Covent Garden, London, by Balthazar Nebot, 1737. When Lady Mary lived there
(1718–1739), Covent Garden was a fashionably risqué artistic and intellectual neighborhood, as well as home to London's fruit and vegetable market. The house where
Charles Maitland inoculated Lady Mary's daughter stood where the Royal Opera
House stands today. (Courtesy of the Tate Gallery, London/Art Resource, New York.)

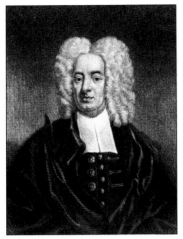

Cotton Mather. (Courtesy of the Library of Congress, Washington D.C., USA/Bridgeman Art Library.)

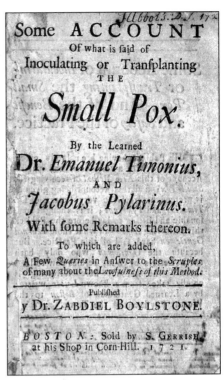

Some ACCOUNT
Of what is said of
Inoculating or Transplanting
THE

Small Pox.

By the Learned
Dr. *Emanuel Timonius*,
AND
***Jacobus* Pylarinus.**

With some Remarks thereon.

To which are added,
A Few *Queries* in Answer to the *Scruples* of many about the *Lawfulness of this Method.*

Published
y Dr. ZABDIEL BOYLSTONE.

BOSTON: Sold by S. GERRISH, at his Shop in Corn-Hill. 1 7 2 1.

The first American entry into the pamphlet wars over inoculation, published by Zabdiel Boylston in Boston, 1721. (Courtesy of the John Carter Brown Library at Brown University.)

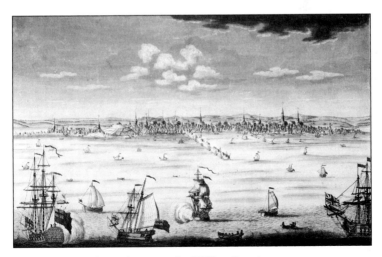

Boston in the eighteenth century, by William Burgis.
(Courtesy of the New York Public Library/Art Resource, New York.)

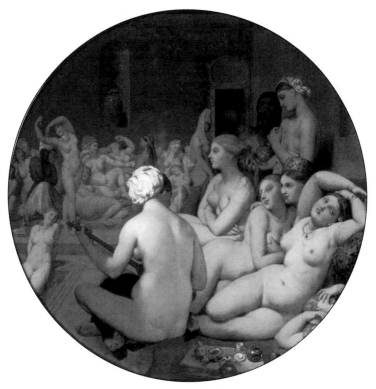

The Turkish Bath (*Le Bain Turc*), by Jean-Auguste-Dominique Ingres, 1862.

In 1717, Lady Mary deemed the women's bath in Sofia a scene worthy of Titian's brush and wished that her friend, portraitist Charles Jervas, could have joined her. "It would have very much improved his art," she wrote, "to see so many fine women naked in different postures." But Titian was long dead, Jervas was far off in London, and in any case the place was off-limits to men. So she painted the scene herself, with words rather than a brush, admiring so much "skin shiningly white"—without the faintest trace of smallpox scarring.

A century later, an exquisitely talented young French painter took notes on what was the most erotic and no doubt most read of Lady Mary's *Embassy Letters*. As an eighty-two year-old man, Jean-Auguste-Dominique Ingres returned to the notes of his hot-blooded youth and at last delivered her scene in paint. His voluptuous masterpiece now hangs in the Louvre. (Courtesy of Réunion des Musées Nationaux/Art Resource, New York.)

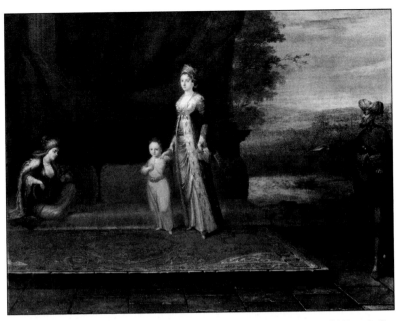

Lady Mary Wortley Montagu and her son Edward in Constantinople (Istanbul), circa 1717, by Jean Baptiste Vanmour. (Courtesy of the National Portrait Gallery, London.)

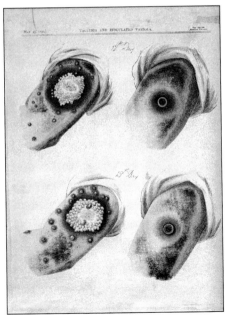

Inoculation (or variolation, using *variola*, the smallpox virus) compared to vaccination (using *vaccinia*, or the cowpox virus) at its height, the twelfth and thirteenth days. Early on, people feared that the sores of inoculation would continue growing until they rotted limbs to the core. By the fourteenth to sixteenth days, however, the sores usually began to heal, though they left much larger scars than the nickel-sized dimpled marks of vaccination. During one of young Edward Wortley's runaway adventures, he joined the Royal Navy and got as far as Gibraltar before he was identified—by his inoculation scars—and returned home. Painted by George Kirtland, circa 1802. (Courtesy of The Wellcome Library, London.)

Photos circa 1908, of patients in London's Smallpox Hospitals, from Thomas Francis Rickett's *The Diagnosis of Smallpox*. (All photos courtesy of The Wellcome Trust, London.)

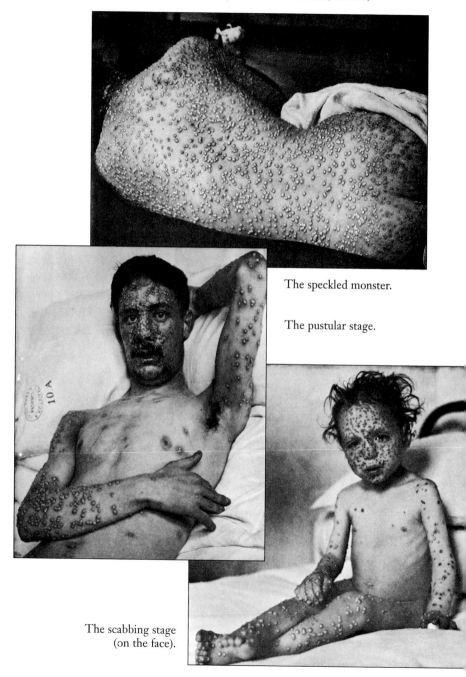

The speckled monster.

The pustular stage.

The scabbing stage (on the face).

A fatal case similar to Mrs. Dixwell's.
(All photos courtesy of The Wellcome Trust, London.)

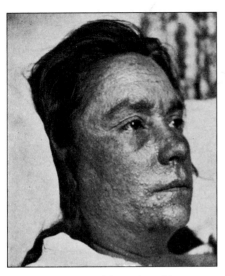

Earliest stage of the rash: red bumps rising.

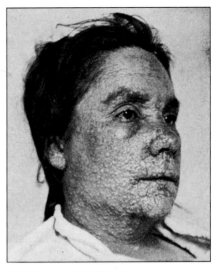

Middle stage: the blistering.

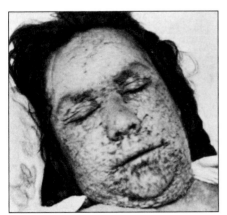

Mature or "pustular" stage: pus-filled pocks running together.

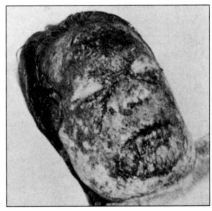

Final stage: pocks bursting beneath scab-crusted skin.

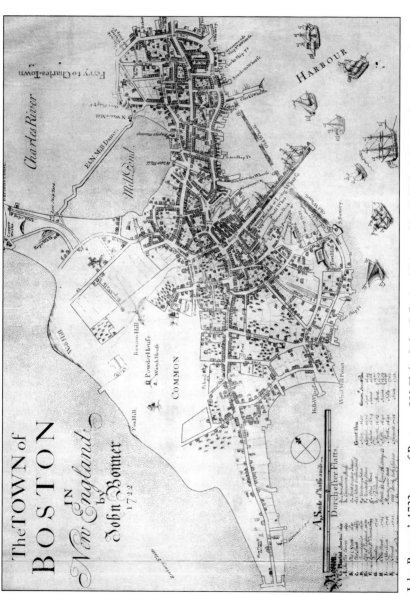

John Bonner's 1722 map of Boston. (I.N. Phelps Stokes Collection, Miriam and Ira D. Wallatch Division of Art, Prints and Photographs, The New York Public Library, Astor, Lenox, and Tilden Foundations.)

before Zabdiel's eyes. He swallowed hard and felt for the vial that had hung on a thong around his neck since he'd first inoculated Tommy. He'd cleaned it out and replaced the old matter with new only that morning, in the course of a regular examination. As he had been doing—*for no reason*, he told himself—whenever he came across a fine distinct case at just the right stage.

Much later that night, Zabdiel finally sat down to write Jerusha. He wanted her to hear the news from him: *Tommy is safe. So are Jack and Jackey*.

But Joshua Cheever was not. Not any longer. Zabdiel ran both his hands up along his head. He could not bear to write that part: that just a few hours before, he had stirred two drops of smallpox into his best friend's blood.

That afternoon over in Cambridge, the House of Representatives adjourned itself without so much as a by-your-leave from the governor. It was the representatives who had first urged Governor Shute to allow the assembly to retreat from the Town House in the center of Boston across the wide expanse of the River Charles, so as to escape the threat of the smallpox. At their urging, the governor had also reluctantly followed Puritan precedent in the face of calamity and proclaimed the following day to be a public Day of Humiliation. He proved recalcitrant, though, in giving the men leave to go home and pray with their families—reasoning that it was their own fault they were huddled too close for comfort in the little town of Cambridge. They had work to do; they could bloody well pray over there.

At the glowering behest of their speaker, Dr. John Clark, the House responded by plucking adjournment from the governor's short list of prerogatives and granting themselves the leave they sought.

The following day, Thursday, July 13, shops and warehouses stayed shut and fishing boats stayed in, as people throughout the province trooped into church to tremble before the wrath of the Lord.

That evening, Dr. Clark directed his carriage to Dr. Boylston's shop. He did not descend, but begged a word with the doctor out in the street.

When Boylston emerged from the purpling dusk, it was not from the house, but from the drive that wound around its side, back toward the garden and orchard; Clark could hear the excited shouts of children in that direction.

"Fine night, Doctor," said Zabdiel with a smile. "How can I help you?"

His greeting went no farther than a nod; he appeared to be holding something in his tightly cupped hands.

Dr. Clark came straight to the point. "It has been brought to my attention, sir, that you are considering spreading the practice of inoculation for the smallpox well beyond the bounds of your family."

Dr. Boylston cocked his head, regarding his visitor with polite but detached curiosity, as if listening to strange, shimmering news from far-off lands.

"I must warn you, sir, against any such step," continued Dr. Clark.

A little crease appeared between Dr. Boylston's eyes. "Do you speak in an official capacity?"

"Let us say that I am delivering a private request, with the sincere hopes of several men of position in this town that it can remain so." Still sitting in his carriage, Dr. Clark leaned forward and rested his chin on the knob of the walking stick he gripped with both hands. "May I have your word, sir?"

Slowly, Zabdiel unfolded his hands; a firefly flickered pale green in his palm. He tossed it into the air. "No," he said with a little shake of his head, his eyes following the drunken, spiraling path of the firefly. "No, I'm afraid not."

"May I inquire why not?" asked Dr. Clark stiffly.

Zabdiel's eyes riveted his guest. "Because I've already broken the promise you're asking me to make."

Dr. Clark felt his face harden. "That, sir, was most unwise."

Dr. Boylston's eyes gleamed with irritating amusement. "I understand you might have concerns," he said, "but I think I can set them to rest, if you'll just step back into the garden, and see my son."

"*No.*" Dr. Clark bristled. "No sir, I will not. I have already discovered more than I wished." He gave a curt command to his driver. "Good evening," he said coldly, as the carriage rolled away.

Zabdiel was still standing there, looking thoughtfully after the carriage, when a woman turned up the street, her broad hips swinging so comfortably through the soft, thickening darkness as to almost hide her hurry.

Moll had come home.

She handed Zabdiel a note, slightly damp and crumpled, and sidled past him, fairly running up the drive toward the kitchen door. By the time he wandered in after her, she already had Jackey curled up in a sleepy ball on her lap while she rocked him, stroking his skin and humming a lullaby in a slow, deep contralto.

Zabdiel paused for a moment to listen, and then he trailed upstairs to sit alone in the parlor with Jerusha's scent skating up from the paper Moll had set in his hands. He gazed for a while at his wife's handwriting spidering over the page, before he actually read it.

I know you will not be pleased, she wrote. *You will protest that Moll has not had the distemper. But Jackey is her only child. At least I have the girls to worry over, here. If I did not, I could not bear it.*

She would, in any case, have come, whether or not I gave permission, so I thought it best to give it.

Send more news, as soon as soon as you may have any to send.

We are all well here.

And then, off by itself at the bottom of the page, the sentence he had wanted to see most.

You have done the right thing.

The days that had crept by so slowly for two long weeks began to reel by in a blur. He inoculated Moll first thing the next morning; he had been prepared for an argument, but when he came downstairs she planted herself in front of him with both feet and fairly demanded it.

That afternoon, John Helyer tracked him down as he was leaving Cheever's and demanded it as well. The smallpox was popping out among the children all up and down Salutation Alley, and Helyer could not bear to think of his own flock penniless and alone in the world, like the three new housefuls of orphans at the other end of the street alone, should he himself succumb.

At home, Zabdiel saw that the boys' scabs were nearly gone, their skin smooth as babies'.

Any impulse he might have had to exult, however, was tempered by the misery swelling around him. The next day, he had to give Cheever the news that his wife's smallpox was thickening ominously; Cheever himself had yet to fall ill. In the streets, the jeering and taunting sputtered back into life; a crowd now followed Zabdiel everywhere, though they maintained a wary distance, as if he himself might be contagious. *Most of the day*, thought Zabdiel, *I probably am.* They could hear the mob's cries from inside Cheever's house: *Poisoner. Pox spreader.*

"Go on the offensive," said Cheever with vehemence, as Zabdiel dressed his incisions; he'd decided to drop the walnut shell, in favor of his tried-and-true dressing of choice: cabbage leaves. Cheever rattled on. "You've got a right to defend yourself. And if you ask me, reasonable people who happen not to have milk toast for livers have a right to hear the truth of the matter, from you."

So that afternoon, a Saturday, Zabdiel sat down and composed a letter for his paper, the *Boston Gazette*. He was no Dr. Mead, he sighed upon finishing, no Cotton Mather whose words flowed on and on with the shake of a pen. But he had managed, he thought, to make his case in plain English, for plain men and women to read. He hoped they would read with their heads, rather than with frightened hearts.

Mr. Philip Musgrave, the provincial postmaster and proprietor of the *Gazette*, was gratifyingly pleased to have Zabdiel's little missive. He needed some draw to keep everyone from deserting to his competition, Campbell's dratted *News-Letter* and its sensational pestilences. The letter would appear, Musgrave promised, in the very next issue: Monday.

On Sunday, July 16, the catcalling thickened. *Raw Head and Bloody Bones!* the crowd screeched after Dr. Boylston. Parties broke off from him to heckle Mr. Cheever and the Reverend Dr. Mather as well. *Murderer,* they shouted at the startled minister on his way into the church.

G.D., Dr. Mather wrote in his diary when he returned home. *At this Time I enjoy an unspeakable Consolation.* It was hard not to puff with some modicum of pride. For the enemy raging against him with dark sulfurous fire was no lesser foe than Lucifer. *The Destroyer, being enraged at the Proposal of anything that may rescue the Lives of our poor People from him, has taken a strange Possession of the People on this Occasion. They rave, they rail, they blaspheme; they talk not only like Idiots but also like Frantics. Not only the Physician who began the Experiment, but I also am an Object of their Fury, their Obloquies, and Invectives.*

He knew, too, with a strong sense of exaltation, the right response: he would turn the other cheek. *My Conformity to my SAVIOUR in this Thing fills me with Joy unspeakable and full of Glory.*

On Monday morning, Zabdiel summoned John home from his uncle Tom's house; when he arrived, Zabdiel inoculated his second son. Visiting Cheever a little later, he found him lightly feverish. His incisions, however, were drying up; perhaps they would not run like the boys' had—though those, too, were finally beginning to heal.

That afternoon, Zabdiel's letter appeared in the *Gazette*, to do battle with the second half of Dr. Mead's treatise on the plague in the *Boston News-Letter*. He got a peculiar and quite unexpected satisfaction from reading his words in print, though they also made him squirm; he instantly saw several places where his prose could have been much tighter.

I have patiently born with abundance of clamour and raillery [he opened] for beginning a new practice here (for the good of the public) which comes well recommended from gentlemen of figure and learning, and which well agrees to reason, when tried and duly considered, viz. artificially giving the Small-Pocks by Inoculation, to one of my children and two of my slaves in order to prevent the hazard of life which is often endangered and lost by that distemper in the common way of infection.

That was a mouthful, he realized, about four sentences in one. Very orderly, very clear, to be sure, but on reflection it made him sound a little rushed, a little too anxious. A little too tied up in knots, he told himself with a short laugh.

And as the thing was new, and for fear of erring in doing, I left it wholly to nature, which needed no help in my Negro man, who was taken ill a day or two before the other two, in which time the symptoms abating, caused me to hope for the same in the others. Until the third day, my little son's fever, with the rage of the people, sufficiently affrighted me, but I no sooner used means but the fever abated and the Small-Pocks came out, and they never took one grain or drop of medicine since, and are perfectly well. And for encouragement, no one need fear in this way of having many pustules, of being scarred in their face, or of ever having the Small-Pocks again. This is fully cleared up by those gentlemen, viz. Doctor Emanuel Timonius of Constantinople, and Fellow of the Royal Society. And Jacobus Pylarinus (a physician as appears by his writing), the Venetian Consul at Smyrna, who have try'd it and known it tried upon thousands—and with good success as they have informed us. And in the three, of whom I have had experience, I find their account just and true. As he himself tried to be just and true, not glossing over the scares or the risks. *And in a few weeks more, I hope to give you some further proof of their just and reasonable account.*

Zabdiel Boylston.

* * *

Officially, Boston's seven selectmen met that same morning. Behind firmly closed doors, they met once again after dinner, joined by the irate speaker of the temporarily adjourned House, who slapped several copies of the *Gazette* down before them.

"We have already failed to contain the disease once," he said, glaring at Elisha Cooke. "The very least we can do is to prevent Boylston—*a doctor,* no less—from spreading it still farther."

"I agree," said Mr. Hutchinson darkly. "This fooling with inoculation must be stopped."

"And if he refuses to cooperate?" asked Mr. Cooke. Like most of the others, he had had a long, informative talk with Dr. Douglass. He had no intention of dissenting; he was just taking the measure of the passions in the room.

"Then," growled Dr. Clark, "I hope you will call him to public account. I have warned him once already. Unofficially, of course," he added as several backs bristled. "I'd be happy to serve you again as a more official messenger," he continued, "but tomorrow morning, as you know, the General Court reconvenes in Cambridge."

"Leave it to me," said the doctor's brother, William Clark. This time, he told himself, no further means of spreading infection would escape his vigilance.

He delivered an official warning, in person, that very afternoon.

Walking by Dr. Boylston's place the next day, Dr. Mather gazed with barely veiled envy at the doctors' boys playing in the yard. But when he tried to cross the street, a crowd skittered out of nowhere, drawing so close that they jostled him. They were possessed, he thought, the very instrument of the devil who was tormenting him by dangling the success of inoculation before his eyes while preventing him from saving the lives of his own children. The press began to terrify him; they would tear him like Bacchus from limb to limb. His heart pounding in his throat, he turned homeward.

On the nineteenth, both Moll and Mr. Helyer were a little shivery with fever. Cheever's temperature, on the other hand, had gone off, and his incisions had almost entirely dried up. As Zabdiel was leaving Cheever's front gate, John and Joseph Webb, brother brewers and distillers who supplied the Salutation, fell in beside him, insisting that he join them at the tavern to taste their latest batch of ale. He had had no more than two sips when they came to the real point, begging him to inoculate their two families.

Zabdiel tried to dissuade them. John, especially—he was getting on in years. They listened politely, and then begged him again. The smallpox was devastating whole families in the area. Reluctantly, Zabiel agreed on a compromise. First he would inoculate the adults: the two brothers and Joseph's wife Deborah. Not till three or four days later would he inoculate the children; that way, while the adults were sickest, Joe's eldest daughter Esther could nurse them. When she, in turn, was sick, they stood at least a chance of being well enough to care for her and the littler ones.

Once they had reached an agreement, the Webbs wanted to waste no time; he stopped in at their place on his way home and performed the operation.

The news did not take long to spread. The next morning as he emerged from the Cheevers' place, it was William Clark who lay in wait; as the alley was too narrow to admit a carriage, he had strolled up with two man-servants. "*Dr. Boylston,*" he said, "as you have repeatedly disregarded warn-ings of a more friendly nature, it now falls to me to request your presence at the Town House this Friday morning at ten o'clock, for the purpose of a selectmen's meeting to consider the hazards of inoculation."

"Will you also be considering the benefits?" asked Zabdiel, unhitching his big old gelding and mounting.

"I have brought a summons, Dr. Boylston, not an invitation to converse at a tea party."

"I will be there, Mr. Clark," said Zabdiel. "I will be there." Before he could say anything he would regret, he rode quickly away.

Moll's fever went off the next day, just as Jack's had, without ever produc-ing a rash. Also like Jack, her incisions were already drying up.

"You've had smallpox before too," Zabdiel told her.

"Don't know 'bout that," replied Moll. "But I've had 'em now."

Cheever, too, seemed to have shaken off the inoculation, but he was certain he had never had the smallpox. By Thursday, though, he was feel-ing so well that he and Boylston both concluded that the operation had not taken. Perhaps he was naturally immune. Sarah, on the other hand, was grossly, terrifyingly ill; never mind inoculation, in caring for her, he had had every opportunity to contract the distemper.

That night, a fire broke out in a chimney up the street, and Cheever ran to help put it out before it could leap to neighboring roofs. By the time the brigade assembled, the flames had eaten well into one house; roaring and spitting, they were fingering greedily at its neighbors. It was not a roof or a house or even a neighborhood that was at risk. Every man there knew that if the fire tore loose, it would surge into a citywide conflagration: other than smallpox, fire was the worst calamity Boston knew. By the time they wrestled it under control and Cheever finally returned home, he was drenched with water and sweat. It was only after he shed his filthy clothing and washed off the soot that he found he could not dry himself off. It was fever, not the fire brigade's water that was keeping him wet. Even as he re-alized this, his head and back exploded with pain.

At dawn, he finally let his servant rouse Dr. Boylston. Zabdiel arrived to find Cheever's temperature high, his pulse hard and quick, his skin dry and inflamed, and his whole body brimming with pain. Either the inoculation had taken after all, or Sarah, close to death in the inner room, had given him the natural smallpox. Either way, it looked grim. Zabdiel shed his coat and went to work, battling through the early morning hours for Cheever's life. Unlike Tommy at the height of his fever, Cheever was still strong, so Zabdiel bled him, blistered him, and gave him a stringent antimonial vomit, hoping against hope to draw the poison up to a boil at the surface of his skin.

As he worked, Zabdiel told Cheever about the meeting scheduled later that morning. "It's an opportunity," he said.

"It's more likely to be another witch-hunt," said Cheever through chattering teeth. "Listen, you sweet fool of a physician: The selectmen made a mighty blunder in the matter of the *Seahorse*. They'll be wanting to redirect blame for loosing this hellfire plague toward somebody else. You probably look like manna from heaven . . . Daniel walking straight into the lions' mouths, never mind the den."

"You're mixing up your stories," said Zabdiel.

Cheever merely grunted. Zabdiel's problem intrigued him; it was something he could think his way through, whereas his own discomfort was mere animal pain. Also, it took his mind off Sarah, whose misery threatened to turn him inside out with grief. So even as Zabdiel drew several pints of blood and painted his back with a caustic ointment that drew blisters bubbling to the surface, Cheever badgered him into planning strategies and preparing arguments, as if he were headed into a trial for his life. He was by no means satisfied with Zabdiel's answers when his own symptoms went off, only a few hours later.

Zabdiel lingered, hoping beyond hope that the rash would dust Cheever with no more than ten or twenty specks and then march off again. It all depended on whether he had had come down with inoculated or natural smallpox. Meanwhile, Cheever went on drilling Zabdiel. His skin was still maddeningly clear when ten o'clock veered close and Zabdiel reluctantly began packing up to leave.

"Take the offensive," said Cheever once more, still lying on his stomach.

"I'll be fine," said Zabdiel. "I'll be back at dinner to tell you all about it."

"Just try not to *be* offensive," Cheever yelled after him.

❧ 2 ❧

PRYING MULTITUDES

Covent Garden, London
April 1721

WELL past midnight, hour dragged by hour up in the nursery. Lady Mary longed to slip up to the bed and hold a lantern over her daughter's sleeping face—like Psyche peering down at Cupid, she thought. She shuddered and gripped the arms of the chair as she rocked, holding herself forcibly in her seat.

Psyche's reckless curiosity had been a mistake. The moment she had seen the truth—that her husband was no monster, after all, but a young golden god—she had trembled with catastrophic relief. A single drop of burning oil spilled from her lamp and splashed her beloved. Startled awake, he had cast one glance of loving reproach her way, and disappeared. To get him back, she had had to brave the dark hollow whispering of Hades—or was that Orpheus and Eurydice? Lady's Mary's mind was thick with exhaustion, and she could not pull the strands of story apart, or make them lie still.

The fire flickered, and she drowsed. Slowly, her grip on the chair relaxed. Sometime later, she watched herself rise, drift to the bed, and draw aside the curtains. Her daughter was encrusted with pearls, tears, roses, and stars. Lady Mary gasped, and all at once they rose from the child's skin in a swarm, sailed about the room in a long shining ribbon like a comet's tail, and then poured themselves onto the floor at her feet.

Sort them by morning, or she will die, intoned a deep voice Lady Mary could neither place nor disobey. She knelt in terror, sweeping at the glimmering heap. But the more frantically she plucked at the tears and the stars, the more nimbly they scattered from her fingers, shivering with high-pitched laughter. Her stomach had drilled a hole deep into despair when the nightingales of Constantinople swooped in to help.

Lady Mary became aware of the sun shining in her lap. Birds were singing, but they were not nightingales. She blinked and found that dawn had slipped in through the windows while she dreamed. She stumbled to the bed and flung back the curtains. Among lace pillows and lacier dolls, little Mary lay fast asleep, her mouth parted in easy breath. On her face burned five—no, six—red flecks.

As promised, the eruption had begun.

Gingerly, Lady Mary reached out to touch her daughter's cheek. It was cool.

She drew in a breath so deep it might have been a sob. Below her, her daughter sighed and stretched; her eyes fluttered, and then she sank back into sleep.

Lady Mary let herself touch her daughter once more, smoothing her fine dark fringe of curls. She was a demure little creature, sometimes tending toward prim. Already motherly—in some ways, more motherly than Lady Mary—and touchingly eager to please. Lady Mary had no notion how she could possibly have produced such a daughter.

Reluctantly, she drew away her hand and went to be dressed. As soon as she was presentable, she would carry the news to Mr. Wortley herself.

By the time Lady Mary retired, this time to her own bed, the six speckles on the child's face had doubled to twelve. An equally small number had sowed themselves across her body. Most wonderfully, they appeared to have stopped spreading in numbers, and were now growing in size instead.

The next morning, Lady Mary ran to her daughter's bed directly upon waking. The rash had not increased by so much as a single speck in the night; the two dozen or so she had were already blistering.

"Looks to be a right light case," confirmed Mr. Maitland a few hours later. Privately, he worried that it might prove too light: however much of a relief it might be at present, surely a mere two dozen pocks could not possibly weave a very strong web of future protection? And what was this dare for, if not that? For the time being, though, he kept his doubts to himself.

By midmorning, the parade of handpicked witnesses began to drift, one at a time, through the nursery. At the far end of the room, Miss Mary Wortley sat on the floor in a patch of hyacinth-scented sunlight and played with her dolls.

"Ignoring the prying multitudes," said Lady Mary.

The girl certainly did not revel in the attention, as her mother surely would have, Mr. Maitland supposed, at her age. At any age, for that matter. On the other hand, the girl did not hide in her new nurse's skirts either. "You invited half the multitude yourself," he countered comfortably.

"I do not count Dr. Mead and Dr. Arbuthnot," sniffed Lady Mary. Her own personal physicians had already arrived and departed. She missed Dr. Garth, she said, now more than ever since he had died two years earlier. *He* would be down on the floor teasing Mary into peals of laughter, not looking her over like a vulture.

The first of the vultures to be admitted was Dr. James Keith, Mr. Maitland's mentor and fellow Aberdonian. He was, however, as different from Mr. Maitland as it was possible to be (and also from vultures, for that matter, as she had to admit): ebullient, cheerful, given to mysticism and seeing the glories of the Lord everywhere.

He made the child smile, at least. Conferring with Maitland, however, his face was grave enough to give Lady Mary alarm.

But Mr. Maitland had only pity for the doctor. "He has lost several of his own children to the worst sort of smallpox," he said.

Dr. Keith was followed by Dr. Walter Harris. On the subject of acute diseases of childhood, among which smallpox was such an eminent foe, he was London's most venerated authority, explained Mr. Maitland.

"You mean he's ancient," whispered Lady Mary behind her fan, as he was announced.

"Antediluvian," agreed Mr. Maitland with irritating calm. Dr. Harris had been one of the nine physicians who had stood helplessly about that bed in Kensington Palace so many years ago, watching Queen Mary die. Since then, he had watched the same disease kill hordes of children. If he seemed reticent, perhaps even reluctant to believe that in inoculation they had discovered a workable shield, it was for no more complicated reason than protection against severe disappointment. Against smallpox, Dr. Harris was accustomed to conceding defeat. "He will not rejoice until he is sure," Mr. Maitland observed to Lady Mary as Dr. Harris departed, "but then he will rejoice indeed. If we can convince him, we will prove the best of allies."

Finally, Sir Hans Sloane, M.D. twice over (once from the dubious Dutch University of Orange, and again from Oxford), Fellow of the Royal Society, Member of the College of Physicians of Edinburgh, President of the Royal College of Physicians in London, and personal physician to King George, was announced. Voracious for knowledge but a stickler for evidence, he had been ferreting out reports of inoculation from all over the Levant for years now. He could not quite decide whether he was miffed or relieved to find a bona fide experiment proceeding right under his nose—

though nearly without him—in the heart of London. It would have been more convenient, certainly, if the persons involved had been slightly less august, and so more subject to his control.

Lady Mary might have enjoyed the curiosity and caution chasing each other across his face, had he not, at his elbow, been towing a second, uninvited guest. Sir Hans bowed deeply, and presented the Hanoverian Dr. Johann Georg Steigerthal.

As it was, she went white with rage, but there was nothing she could do about it. She could not very well send the king's two favorite physicians packing from her house. As Mr. Maitland meekly put it to her in a pill both sweet and sour, this visit amounted, more or less, to a sickroom visit by the king himself.

Sir Hans proved quite interested in the incisions, and wished for a closer view. With a curt little nod, Lady Mary marched across the room before him. During the whole inspection, she stood over her child like a lioness.

The two men were gentle, but they spoke of Mary as if she were as inanimate as one of her dolls. The blisters, noted Dr. Steigerthal somewhat dubiously, looked more like chicken pox than anything else. The matter within them, agreed Dr. Sloane, looked to be too light and thin to be the true smallpox.

Never mind that Dr. Harris had made the same observations. Lady Mary regarded their doubt as a personal affront. After no more than ten minutes, Mr. Maitland hurried the two men out.

"They might at least *pretend*," she shrilled as he returned, "not to expect that they're practicing for her funeral procession."

Across the next two days, Mary's pocks filled as much as they ever would, which was not much. Truthfully, they gave Mr. Maitland pangs of concern to the point that he found himself in the strange position of rooting for a case of the smallpox to get worse. *Slightly*, he emphasized to himself.

Had he done something wrong? he wondered. Countless times, he reviewed the inoculation in his head, as if he could have forgotten a step, though he knew this was impossible. In the end, he accounted for the lightness of her case by regarding the difference between the climates of London and Constantinople. Perhaps the pocks would not ripen so fully in the chillier air of England, especially during a spring that had been more than usually dank. This explanation had the added bonus of easing his mind about the operation's effectiveness too. The Circassians of the Caucasus practiced inoculation to astonishingly beautiful effect, as did other peoples along the banks of the Caspian Sea, in climates much colder than that of Constantinople. Much colder than that of England and Scotland, too, for that matter. Manifestly, they made it work: did their daughters not stock the finest harems in all Turkey?

Lady Mary did not share Mr. Maitland's caution or the physicians' doubts. As soon as Mary's blisters thickened into pustules, and it was clear that no more new pocks would appear, she gathered her daughter in her arms, and wept. *It is over,* she thought.

It was not over.

No sooner had she dried her eyes, and let her daughter wriggle free, than a line of curious friends and powerful connections appeared at the nursery door. At least, that is what it soon began to seem like.

Lord and Lady Townshend came several times: Dolly because she was a child at heart and loved little Mary almost as much as she loved her mother, and Lord T because he loved to see Dolly happily at play with babies. Also, he quite liked Lady Mary in her own right. *Damned fine woman,* he rumbled to himself. *Startlingly intelligent. Can actually talk political sense.* Besides, he owed her an infinite debt for bringing a once-reluctant Dolly around to the point of marrying him. As a result, he was permanently on the lookout for indirect means by which to repay her.

In any case, even without Dolly, he would in all likelihood have made a visit, though doubtless one of a stiffer nature, in his capacity as secretary of state. For he and his formidable ally in Commons, Sir Robert Walpole (Dolly's brother)—not to mention the entire Whig ministry—had staked everything on the ascendancy of the German family now occupying the palace of St. James. Smallpox, you might say, had set the House of Hanover on the British throne; it was unthinkable that the foul disease should swat them off again. Unthinkable, but not impossible, apparently, Lord Townshend sighed to himself. The ministry had thought the family strong against this particular distemper until Princess Anne—then just three lives away from the throne—had had such a terrible time battling it last spring; she had been quite touch-and-go for a week. And really, she had been sadly marred by its grinding tracks, he clucked. There was now one new prince, to be sure, but two princes and three princesses still seemed a paltry force with which to face a speckled demon that could dispense with thousands with a mere breath.

A viable shield against this ravager was potentially a defensive weapon of power that no one at the highest levels of realpolitik could afford to ignore.

He was not the only person to draw such a conclusion. Another day, the duchess of Dorset arrived with Charlotte Tichborne. Both ladies officially belonged to the Princess of Wales's household, but they were also genuinely her friends; not coincidentally, the pair had been childhood friends of Lady Mary as well. "The princess," said the duchess, trying to find the right tone between grandeur and familiarity as she swept up the stairs, "is quite keen to know how your Mary does, my dear."

At the door, she raised a perfumed scarf to her nose and peered in. Her hand dropped, and then her jaw followed. This was no malodorous room holding a wailing, shivering child covered in sores. The girl was hopping about, trying to coax a canary into singing. On her face were a few small pimples. No more than the chicken pox.

The duchess left at something very close to an undignified run: not out of terror, but out of excitement.

Charlotte Tichborne was both more relaxed and more relaxing. As a woman of the bedchamber, Charlotte had the ear of the princess as often—possibly more often—than the duchess did, but as a commoner and a widow, she was not such a fierce guardian of either the princess's dignity or her own. The duchess could claim that as her duty; Charlotte thought hers was to fill any room she was in with cheerful chatter.

In Lady Mary's nursery, she stayed long enough to teach little Mary a new game. But not much longer. She, too, wanted the pleasure of reporting this sight to her royal mistress.

The parade of visitors would have stretched on to the crack of doom, thought Lady Mary, if the disease had not been so mercifully quick. Within no more than three days after ripening—if it could even be called that—Mary's small dusting of pocks had already scabbed over. Only a week after the first fleck had appeared, she was shedding her few small scabs.

A week after that, there was nothing more to see.

Having lost his two elder sons to the flat pox and the purples, Dr. Keith came to his conclusion about inoculation more quickly than the others. On May 1, he had Mr. Maitland drain five ounces of blood from his last surviving son, Peter, who was not quite six. Ten days later, Mr. Maitland returned to inoculate the boy. Peter's fever and rash appeared earlier and a little thicker than little Mary's had, but his bout with the smallpox, too, was marvelously light. By the end of the month, he had dropped all his scabs.

At the same time, a month shy of her eighth birthday, the Princess of Wales's youngest daughter and namesake, Princess Caroline, flushed with an illness that Sir Hans Sloane feared might be the purples. For several days, the beating of drums and the piping of music was forbidden throughout the grounds of St. James's. Even Mr. Handel prayed for the little princess in silence.

After four terrible days and many close consultations, Sir Hans shifted his diagnosis to scarlet fever. The little girl was still gravely ill, but even so, both the Prince and Princess of Wales wept with relief. Their plump, dark-haired little Caro had been spared.

With this second success of inoculation and this second close call within the royal family, the physicians, the Princess of Wales, and the Whig ministry began to scheme among themselves to bring the operation into still greater repute. They never all sat down at once; their maneuverings followed more devious and meandering indirections—a scribbled note here, a book borrowed there, a stolen and hurried conversation or two elsewhere. From time to time, they skimmed through Covent Garden to include Lady Mary.

She had, after all, taken the first and therefore the greatest risk. It had been wonderful to watch her daughter sail through the smallpox so easily, the others all agreed. But that was not evidence enough: not, in any case, for what they now wished to do. It was one thing for a private lady to submit her children to such a hazardous operation. It was quite another for a new dynasty to risk its heirs. More proof was paramount.

But where to find it, and in abundance?

Lady Mary never discovered who first realized that there was in London an almost infinite source of already lost lives, chained in darkness within the prisons that had been built in and around the ancient gateways through the city's medieval walls. Perhaps someone in the ministry had a thought jogged by a conversation, of an evening, with the Tory scribbler turned Whig propagandist, Daniel Defoe—hard at work, as he put it, on a grand new tale about the fortunes and misfortunes of a jailbird. A woman, no less! Moll or Doll or Poll, the minister thought. With a country for a surname. Not France. Flanders. That was it: *Moll Flanders*.

Perhaps Dr. Keith dreamed it up, in concert with his friend, the pastor of St. Sepulchre's, the church that tolled its funeral bell as the condemned prisoners of Newgate clattered past on their last ride from the dungeons to the hangman's noose at Tyburn. Perhaps it was Dr. Sloane, who knew that the French king had used prisoners from the Bastille to test the effectiveness of quinine in fighting malaria and a certain delicate surgery in closing anal fistulae. Or perhaps it was the princess, who knew of the same French experiments.

No one owned it, this notion that they might experiment on condemned prisoners. The idea was just suddenly in the air, in the messages and whispered conversations that crisscrossed the western fringes of London from Leicester Square to Covent Garden, from Great Russell Street in Bloomsbury, where Sir Hans lived, to St. James's and Westminster.

At last, the princess did convene what she called a council of war, and a plan took shape. Sir Hans and several other physicians from the Royal College would approach the king; Lord Townshend would approach the lawyers, and the Princess of Wales would remain uncharacteristically quiet. This was not a battle in which she meant to score points in the public eye, by trumping the king. This was a battle in which all that mattered was to get her children inoculated—if, indeed, inoculation worked. She did not care who took the credit.

The obvious assumption that what was good enough for her children was by no means good enough for the royals irritated Lady Mary. All those physicians with their grave jowly shakes of the head that intimated that she was a rash mother made her cheeks flame. They would trust felons, God forbid, but not her!

She was not, however, so cross as to refuse any help they required of her. Up to and including sacrificing much of the time and attention of the man she had come to regard as her own private surgeon: Mr. Charles Maitland.

On June 14, Lord Townshend wrote to both the attorney general and the solicitor general, asking *whether His Majesty may by law grant his gracious pardon to two malefactors under sentence of death upon condition that they will suffer to be tried upon them the experiment of inoculating the smallpox?*

By June 17, he had an answer: *The lives of the persons being in the power of His Majesty, he may grant a pardon to them upon such lawful condition as he shall think fit; and as to this particular condition, we have no objection in point of law, the rather because the carrying on this practice to perfection may tend to the general benefit of mankind.*

His satisfaction might have been complete, if he had not also attracted the attention of the press: someone had leaked a (thankfully) garbled story about two prisoners volunteering, out of the blue, to undergo the experiment, in return for pardon. It was preposterous, of course—*did the newspapers really imagine that a couple of felons in Newgate had somehow divined this possibility in the dark?*—but the press gleefully devoured it nevertheless, especially the Tory press, which was, as a matter of course, hostile to the Whig ministry.

At least the prince and princess had been left out of it. The mere thought of it made him sweat. Never mind that the prince had almost nothing to do with inoculation, except to follow Caroline's lead in believing it was a good idea. Should either of their names—especially the prince's—reach the king before he could be brought to think that the prison experiment was his own idea, he might well reject it out of hand, merely because his son was for it.

Sir Hans did his best to dangle the notion of a Newgate experiment like a bright lure before the king. George I was intrigued, but he did not snap at the bait. He did, however, ask his two Turkish servants, Mehemet and Mustafa, what they knew of this inoculation nonsense. Unfortunately, they had been captured from Turkey too young to remember anything of use.

Sir Hans did not concede easily. "His Majesty is thinking about it, Your Highness," was the best he could report to the princess, however.

June veered into July, and still the king considered.

The weather warmed up, and the palace staff began packing for the annual summer trip west to the clean air of Kensington. Around St. James's, a flurry of farewell parties gathered, before everyone dispersed for the summer—though they were quieter than usual, due to the smallpox. Lady Mary was summoned to one last weekly supper party for the king in the countess of Darlington's apartments at St. James's. With the scrupulous formality for which the palace was famous, she was handed down from her carriage and ushered inside by a footman.

At one moment, they were following the route she could have followed blindfolded. The next, they were in passages she had never seen before. A door whispered open, and she was whisked into a small parlor with light from a small fire laughing as it skated off the polish of oak paneling. Only then did she realize that the servant she had been following was no mere royal footman but the Turk Mehemet, the king's most trusted personal servant. He poured her a goblet of wine soft as black velvet and left her staring up at a portrait of the countess of Rochester, whose ravaged beauty had once made Samuel Pepys weep. She had not drunk half her wine when behind her another door sighed open, in paneling in which she had not seen any door.

She froze. The scent was familiar, the voice even more so.

"*Ah, ma très chère Marie,*" said the king as she turned and sank into a deep curtsey. The squabbling of the last few years had marked him, she thought; his face looked tired and lined. But his eyes still snapped a mischievous blue. "I can send you to the ends of the earth, my dear," he said in his German-accented French, "but I cannot distance you from controversy, it seems. What is this we hear about you having hauled home from Turkey some strange—might I say revolting?—remedy for the smallpox?"

❧ 3 ❧

AN INFUSION OF
MALIGNANT FILTH

The Town House, Boston
July 21, 1721

JUST past noon, the doors of Representatives' Hall swung inward. Set like a lantern into the top two floors of the Town House, the place was sweltering, though all the windows were open. *Dr. Zabdiel Boylston*, thundered the steward, sending echoes spiraling heavily into the dome overhead, rousing a few sleepy doves.

Standing at a podium across the circular room, Dr. Douglass frowned. He had expressly instructed that infernal steward to announce Boylston correctly, as "Mr."

The servant did not behave as desired, but at least Boylston did, jerking in a gratifying double-take as he registered Dr. Douglass in position as chief interrogator.

"Ah, Dr. Boylston," said Elisha Cooke from the vicinity of Dr. Douglass's left elbow. "Have a seat." He motioned toward something much less grand than his own chair—shabby, in point of fact—marooned alone in the empty center of the floor.

"I prefer to stand, thank you," said Boylston.

"As you wish," said Mr. Cooke, though the tone of his voice was at odds with his pleasantry. Mr. Cooke had assumed the second-best seat in the room, along with the controlling gavel. Next to him, John Clark was occupying the speaker's chair. It wasn't quite correct, Dr. Douglass sniffed to himself, since the governor had just yesterday dissolved the General Court, necessitating new elections—mostly to try and rid himself of the chronic irritation of Dr. Clark as speaker of the House. Dr. Clark, however, was glaring about as if daring someone to challenge him for the seat;

he had probably lain awake all night concocting some brilliant answer to the governor's opposition, and now wanted nothing so much as an opportunity to unsheathe his speech like a sword of vengeance.

Dr. Douglass smiled inwardly. He had already gone a good way in redirecting Dr. Clark's overflowing anger toward his own foe. *Mr.* Boylston. Had he not accepted the stolen story of inoculation from Dr. Mather? And begun to try to pawn it off as his own? Had he not begun advertising— *advertising!*—the operation as safe, to boot, when clearly it was so malignant as to be nothing short of wicked? Well, Mr. Boylston was about to be made to pay.

He scanned the rest of the room. Curved around him in three tiers of seats lining the room's perimeter, nearly thirty grave faces peered out from the luxuriant curls of full-bottomed wigs. All the selectmen were there, their number recently restored to seven with the election of Captain Nathaniel Green—another of Cooke's yea-sayers—in the place of the hapless man who had died only two days after victory in the regular yearly election last March. Scattered among the politicians were five or six justices of the peace. Most important, Dr. Douglass saw every last man in town who might make any claim to practicing medicine, right down to part-time apothecaries. The hall was as dense with power, wealth, and intelligence as could be hoped in provincial Boston.

Furthermore, the men who mattered had recognized the seriousness of the situation by donning hues even more somber than their faces. With fastidious satisfaction, Dr. Douglass noted that despite the heat, most of the fabric was sumptuous and the tailoring stiffly formal. Boylston, on the other hand, was wearing the dun-colored everyday suit he probably practiced in. On his head was a lightweight tiewig of the sort meant for riding, its long dark hair drawn into a single queue at the back, where it would stay safely out of the way during even the most breakneck of gallops.

Mr. Cooke banged down the gavel. "Dr. Douglass, I believe we may proceed?"

Dr. Douglass bowed, first to Cooke and Clark, and then to the assembly. "We have gathered here today, gentlemen, to discuss the hazards of Mr. Boylston's newfangled operation of inoculation—"

"Oh, it's not mine," Boylston cut in.

Dr. Douglass glanced over sharply. Boylston was resting one hand casually on the back of the chair he should have been sitting in; an impudent smile hovered around his mouth. "Give credit where it's due," he said. "If inoculation belongs to anyone, it is to the Royal Society."

"But you admit, sir," countered Dr. Douglass, "that it is you who have put this hazardous theory into practice?"

"I'll own having put it into practice," said Boylston. He straightened and shifted his gaze to the men assembled around them. "Whether it is hazardous, however, is surely not an established premise, gentlemen, but one of the central questions we've come together to debate. I hope to convince you that far from being a hazard, inoculation is a blessing for which we owe the Royal Society our deepest thanks."

"Since you have begun by citing the Royal Society," said Dr. Douglass, "perhaps we could begin by investigating your sources." Boylston nodded, and Dr. Douglass went on. "The *Philosophical Transactions of the Royal Society*, sir, is a most illustrious and learned journal. Are you in the habit, may I ask, of reading it?"

"No," said Boylston.

Dr. Douglass had hoped for consternation or a little defensiveness. But the man actually *grinned* at him.

"Not at all," Boylston continued. "Even in this instance, I cannot claim to have read the original, but only Dr. Mather's transcription. The original, you know," he went on, "isn't so easy to come by."

Smiles rippled around the room. Everyone knew that Dr. Douglass was the only man in town with a subscription, and that he had recently put his copies under lock and key.

Dr. Douglass grimaced. By hinting that he, Dr. Douglass, was out of line in protecting his own property, Boylston had eviscerated the argument of theft before he even had a chance to deliver it. Boylston, he thought, might have to be given credit for rather more cleverness—perhaps *cunning* was a better word—than he had originally supposed. Cunning, however, was not the same as learning. "Perhaps you are not aware, then, that this journal is often full of *jeux d'esprit*," he said, savoring the French.

"Glad to hear it," said Boylston comfortably. "I'm sure even great scholars deserve to amuse themselves now and then. But as for the two articles in question, Dr. Mather does not regard either one as a jest. Since he is a Fellow of the Royal Society as well as the most learned man in the province, I trust his judgment."

More than I trust yours. The implication shimmered in the air between them.

Dr. Douglass bristled. This perpetual awe accorded Mather's learning irritated him no end. "Dr. Mather's erudition," he said, "is not in question. He did not, however, write the articles. It is their sources I wish to examine."

"If you mean their authors, it's my understanding that Emanuel Timonius and Jacob Pylarinus are physicians of high standing in Turkey and the Levant."

"Italians!" sneered Dr. Douglass. "Exiled in infidel territory and letting themselves be led into folly by a gaggle of old Greek women."

"The Romans and the Greeks," said Boylston, "have been counted wise before now. In any case," he added, "Dr. Timonius may be Italian by birth, but he's part British by training. He possesses a degree from Oxford, I believe, and he, too, is a Fellow of the Royal Society."

Dr. Douglass drew every inch of his dignity together. "Every other medical practitioner in this town, sir, has rejected the operation as a dangerous bit of Oriental quackery. Are we to understand that you regard your judgment as trumping such a heavy weight of opinion?"

Boylston folded his arms and considered Dr. Douglass. "I regard it the right of every doctor in this town," he said at last, "to weigh the evidence and draw his own conclusion."

"And on what did you base your conclusion?"

"Experience," said Boylston.

"What experience?" challenged Dr. Douglass.

"There's a small army of people right here in Boston who've undergone the operation in Africa—"

"*Africans!*" snorted Dr. Douglass. "Idiots!" He snapped his fingers. "The greatest race of liars on the earth."

Chuckles sputtered around them. "Anyone who can talk may lie, sir," said Boylston quietly, and the amusement dropped out of the air like lead. Somewhere in the brightness, a bee buzzed. "I have made it my business to speak to as many of these African inoculees as I could discover, and I am satisfied that they are not lying."

"They can barely blunder their way through English," said Dr. Douglass, exulting in incredulity. "And yet you trust them when they tell you that they possess medical knowledge of the utmost importance and intricacy?"

Rustling and scraping filled the air as chairs were drawn closer, men leaned forward, and necks swiveled and craned. Boylston held Dr. Douglass's glare until the fidgeting settled down.

"Do you believe there are lions in Africa, Doctor?"

Dr. Douglass shrugged. Perhaps the man was mad. "The merest schoolchild knows that to be true."

"Have you been to Africa?"

"No."

"Then on what grounds do you believe such a preposterous claim as that there are cats as large as ponies there, scampering about in packs?"

Once again, snickers crackled around the edges of the room.

"On authority," said Dr. Douglass coldly. "*Learned* authority. Not the hearsay of slaves."

"I don't consider either personal or eyewitness experience to be hearsay," said Boylston, "regardless of the accent it's delivered in. Especially when backed with physical evidence, like the scars of inoculation incisions, lack of scarring elsewhere, and apparent immunity." He leaned on the chair back and smiled. "I've got at least as much evidence that inoculation is not only common but successful in Africa, Doctor, as either of us has that there are lions there."

The crowd's amusement bubbled into open laughter. Boylston turned his attention to his audience. "Why should it be any more unlawful to learn of Africans how to help against the smallpox, than to learn of our Indians how to help against snakebite? Shouldn't we have the humility to take knowledge where and how we find it?"

Heads began to nod.

"In any case," added Boylston, turning back to Dr. Douglass, "if you absolutely refuse to consider the evidence of African experience, I can now offer you my own."

"Yours, sir!" exploded Dr. Douglass. "I was not aware that you risked your own life. I heard only that you had risked your son's." *Ha!* he thought. *That struck home.*

"It is a lasting regret," said Boylston, "that I could not test the safety of the operation on myself first. As you no doubt can see, sir, that was not possible."

The first true thing the man has said all morning, thought Dr. Douglass. Boylston's face was as cratered and pitted as a battlefield.

"I wrestled with doubts, I assure you. In the end, I decided that the danger of my son contracting smallpox in the common way was far greater than the danger of inoculating him." Again, Boylston turned his attention to the men around them. "So as you know, I inoculated my youngest son and two slaves. I'm happy to report that on all three of them, the experiment has succeeded."

Surprise rose in swelling murmurs.

"I must say, sir," interjected Dr. Douglass, "I have heard otherwise. One of your slaves had no reaction whatsoever, is that not true?"

"He had a slight reaction. We have since decided that he must have had smallpox before."

"How convenient," said Dr. Douglass. "I have also heard that you yourself admitted that your son was at death's door."

Boylston glanced at George Stewart, who looked as if he had been sucking lemons and enjoying it. "My son had a high fever," he acknowledged. "Higher than either Dr. Timonius or Dr. Pylarinus led me to expect."

"So high, in fact," retorted Dr. Douglass, "that neither vomits nor purges could control it. Nor did blistering, saffron, hot cordials, or *suppedanea*." He threw down the Latin like a challenge.

"I don't know who fed you that nonsense," said Boylston, "but I hope that no one who knows me well would credit such a cluttered course of treatment. Besides, I have never found that laying fresh kidneys to the soles of the feet really helped to draw off fever. Have you?"

"The evidence," growled Dr. Douglass, "is inconclusive."

Boylston shrugged. "I dosed Tommy with nothing but a little ipecac, and sure enough the fever went off. Within a day, the rash had come all the way out, as kind and distinct as you could wish."

"But it did not come all the way out, did it?" asked Dr. Douglass. "Your son's rash was anomalous, was it not? So light and superficial, in fact, that it must be seriously considered whether it was the proper smallpox at all, or something more akin to the chicken pox."

"It was the smallpox," said Dr. Boylston.

Crowing in his soul, Dr. Douglass pounced. "And how could *you*, sir, possibly know?"

Confusion crinkled Boylston's forehead. There was a moment of uncomfortable silence, and then, off to the left, Dr. Clark cleared his throat. To no one in particular, the once and would-be future speaker of the House said, "Let us confine ourselves to the facts. Dr. Boylston has more experience with that distemper than any medical man in this town, with the possible exception of myself."

Dr. Douglass threw a look of reproach in Clark's direction; if he wanted Dr. Douglass to win this battle, he could at the very least keep from helping Boylston back up, just when Dr. Douglass had pinned him. "Dr. Boylston, sir, told me himself that he had not seen so much as a single case of smallpox before he inoculated his son."

Boylston stepped forward, looking oddly stricken. "I believe, sir, I owe you an apology. A few weeks back, you asked me very particularly whether I had yet seen one case of the smallpox. I was in the middle of saying, no, *one and twenty*, when the conversation went elsewhere. We parted before I could correct the error. I must beg your pardon for having forgotten it till now."

Cold needled Dr. Douglass's face, and nausea twirled through his stomach. *How had he gone so wrong in estimating the cunning of this charlatan?* He reviewed his strategy of attack and made a quick decision. He was not without mercy. If the man had shown the slightest respect for his betters, the least meekness in owning his ignorance and allowing himself to be taught, Dr. Douglass assured himself, he would have dealt with him gently.

As it was, he would destroy him.

He bowed stiffly. "Let us move on to discuss the procedure itself," he said smoothly, "since that is something that we can both agree occurred." Boylston nodded. "Perhaps," continued Dr. Douglass, "you could oblige the company by describing exactly what you do."

Boylston obliged better than he had dared to hope; apparently the credulous fool followed Timonius to the letter—even down to the preposterous barbarity of the nutshell, though latterly he had at least replaced that joukerypawkery with the more proper dressing of a cabbage leaf. As Boylston finished, Dr. Douglass gave him a genuine smile: he had set up his own annihilation almost perfectly.

Clasping his hands behind him, Dr. Douglass paced in front of his prey. "You admit, then, that you deliberately infect your patients with a lethal substance?"

Boylston frowned. "That's an exaggerated way of putting it, sir."

Douglass dismissed this objection with a wave. "Accurate, sir. No more than accurate. I have it on the authority of the Royal Society's own experiments that the insertion of foreign matter into the mass of the blood causes terrible disorders, and not infrequently, death."

"*What experiments?*" said Boylston. "What sort of matter?"

Dr. Douglass spread his hands. "It does not matter what sort of matter, sir." *There. If he wanted jests and jibes, let him eat that pun.* "They have tried snake venom and tobacco oil, known noxious substances, but they have also tried the agreeable balm of new milk to equally injurious effect. So how are we to suppose that death itself can be avoided when such malignant filth as smallpox is injected into the blood?"

"I do not inject smallpox in quantity into the blood," insisted Boylston. "I apply a single droplet externally, by incision."

Douglass waved off these qualifications. "After injecting your patients with purulent smallpox, do you keep them under quarantine?"

"I have no power to declare or enforce quarantine. I can only advise."

"And what is it you advise?"

"That they should keep a clean, cool diet and a quiet life until the fever rises, and then they should keep to their chambers, if not to their beds, to avoid infecting others."

"So you inoculate, and then let the infected wander freely about?"

"Do you let your patients wander freely about, Dr. Douglass?" retorted Boylston. "Or do you station guards from some private army at their doors?"

"I am not responsible for infecting them in the first place," snapped Dr. Douglass. "In short, sir, you admit that you inject your patients with smallpox and that having infected them, you allow them to wander about infecting entire unsuspecting neighborhoods." He stopped his pacing, glaring at Boylston with contempt. "Are you aware that these actions are perilously close to the definitions of poisoning, and of spreading infection?"

He took a step toward the man. "Are you aware that both acts are, by the penal laws of England, felonies?"

Another step brought him menacingly close to his foe. "If anyone should perish from your work, it is hard to see, sir, how you will avoid a charge of murder."

Sepulchral silence settled upon the room, except that one of the doves high up in the dome suddenly flapped her wings in a flutter of pink and gray, before subsiding into a steady drip of anxious cooing.

Boylston stared down his nose at Dr. Douglass. "Do you use antimony?"

"It is not I who am on trial here."

"Nor," said Boylston, "am I. I am merely trying, as you have done, to determine certain standards and definitions. Do you use antimony?" he repeated.

"Yes," scowled Dr. Douglass.

"How about spirit of vitriol, sir? Sulfuric acid?"

"Yes."

"Aren't these both strong poisons?"

"In quantity, yes."

"So you, too, poison, at least by your standards. Do you let blood?"

Dr. Douglass grunted assent.

"Where do you make your incisions, sir?"

"In the arms or wrists. Occasionally in the neck."

"But isn't the cutting of wrists and throats, sir, murder?"

"Not when done in measure."

"Precisely. Not when done in measure. Inoculation is no different."

"*No different!*" exclaimed Dr. Douglass, whirling away. "You inject filth—"

Boylston cut him off. "I make no claim that smallpox matter is not poisonous. But inoculation uses only a tiny drop of what fills the whole skin in even the lightest case of natural smallpox. There is good evidence that in such minute quantity it may prove one of mankind's greatest benefits. To my son, and two of my slaves, it already has."

"It *may*," snarled Dr. Douglass, feeling the situation bucking away from him. "In three cases, you say, it has. But is it infallible, sir? May it not ever cause harm?"

"A purge or a vomit may harm," said Boylston, his voice like steel. "Do you plan to give up those remedies on the same basis?"

"But is it infallible?" cried Dr. Stewart, jumping up from his seat in the back row. "Can you give your word that no one will die from it?" Around him, several others took up the cry. Hugh Kennedy, Francis Archibald, John Gibbins. Dr. Cooke had to bang on the desk with his gavel several times to silence the room.

Boylston's eyes singled out Dr. Stewart. "It is medicine, George," he said. "Not divinity. If it's practiced long enough, no doubt it'll harm someone. Can you—can any of you—give your word that you've never once known a patient to die from a purge or a vomit?"

He swept his eyes across the crowd, most of the men at edges of their seats, a few standing. "You have heard Dr. Douglass make a mighty bustle about malignant filth being infused into the mass of the blood, as if there were no difference between injecting a quart of poison into a large artery and applying a drop small enough to fit on the point of a needle to a scrape in the skin.

"The degree of difference, Dr. Douglass claims, is immaterial; I believe it is crucial. It is not just in quantity, though, that inoculation differs from poisoning, but in intent. Poisoning aims to cause death. Inoculation aims to prevent it.

"I will not do you the disservice of claiming that we have sailed into safe harbor. I will not tell you that nothing will ever go wrong. We are yet but learners, after all—starters, really—imperfect in knowledge and practice. So far, I have to admit that the fever has proved more intense than advertised, and in some cases the pustules more numerous.

"In the main, though, inoculation falls out just as Timonius and Pylarinus report. Just as they have written, the worst case of inoculated smallpox I have witnessed—my son's—has proved far, far better than the least case of that distemper received in the common way."

Boylston took a deep breath. "Inoculation, gentlemen, is the first real weapon we have ever discovered in the fight against the speckled monster. Should we toss it away because we don't yet know how to wield it perfectly? Or should we run to learn its secrets?" He paused and again scanned the room.

"I cannot tell you what to think in your heart of hearts. But I can tell you what I know, in mine: if only we can steel ourselves to accept this blessing and make ourselves more expert in its practice, we may save hundreds, even thousands, of lives."

Behind his desk, Mr. Cooke sighed. His belly was rumbling, but they were nowhere near ready for any vote whose outcome he would appreciate. Dr. Douglass had promised the selectmen an easy victory. Easy was clearly out of reach. At this rate, victory itself was no certainty. It would do no harm to give the doctor some time to settle down and review his strategy.

He brought the gavel down and announced a dinner recess. They would reconvene, he said glowering at Dr. Douglass, at four o'clock.

As he stepped into the street, Zabdiel plucked off his hot, scratchy wig and thrust it in a saddlebag. Without pausing to chat, he mounted his horse and rode north to Salutation Alley.

Cheever's house was on the left, on the southern side of the narrow lane. In the cauldron of summer, the coolest rooms were those downstairs, right at the front. Even so, it surprised him that Cheever answered the door himself. He must have been watching out for him. "Apparently," said Zabdiel, "you're feeling better."

"I'd be good as new if you hadn't blistered my back into tatters this morning," said Cheever. His eyes betrayed him, though; his good cheer was nothing more than a thin, forced mask.

"Or you might still be broiling," said Zabdiel. "Sit still, man, long enough for me to take your pulse. You're worse than a two-year-old." The fever had entirely gone off; his pulse was normal. He drew his friend to the window to inspect his face: there were three or four flecks on his forehead.

"The eruption's begun," said Cheever.

"It has," nodded Boylston.

"How long before you'll know whether it's from the inoculation?"

Or from Sarah. They both recognized that implication.

"A day or two," said Zabdiel.

Cheever gave him a wan smile. "It's not me I'm worried about," he said. His face pinched. "Come and see Sarah."

In a darkened chamber upstairs, she lay moaning on the bed, her breath rasping in her throat. Her blisters had begun thickening into pustules two days ago, but still they were filling and spreading. If it went on much longer at this rate, thought Zabdiel, she would certainly flux in her face, and possibly over her body as well. Worse, he discovered that the sores in her nose and mouth had fluxed that morning, while he was stuck chattering in the Town House.

"I thought I could help," said Cheever from the doorway. "But I can't touch her, I can't even breathe near her, without putting her in agony." He stopped and looked away. When he started again, his voice was harsh and low. "When I come near her now, she shudders. When I drip water down her throat, she screams. But if I don't give her water, she'll die. *I can't help her, Zabdiel.*"

Zabdiel laid his hand on his friend's shoulders. "You're doing all any man can do," he said quietly. "Far more than most would dare."

It was all the comfort he could give.

* * *

At 4:00 P.M. sharp, Mr. Cooke called the meeting back to order and gave the floor once again to Dr. Douglass.

"This afternoon, gentlemen, I should like to begin by offering a case of conscience—merely as food for thought, since it is properly the purview of ministers. Smallpox, now, has been recognized for many thousands of years as a divine scourge, revealing the wrath of God Almighty and goading the wicked into repentance. Is it a Christian's endeavor to wrest that rod so lightly from the hand of Providence?"

Boylston studied Dr. Douglass for a moment. "May a Christian not employ new medicines, humbly giving thanks to God for his good Providence in revealing new discoveries to a miserable and suffering world? By your argument," he said, "you condemn all of progress in medicine as unchristian."

Behind his desk, Mr. Cooke sighed. "Let us set aside theology for the moment, until we might convene a more appropriate gathering of experts."

Dr. Douglass did his best to keep his scowl to himself: would both Cooke and Clark undercut him all day? "My intent exactly," he said, shifting directions. "Let us return to the subject of more worldly experience, on which Mr. Boylston has based much of his evidence. I now offer you the testimony of another man with firsthand knowledge of the operation."

Some men had been drowsing, and two had frankly sunk into postprandial naps. Now heads swiveled; eyes snapped to attention. *Who else was messing with inoculation?*

"*Monsieur le docteur Laurence Dalhonde*, may I ask you to step forward?"

A coolly elegant man rose and made his way onto the floor in a gentle cloud of lavender. The heat had wilted many of the men in the room, staining their dark suits even darker with perspiration. But Dr. Dalhonde did not appear to have sweated so much as a drop.

"Dr. Dalhonde, how long have you been practicing medicine?"

"*S'il vous plaît,*" he said with icy hauteur, "*je préfère parler le français.*" *If you don't mind, I prefer to speak French.* A refugee from the religious persecution in France, he kept close within the French community. He had never bothered to learn much English, which he regarded as a boorish language.

"*Très bien,*" said Dr. Douglass smoothly. "I will translate." Not for nothing had he spent those years studying in Paris, he thought. He repeated his question.

"I have been practicing for thirty years or thereabouts," answered Dr. Dalhonde.

"Have you ever practiced inoculation?"

The doctor's look of horror needed no translation. *"Non,"* he replied with contempt. *"Jamais."*

In spite of himself, a small smile tickled the corners of Dr. Douglass's mouth. "When did you first encounter this infamous practice?"

"Twenty-five years ago," said Dr. Dalhonde.

"That's not possible," cried Boylston. "It had not—"

The room erupted into a buzz of chatter. Mr. Cooke rapped the desk his gavel.

Boylston took a step toward the selectman. "But—"

Mr. Cooke cut him off. "Dr. Boylston, you had your say this morning. You will have your say again later this afternoon. Just now, however, we wish to hear Dr. Dalhonde."

Dr. Boylston made one more move to speak.

"Uninterrupted, if you please," specified Mr. Cooke, waving him back to his place.

Boylston gave him a curt nod, and stepped back.

"Proceed, *s'il vous plaît*," said Mr. Cooke.

With a smug bow, Dr. Douglass turned back to Dr. Dalhonde. "Perhaps, M. le Docteur, you could be so good as to describe those events."

It was delightfully damning testimony. Not from an unknown Italian Papist whiling away the years among Turks. From a respected French Calvinist standing there, flesh and blood, in front of them.

Twenty-five years earlier, it transpired, Dr. Dalhonde had been with the French army in Italy, near Cremona, when this very operation had been attempted upon no fewer than thirteen soldiers. On three of them, said Dr. Dalhonde, the operation had had no effect, but on the other ten, the results had been horrible.

"And what, monsieur," asked Dr. Douglass, "were these horrible results?"

"Death, sir. Death and destruction."

Another buzz stirred the room; again, Mr. Cooke pounded it into submission.

"Four men died in agony. Another six barely recovered, troubled for life with swellings and tumors in the glands of the throat."

"And was that your only experience with inoculation?"

"Mais non. I experienced it a second time twenty years ago." That had been in Flanders, said Dr. Dalhonde, when the duc de Guiche had consigned a captain of the dragoons to his care. The man had been suffering terribly from the smallpox, truly terribly, covered not just with pocks, but with boils and ulcers. "He grasped my coat," said Dr. Dalhonde, shaking

his head at the memory, "and cried out piteously in these very words: 'Ten years ago I was inoculated five or six times'—"

"*That's impossible,*" Boylston burst out once more, loosing catcalls from the rim of the room.

"*Silence,*" roared Mr. Cooke, rapping furiously with his gavel. "One further peep, Dr. Boylston, and you will be dismissed from this meeting. Is that clear?"

Boylston bowed, and Dr. Dalhonde picked up the thread of his story. " 'Ten years ago,' said this poor captain, 'I was inoculated five or six times, but the cursed invention had no effect. Must I therefore perish? Can you do nothing for me?' "

Revulsion chiseling his face, Dr. Dalhonde paused to glare at Boylston.

"Alas," he continued, "I could not. The man survived: but some of the ulcers never left him. One of them, on his arm—just where he said he had endured this diabolical operation—lamed him for life."

A sigh trailed through the room.

Dr. Dalhonde did not wait for Dr. Douglass's next prompt. "I had one final encounter with this diabolical procedure, only a few years afterward. In Spain, at the Battle of Almanza in 1707. Smallpox was eating through the army with such speed and strength that veteran soldiers who scorned to fear battle were quaking in their boots. At last, terror drove two Muscovites to dare this operation.

"One had no reaction at all. The other had a light smallpox and then recovered. Six weeks later, however, he was seized with a frenzy. His entire body swelled until he died. At first, they believed it was poisoning, so two of the personal physicians of the king of Spain, and a third who was in the entourage of His Royal Highness, le duc d'Orleans, opened the body. His lungs had ulcerated, which convinced them that it was no new poison, but the slow working of that previous infection."

"*Merci,* M. le Docteur," said Dr. Douglass, through the muttering swirling around them. "*Merci beaucoup.*"

Dr. Dalhonde bowed and retreated to his seat.

Dr. Douglass, meanwhile, fixed the company with the glare of a falcon. "Let us review the salient points of the doctor's eloquent testimony.

"Manifestly, inoculation maims and kills. Not always, you will notice, immediately, but sometimes as much as six weeks, or even years, later. Mr. Boylston has painted grand dreams of success, but all he can really tell you is that he has not killed anyone yet—though by his own admission, he has come close. His son and two slaves are alive a month later. But who can say where they will be in another month's time? In a year? Ten years?"

The company was silent; Boylston stared rigidly forward.

"And what profit is promised in return for this risk?" Dr. Douglass continued. "It is a shield, the inoculator has said, that may save extravagant thousands. But Dr. Dalhonde has given eyewitness testimony that it is not: one of his own patients who suffered the operation numerous times came to him deathly ill of the natural smallpox. By which we may conclude that it not only leaves one as vulnerable as a newborn, but considerably worse: covered with ulcers that rot limbs to the core."

He paused for a breath, and Boylston jumped in. "If people had had their limbs rotting off, sir, or had been dying, or proved liable to smallpox after inoculation, I ask you—I ask you all—is it conceivable that this operation could have grown in popularity in such a great city as Constantinople for forty long years?

"Against this practice, you recount secondhand stories that make no sense with respect to the evidence given by no lesser body than the Royal Society. Let me make a counteroffer: In addition to the three patients you have heard about, who have already recovered, I have inoculated seven more persons, whose rashes have not yet come out."

Gasps of outrage shivered through the room like arrows, but he ignored them till they fell away. "I invite all you to visit these inoculated patients as they progress through their illness." Jeers and gibes tossed upward into the dome. Boylston glanced at Mr. Cooke, but he made no effort to quell the noise, so Boylston raised his voice to speak through it. "What makes this practice so valuable, in my opinion, is that it offers an escape from the violence, rage, and hazard of the disease taken in the natural way."

Around him, the hooting died. "Before you condemn inoculation out of hand, compare for yourselves the experience of these patients with that of the many poor souls suffering smallpox in the natural way."

"I cannot say I recommend such a course," said Dr. Douglass from behind Boylston, "due to the danger of spreading infection."

"How?" cried Boylston, spinning around in frustration.

Dr. Douglass smiled. "Let me explain: Dr. Dalhonde has testified that inoculation produces many kinds of sores, beyond pocks. It is not just the existence of such sores that must concern us, but their location, their nature, and their consequences." He lowered his voice, so that men had to crane forward to hear him. "Some of the sores are not pocks, but swellings and tumors in the glands of the groin, armpits, and neck."

He imagined his voice stretching long and razor sharp; he cooled it to ice to deliver the coup de grace. "The very places," Douglass continued, "where one finds the sores of the black plague."

A sigh, a little breath, came out came from all thirty men ringed around him at once. Fear shirred the air with a vision of streets stacked with flyblown corpses gnawed by starving dogs, of children turning their backs on parents and parents thrusting children from their doors. The smallpox, true, could kill whole villages and towns with equal virulence, especially in this new world, but smallpox was a disease they knew. The plague, in Boston, was unknown save in nightmares.

Not in France, though. Was it not devastating Marseilles and Aix-en-Provence? *And wasn't France the very place that Dr. Dalhonde had encountered inoculation? Were the two indeed connected?*

Two clouds of death, one of yellow-white sores, the other purple-black, seemed to take shape and hover in the dome overhead; slowly, they began to stream and stretch toward one another, in a perfect, whirling storm of devastation.

Dr. Douglass kept his eyes on Boylston. With mounting glee, he watched him fit the steps of Dr. Douglass's masterful argument together. Watched him link this assault with the carefully laid trail of articles in the *Boston News-Letter*. Watched him move from the paper to its owner, editor, and chief writer, John Campbell, another Scot. Watched him surmise the sly ease with which Dr. Douglass had slipped such "news" into Campbell's insatiable maw during the half-drunken cheer of the Scots Charitable Society, meeting in an upper room at the Green Dragon.

"Are you suggesting, sir" croaked Boylston, "that the operation of inoculation *causes* the plague?"

"You have made the leap yourself," said Dr. Douglass.

"Ridiculous!" exclaimed Boylston. "Excessively ridiculous!"

"Not according to Timonius and Pylarinus, in whom you have otherwise put such trust. Both say that inoculation can produce the very abscesses, swellings, and tumors that Dr. Dalhonde has witnessed."

"And they both insist they are rare," Boylston retorted. "And neither makes any mention of the plague whatsoever."

"Perhaps," said Dr. Douglass, "they did not need to in Constantinople, where the plague can kill as many as a hundred thousand people in a year."

The intake of breath was audible. Of all the world's queenly cities, Constantinople was the one most haunted by the plague. It was also the city where inoculation had originated. Was this not further evidence that the two were linked?

"One disease does not transform into another," said Boylston, his anger at last making him reckless. "You might as well say that inoculation turns men into women."

This time, Dr. Douglass noted with satisfaction, his flippancy was greeted with silence.

"Indeed, sir?" Dr. Douglass smoothed his voice to glassy calm. "On what grounds do you say so?"

"Lots of diseases cause glandular swellings," said Boylston. "If you begin shouting *plague* at every glandular swelling in the country, you'll be chasing a thousand people a week."

"Have you ever seen a case of the plague?"

Boylston caught his breath. "No, I have not."

"Not one? Not one and twenty?" sneered Dr. Douglass.

"None," said Boylston.

"Then you have no grounds for making such a statement," said Dr. Douglass briskly. "A spark in one of your inoculated patients might escape your attention until our whole town was burning with a fire that would make this plague of smallpox look like a child's bonfire on the beach."

He turned from Boylston to the men. He began his final assault quite gently, as if he regretted what he must say. "Unfortunately, as you have seen, Mr. Boylston's experiment proves to be quite flawed. He has based it, as he admits, on articles that appeared in the Royal Society's *Philosophical Transactions*. Unfortunately, he failed to recognize that they were meant as no more than virtuoso amusements.

"I do not blame Dr. Mather in this," he added. "No doubt the reverend has operated all along under a pious and charitable design of Doing Good." He inflected his voice in the merest shadow of a Mather imitation. *Yes—a smile or two lifted at the mockery, and not just among the Scots.* "Even the best of men have some foible, and that of Dr. Mather is credulity in his amateur zeal for medicine." He hardened his voice.

"But what should we say of Mr. Boylston, who professes to practice the medical arts?" He shook his head. "Mr. Boylston has displayed not only credulity but criminal rashness. This sort of quackery is only fit for a stage in a country market town; he defends it with nothing more than the hearsay of old Greek women and African slaves.

"In short, he is mischievously propagating infection, not just anywhere, but in the market square at the very heart of town. Already he has convinced seven hapless souls to risk their lives and health on the basis of a few scanty experiments. How many more can we let him infect? *And with what?*"

Boylston opened his mouth to speak, but Mr. Cooke brought his gavel down. "Gentlemen," he said, "I think we have heard enough. The time has come when I must beg you to consult among yourselves, weighing carefully all the evidence you have heard here today. The selectmen would like to have your recommendation in deciding a proper course of action."

Politely but firmly, Boylston was requested to withdraw to the anteroom. Barely a quarter of an hour passed before he was recalled.

Dr. Douglass could not look at him, for fear of trumpeting his triumph aloud. Instead, he watched Mr. Cooke smooth the sheet he had written out with such care and forethought the day before. It had passed, with no emendations.

Fixing Boylston with a baleful stare, Mr. Cooke announced, "On the subject of inoculation, sir, the doctors of this town have made the following recommendation to the selectmen." He looked back down and read:

"In considering the operation called inoculation: it appears by numerous instances first, that it has proved the death of many persons soon after the operation and brought distempers upon many others which have in the end proved deadly to them.

"Second, that the natural tendency of infusing such malignant filth into the mass of blood is to corrupt and putrify it, and if there be not a sufficient discharge of that malignity at the place of incision, or elsewhere, it lays a foundation for many dangerous diseases.

"Third, that the operation tends to spread and continue the infection in a place longer than it might otherwise be.

"Fourth, that the continuing the operation among us is likely to prove of most dangerous consequence."

Mr. Cooke looked up at Boylston. "Your fellow physicians, in other words, have deemed the operation so wicked as to be criminal. In consideration of which, the selectmen have unanimously agreed that should you persist in this practice, we will have no choice but to charge you with felony poisoning and deliberate spreading of infection." Boylston's face could have been carved from stone. "Furthermore, should any of your patients come to grief, we will be forced to pursue a charge of murder."

The last word rang through the silent room.

In the speaker's chair, Dr. Clark stirred and stood. "You have, sir, put this town at the gravest risk. Some might say you have betrayed the noblest goals of our profession, to heal and not to harm. It is fervently to be hoped that you will abide by these resolutions."

At last Boylston stirred. With stiff courtesy, he bowed to Mr. Cooke and again to the gathered company. "Thank you, gentlemen," he said stonily, "for your consideration. Should any of you wish to gather further information at first hand, my offer of visitation still stands." The recoil was visible. "Good day." With that, he turned on his heel and strode out.

Zabdiel drove himself down the stairs the way he had once, as a boy, driven himself up from deep water toward air and glittering light just as his lungs were on the point of explosion. Down, down, down, he went, through a gauntlet of waiting men whose silence turned to the hissing of serpents as he passed; the news was spreading fast. Down through the doors and into the street.

The late afternoon light was fading under the burden of ever longer, thicker shadows. Thankfully, there was no mob lying in wait outside. A side effect, he thought wryly, of the selectmen's need to keep this meeting secret, so as to heighten the ambush. At this point, he would take whatever accidental good he could find in the world.

Across the street, though, one woman did turn and step toward him. Esther Webb, whose parents and uncle he had inoculated three days before. Her face lit with hope as she hurried across to him.

He thought of Cheever's early flecks, and Sarah's grotesque agony.

"Esther," he said, seizing by her shoulders, "listen to me. I cannot inoculate you as we planned." He saw her hopes fall again, as she read disaster on his face. "They will try me for murder," he rasped. "You must take your brother and sister and leave now. Anywhere. Tonight. It may not yet be too late." She felt limp in his hands. He shook her. *"Do you understand?"*

How could she? The full weight of understanding was only now beginning to settle on him. The selectmen had threatened him with a death sentence if he were to continue inoculating. But others faced a death sentence if he were not to inoculate. *Others.* Not just a faceless ten or twenty, or even a hundred, who might have been saved: The young woman who stood there in front of him. The young woman whom he had refused to inoculate earlier, who had undertaken to nurse her parents through the inoculated pox with the full understanding that she, too, was to be inoculated in turn, tomorrow.

Terror winged across her face. Pulling away from him, she spun on her heel and melted into the shadows.

He stood there for a moment, empty and shaking, and then he turned for home.

Up in his bedroom, he stared dully out the bedroom window, watching the boys at play in the garden. An hour later, he was still there, though the boys were not.

Jack knocked and rescued the untouched supper tray. On his way out, he paused at the door. "I heard what they said in the Town House," he offered.

Oh, yes, he'd heard it: "The greatest race of liars on the earth." That had whirled through the entire black community about five minutes after the steward—a man who had worked fifteen scrupulous years to buy his freedom, and another ten to rise into the stewardship—had managed to snort it out over his own dinner.

"I heard they don't like your evidence," Jack continued. "I hope you remember, you got plenty of more evidence coming. It just ain't all the way cooked yet. So I hope you consider your own advice."

"What advice?"

"Now we wait," said Jack.

"Now we wait," repeated Zabdiel, as if they were words he'd never heard before. At the dim end of a long summer dusk, the garden was mysteriously pale, a world of gray and silver, of columbine and gillyflowers and tall foxglove, all glowing like will-o'-the-wisps caught out of time. It would do Esther no good to wait, unless she could be pressed upon to do it elsewhere. Or unless he went ahead and inoculated her anyway.

Traces of citrus and anise from his patches of lemon balm and sweet cicely drifted through the casement. He smelled, too, the rich brown fragrance of his horses. And there—fainter but still pungent, a too-sweet scent of nausea that took him a moment to place. He had been riding, when he smelled it. Thinking of little but wind and the sound of thundering hooves. And smallpox. *That was it:* the night ride, when he had decided to inoculate Tommy.

Just beyond the gate that led out onto the Neck, he had passed by the creak and clank of the gallows. And he had smelled Joseph Hanno, rotting in the gibbet after being hanged for murder.

⚜ 4 ⚜

THE CASTLE OF MISERY

Newgate Prison, London
July 24, 1721

SHE had been dreaming of a green place, filled with the sound of sweet running water. She did not want to wake up. Refused to wake up, until someone kicked her in the ribs for the third time, seized the irons shackling her legs, and began dragging her toward the door, scraping her skin raw against the lice layered like thick crawling seashells between her body and the floor.

She fought like a wildcat in the first few minutes of wakefulness, blinking in the glare of the stinking torch. This place was hell, but the place they were taking her to was worse. Pawnbroker's daughter, pickpocket, whore—native of London's infamously fetid and windowless tenements—nineteen-year-old Elizabeth Harrison was no green girl. She was not queasy about turning tricks, especially when it would buy her a hot meal, a few hours' sleep in some clean, safe place, or at the very least, the oblivion of gin.

Her father, her mother, and one, possibly two, brothers—she wasn't really sure—had preceded her in this evil place, ending their days with a drunken ride out to the gallows at Tyburn. By the time she had followed in their footsteps, she knew a thing or two about making the best of this fearsome place. She'd been happy to attend to the needs of John Cawthery, the blustery highwayman turned jailer's toady. Wardsmen, they called the felons who were part guard, part prisoner. He, too, was a felon, eventually bound for Tyburn, but meanwhile he had been given relatively clean, airy cell, all to himself, on the top floor, and a tab at the bar, in exchange for duty as a turnkey.

But the night before, he had played cards too hard and too long in the cellar taproom, and had lost her to a mean-eyed lout who was playing for his entire ward, Stone Hold, the deepest, meanest dungeon in the prison. As Cawthery steadily lost, she steadily drank enough raw gin to cast her so deep in the tapsters' debt that she'd never climb out. At the time, she hadn't cared for anything but some way to forget that that she was being bet—being sold—by a jailer to a roomful of murderers to do with as they pleased in a crowd. It did not help to know that the man who had won her had won his spot on the floor of the Stone Hold by slitting the throat of a whore in the very midst of country matters.

So she fought.

In the scrabble, a thumb came her way; she bit down hard. "Lizzy!" roared Cawthery, walloping her across the cheek. The blow momentarily blinded her and dissolved every bone in her body to jelly. "I ain't taking you to the boys, you damned 'ellcat," he whispered in her ear. "I found us another way out. Maybe all the way out, if you get my drift. Any more of my blood spills, though, an' I waltz out o' this room without sayin' another word."

She shook the floating sparks from her eyes and tried to glare at him.

He went on. "There's a doctor wot wants to see some likely-looking prisoners—for some scheme that may earn them as partakes a pardon."

She shook her head again, this time to jostle his words into sense.

"A pardon, Lizzy!" he snarled. "Rumor has it, there's royal highnesses involved."

"Royal highness of what?" she said thickly. "Rotgut?"

"Aw, Lizzy, shut up. The king 'isself want you at Kensington, for all's I know. Just tell me: 'ave you 'ad the smallpox?"

"Who is it wants to know?"

"I'm doin' you a favor, silly bitch. Or tryin' to. But it all rides on you bein' unbit as yet by the smallpox," he said, reaching toward her cheek. She snapped at him again, and he snatched his hand back. He stood over her, wrestling with his temper, his fists clenching and unclenching. After a moment he spat. "You can follow me to it"—he shrugged—"or you can stay 'ere and wait for one o' the boys to fetch you to the Stone Hold." He bent and unlocked her shackles. "Your choice," he said, and turned to leave.

She frowned, searching about in her mind for the trick she was sure was there somewhere. *What could the king possibly want with a ravaged soul like her?* Whatever it was, it could not possibly be as bad as this castle of misery. She pushed herself up to a stand, and stumbled after him.

* * *

The warden himself looked on as the head jailer lined a dozen women up against one wall of a large sunny room; the sudden burst of sweet air made her a little dizzy. She squinted against the glare, and became aware of dark figures huddled in the far doorway.

"Her," said a peremptory Scottish voice, pointing at poor Mary North with a long, stiff demon claw that she only later realized was a walking stick. Mary was hustled off wailing through another door in the side wall.

"And her," said the voice. The second woman, whom Lizzy didn't know, fainted and had to be carried away.

"That's it, then," said another voice, sounding of velvet and sweet English plums. Lizzy managed to gasp in a small bit of air.

"No," said the Scottish voice. "One more," and then slowly, ever so slowly, as if it might take as long as the entire previous eighteen years of her life, she watched that claw rise to point straight at her. She went cold with fear, and lost all power to move. It did not matter; she was shoved through that door in the wake of the other two women.

It opened onto a stone corridor; holding her up between them, two guards half dragged, half carried her down the passage and into another room, empty save for a washtub, five steaming basins of water, and a short, squat bundle of disapproval that turned out to be a woman jailer. Lizzy's clothes—no more than rags, really—were removed and burned. Under the jailer's watchful eye, Lizzy scrubbed herself with harsh lye soap until her skin burned. She rinsed every hair on her body with tobacco juice—twice—and then topped it with the strange luxury of lavender oil. She was handed a lice comb, and most degradingly made to use it, naked, while the warden watched in disgusted silence.

Finally, she was bundled into a clean set of clothes, almost new, and hustled back down the passage, this time to a smaller room. This time, the watchers entered the room with her, though she was still made to stand in the far corner.

She had not known the prison contained any room of such luxury: the walls were several feet thick as they were everywhere else, but here they were pierced by tall windows streaming with golden light. Carpets softened and warmed the walls, fragrant rushes strewed the floor, and two plush armchairs huddled in the far corner near a fireplace crackling merrily with a fire that drove away the damp.

"Now, madam, here is your choice," said the Scot from one of the armchairs. "You are a convicted felon, condemned to the gallows at Tyburn. You may choose to go that direct way to your maker, or you may avail yourself of the king's mercy."

"Wot's the catch?"

The warden cuffed her from behind. "Mind your manners for the gentlemen," she growled.

"Well, 'e ain't goin' to pardon the likes o' me for no catch," she said.

Across the room, the gentleman laughed and held up a hand, staving off the warden's next blow. "The catch," he said, "is that you must allow yourself to be inoculated."

Lizzy's face furled into thought. "Wot'zat?"

"A remedy for the smallpox."

Her eyes narrowed.

"Give the gentleman your answer," said the warden impatiently.

She looked at the Scottish man. "Not meaning to be ungrateful, sir, but I wants to know wot it is you want to do to me," she said, dodging the next blow. "'Aven't I got a right to ask such a question?"

Across the room in the stiff, shabby armchair that he fervently hoped was not crawling with lice, Charles Maitland considered Mrs. Elizabeth Harrison. She was not, like so many of the others, out to trick him just for a brief crow of victory, he thought. Or perhaps she was, and just hid it better behind a pretty face—for her face was surprisingly pretty, minus the grime. At least he had been right about the light of intelligence in her eyes—which was what had drawn him to point her out of that dismal crowd, in the first place.

"I will scratch you on each arm, and insert a tiny bit of smallpox matter," he said.

Most ladies he knew, unprepared, would have shrilled in horror, and many would have fainted dead away. True, she was no lady. But she was nonetheless a young—touchingly young—woman, and her reaction surprised him. She just cocked her head and considered.

"If it works," he continued, "you'll come down with a light case of that distemper, rendering you secure from catching it in the natural way for the rest of your days. Which, if you accept the bargain, stand to stretch to a considerably greater number than if you don't."

"Wot makes you think it'll work?"

He sighed. It was a good question, to which he had no good answer. "I have seen it work on two children of the quality."

Her eyebrows shot up. "Then why should the king in 'is castle want to know about 'ow it works on the nonquality?"

"The king in his castle"—*how had she known that?*—"wishes to know whether it works steadily." He watched her register the implications—yes, she was a smart one. Much braver in the face of knowledge, he suspected, than drowning in the miasma of ignorance. She had looked skittish as a deer when first shoved in the room, but none of his revelations, stark as they were, had made her flinch. Far from it; she was growing more sure of herself with every tidbit of fact he gave her. "The king, you see, cannot in good conscience ask free men and women to risk death to satisfy his curiosity. You, though, have already been consigned to death. In his mercy, he offers you a gamble at life."

She smiled; she still had most of her teeth. "I like you, guv'nor," she said. "I thinks yer honester than most. I'll try yer med'cine."

"Straight from the fryin' pan into the fire," she growled to Cawthery later, as the six chosen felons had gathered in the Press Yard hall—as grand a place, really, as she had ever dwelt in. Clean, at least in comparison to the tenements she had grown up in. As for the wards on the common side of the prison, there was no comparison.

There were six of them in all: three women, and three men. All convicted felons, facing the gallows. Cawthery was one, she was glad enough for that, though she had little doubt that he'd trot his pardon straight back to the excitement of robbing the king's highways. Twenty-five was too old to learn new tricks, he said, and too young not to need the easy money of the old ones.

He was by no means the oldest of their little company, though. At thirty-six, Mary North granted herself the position as matriarch of their new little clan. She was to be hanged for returning to London after being transported overseas for robbing a linen draper near Cripplegate; Maryland had not agreed with her, she sniffed. She was not born to be in service, especially in such wilting heat, so she had slipped away to the docks and worked her way back home as a sailor's dolly. Unfortunately, her husband had found the bounty on her head more to his liking than sharing her widely shared bed. So here she was.

Ann Tompion was twenty-five, same as Cawthery; like Lizzy, she had been convicted of theft. Of all of them, she had taken the steepest tumble down the long stair of Fortune: her husband had once been watchmaker to old King William himself. But Mr. Tompion had died nigh on ten years ago, and his widow, who was no good with watches, had found it hard to make ends meet. So she had met her end, as the gibe went, by stealing it. John Alcock, at twenty, was in for horse theft. Richard Evans, just Lizzy's age, did not deign to give them his story.

He did not fit in with the others in any case. They had all heard that not having had smallpox was a condition of the bargain: but Evans's face had clearly been cratered and gnarled by its claws. He sat alone in a corner, sneering at the rest of them.

"As if it took talent to put pocks on your own face," needled Mrs. Tompion.

Evans responded by drinking himself into a solitary stupor.

The Royals, as they soon came to be called, were not the only prisoners in that exalted part of the prison, of course; they mingled with the lucky few who could afford to remain in the Press Yard. As space had got tighter, what with the beds reserved for the Royal Experiment, the price of the other Press-Yard beds had risen considerably. It did not endear the Royals to their fellows. Nor did the specter of pardons.

That night in the Press Yard taproom, one of the women from the women's ward taunted "Their Highnesses" mercilessly. "I'll tell you the meaning of nockle-ate, you knuckleheaded fools," she said, staring hard at Lizzy. "Them gentlemen'll drain yer blood and then drink it." She took a long, gurgling suck on her gin, for illustration. "The rest of us ain't such want-wits as to believe blabber about remedies for the smallpox. If there was such a thing—an' I ain't sayin' there is, mind you—but if there was, would they be trying it on the likes of us?"

She put both palms on the table and leaned forward. "It's virgin's blood they'll be needing—an' 'tis their own great pox they'll be curing. On'y, ain't a maid among the lot o' you, is there? So it'll all be useless." She cackled with delight and drained her gin.

"Have you seen what they done to the common room?" said someone else. "Set a rail acrosst it, like an altar rail, and lined up benches on the far side."

"Just like I tole you," said the woman, slamming her empty cup down on the table. "Them gentlemen'll hold a black mass and drain yer blood."

Lizzy ushered a pale and shaking Mary North back to bed; Ann Tompion followed, her face hard and blank. Their chamber was a plain stone room with three beds, tables, and chairs; the walls were bare but for biblical passages and scraps of verse written in charcoal. She couldn't decipher them, but Mrs. Tompion could.

"See that one?" said the watchmaker's widow, pointing. "It says, *Abandon all hope, ye who enter here.*" Then she closed her eyes and went to sleep, still tense and unmoving.

Clinging stubbornly to hope and the memory of the doctor's kind eyes, Lizzy lay awake until dawn.

❧ 5 ❧

SIGNS AND WONDERS

The North End of Boston
August 1, 1721

AT the top of his house on Ship Street, Dr. Cotton Mather stood
at his library window, glaring at the people scuttling by below and
the masts bristling along the wharves across the street. Beyond that
brooded the ocean, from whence had come so many of Boston's fortunes
and misfortunes. The contagion that was its most recent curse was spreading with gathering speed, and so was the fear of it, like a rolling black fog
that made old friends stumble blindly past one another in the street.

Already, the town lay under dreadful judgments, but it was ripening for
more, with its monstrous and crying wickedness, the vile abuse that it
hurled at him. And for what? He had done nothing but instruct the physicians how to save many precious lives. He smiled in vengeful triumph: they
meant to frighten him, no doubt. But all they did was to give him the glory
of being crucified with Christ.

A knock jarred him from his reverie. "Come," he rasped.

The door cracked opened slightly, but no one entered. He strode over
and swept it back against the wall. Sammy stood ghostlike in the doorway,
his face pale. Tears coursed silently down his cheeks.

He pulled the boy inside and made him sit down.

"It's Will," his son stammered at last.

Cold prickled over Dr. Mather's neck, followed by waves of heat. Will
Charnock was Sammy's seventeen-year-old best friend, his chamber mate
at Harvard. John Charnock's second son, just as Sammy was his second
son. Even after returning home from Cambridge, the two boys had spent
almost every waking moment together.

"He broke out in a fever last night," Sammy said miserably. "Dr. Clark says it is the smallpox." Something fell through the pit of Dr. Mather's belly, and the world went dark for a moment. When his eyes cleared, he found his son on his knees before him. "I want to try your new operation, Father," he begged.

Dr. Mather recoiled. *"Not mine."*

"Please, Father," wailed Sammy, his voice breaking with terror. "Let me be inoculated."

How could he refuse? How, on the other hand, could he agree? Searching desperately for some way between yes and no, he dropped one hand on his son's head. "Let us pray," he said. As he once had with Lizzy, he now spent hours on his knees with Sammy, supplicating the Lord. When the trembling and weeping had finally subsided, he stood.

Sammy, still on his knees, awaited his father's blessing. "May I send Obadiah for Dr. Boylston?"

"No." Dr. Mather drew in a sharp breath and said with more calm, "Not yet."

Sammy opened his mouth to protest, but Dr. Mather raised a warning hand. "I will take it into consideration," he said.

Sammy bowed his head, and rose to go. At the door, he paused. "Please hurry," he whispered, without looking back. Then he was gone.

After giving his son just enough time to withdraw to his own chamber, Dr. Mather clapped his wig on his head, tugged it straight, and departed.

Perhaps Sammy is mistaken, he thought as he strode toward the Charnocks'. *Perhaps Will's malady is no more than a headache and a stomachache. A short, sharp joust with bad oysters or spoiled meat.*

It was not. Sammy had been right.

Dr. Mather left the Charnocks' in a daze, hardly knowing what he was doing or where he was going, aware only of Sammy's cry spiraling through his mind: *Please, Father, let me be inoculated.*

If he should die by receiving it in the common way, thought Dr. Mather, *how can I answer it?* He resolved to allow it. Two strides later, a curse hurled from a high window across the street cut through his resolve: *On the other side, if I suffer this Operation upon the Child, our people—who have Satan remarkably filling their Hearts and their Tongues—will go on with infinite Prejudices against me and my Ministry. If he should happen to miscarry under it, my Condition would be insupportable.* Round and round these threats chased each other, until his feet took him, almost of their own accord, to the house of his father, Increase Mather.

The encounter was not one of their best. He went for advice; he was showered with icy disappointment instead.

Back at home Dr. Mather shut himself in his library as the light waned and rain spattered the windows. *Full of distress about Sammy,* he scrawled into his diary. The whole argument seesawed once more through his mind. On the verge of hunching beneath a load of despair, he straightened his back and stabbed at the paper. *His Grandfather advises that I bring the Lad into the new Method of Safety, and that I keep the whole Proceeding private.* He sighed and rubbed his temples. How did his father expect him to arrange this? Getting Dr. Boylston to operate in private was the least of his problems. First, he would have to get him to resume inoculating at all.

My GOD, I know not what to do, but my Eyes are unto Thee!

His eyes were also upon Dr. Boylston: for nearly three weeks now, Dr. Mather had kept a close watch on the doctor and his inoculated patients. It had not been hard; John Helyer was one of his parishioners. It was no more than Dr. Mather's duty to visit him every day. If he chose to head north each morning the very moment that he saw Dr. Boylston ride by the house on his own way to Salutation Alley, his man Jack in tow, who was to know or care?

Dr. Boylston was a man of habit; he usually stopped first at Mr. Cheevers's house. By dawdling either at the Helyers', or on his way there, Dr. Mather now and again met the doctor, coming or going. Always, the minister asked about the progress of the experiment. No one need search any farther than his transcriptions of Timonius and Pylarinus to explain his eager interest. Furthermore, every last one of the inoculees was either currently his parishioner, or had once been, until swarming off to form the upstart New North: of course he would ask about them. Nothing could be more natural.

Mr. Cheever sped through the distemper with startling speed; his inoculation had been an unequivocal success. Most of his sparse scabs had already crumbled away. Under his unceasing care, Sarah Cheever had clung to life; against all expectation, she had turned a corner, and her distemper was subsiding. Quietly, Dr. Boylston said that he thought her chances of surviving were strengthening.

John Helyer's main problem was nerves; he had had palpitations as the eruption broke out, but the spread had slowed and stopped at no more than half a hundred pocks. Since then, he had subsided into calm, if not downright smug, cheer. One street over, old Mr. John Webb had rebounded from an early bout of faintness, probably also attributable to nerves. Mrs. Deborah Webb remained fretful and fragile, to be sure, but even the family rolled their eyes at this, at least when she wasn't looking: that was Mrs. Webb's normal state of being. Except for Mrs. Esther, her daughter; much against Dr. Boylston's advice, she had tended her mother and father with stubborn gentleness from beginning to end.

At home in Dock Square, reported the doctor, his son John's light sprinkling of pocks was scabbing over. Having been forbidden milk after it gave him nosebleeds, the boy was grimacing his way through teas of all kinds that his father and Moll could dream up, while concocting more and more outlandish schemes to steal slices of ham and chicken from the kitchen. The decree of meatlessness rankled even more than the ban on milk. Unfortunately, after the first two nosebleeds, nothing escaped the kitchen without Moll's notice.

Moll, of course, was perfectly well and had been for some time. Her incisions, like Jack's, had quickly dried up, leaving only the smallest of scars.

Dr. Mather was by no means Dr. Boylston's only observer. Ambush over, Dr. Douglass had hurled his accusations of poison and plague into the press, writing a letter to the *Boston News-Letter* and signing it W. Philanthropos—William, lover of mankind. Dr. Mather winced just thinking about it; there had not been a single line in the whole missive that had the least pretension toward love or charity. It was not even useful as a mask of anonymity: everyone in town recognized the rant as Dr. Douglass's.

It was not so much an argument against the operation as one long snarling mockery of Dr. Boylston. *A mere operator*, Dr. Douglass had called him, *an undertaker, a cutter for the stone*. As if there were something shameful in that! *Illiterate*, he'd sneered, *ignorant, confused, rash, mischievous, negligent, inconsiderate*. Why Mr. John Campbell had agreed to print such unmannerliness Dr. Mather couldn't fathom.

Kind Reverend Colman, usually tolerant to a fault, had crackled with righteous indignation. He composed a dignified reply to Mr. Misanthropos—he did not deserve the name Philanthropos, said Mr. Colman—and canvassed Boston's other ministers. If they agreed with his defense of Dr. Boylston—a man whom heaven had adorned with remarkable gifts of tenderness, courage, and skill, as well as a gentle and dexterous hand—they could join him in signing it.

Not surprisingly, the pastors of the First Church and King's Chapel— Mr. Cook's and Dr. Douglass's parishes, respectively—declined. But the pastors of three other churches—the Old North, the New North, and the Old South—consented. Dr. Mather's father graced it with his signature, *Increase Mather*, right at the top, passing the pen to his son and pointing right where to sign. Then came Mr. Colman, followed by Thomas Prince, pastor of the Old South Church, and John Webb, pastor of the upstart

New North. Mr. Webb's father, uncle, and aunt had trusted in Dr. Boylston; his nieces and nephews had been barred from the operation by the selectmen's ban. He looked as if he would prefer to sign in fire and blood, but had settled for a great flourish. Right at the bottom, William Cooper, Mr. Colman's assistant pastor at the Brattle Square Church, squeezed in his name.

Mr. Musgrave published Mr. Colman's letter in his *Boston Gazette*—rival of Mr. Campbell's *Boston News-Letter* and the closest thing there was to an official newspaper. Just above it appeared Dr. Boylston's open invitation to the justices, selectmen, and other gentlemen of the town to visit his inoculated patients at their convenience.

In answer, Mr. Campbell's paper went silent. Dr. Mather smiled to himself. A discreet delegation had gone to the governor, intimating just how dangerous it was to allow this sort of defamation in print: if it could be directed at Dr. Boylston, who might be next? The governor had taken the point. It had hardly been necessary to hint that Dr. Clark, Mr. Cook, and the other selectmen were behind this attack—or at least in tacit support.

To make his point, in turn, the governor had not had to do anything other than shut his mouth: official news in the form of unofficial gossip was the lifeblood of papers like Mr. Campbell's. The next time the publisher had stopped by the governor's office for his weekly exchange of gossip, the governor treated him to polite silence. A few days later, when Dr. Douglass had slapped another Philanthropos letter into Mr. Campbell's hands at a meeting of the Scots Charitable Society, Mr. Campbell wordlessly handed it back.

He could not, however, call back the fear his paper had already sparked: having devoured Dr. Douglass's lies, the whole town was muttering about the plague.

On August 4, Dr. Mather ran into Dr. Boylston at the house of Samuel and Mary Hunt at the foot of Salutation Alley, next door to the inn owned by Mary's father, John Langdon. The Hunt children had fallen ill in the night, and Mrs. Hunt was distraught; she did not want to leave her babies in anyone else's care, but she had never had the distemper herself. Dr. Mather owed the Hunts a debt of loyalty; Mary and her husband Samuel had both refused the familial pressures to shift their worship to the New North Church when it had splintered off from his congregation. He spent a great long time with her that morning, instilling a proper sense of resignation to Providence.

Dr. Boylston instilled some drops of laudanum in a small glass of wine and had her drink it down, which no doubt also helped restore calm.

"How does the experiment with inoculation proceed?" asked Dr. Mather, as they were leaving.

"I am all but certain that all ten of my inoculated patients will survive," said Dr. Boylston with obvious relief and a little whiff of pride. "Unscathed, no less. I am not ready to shout it from the rooftops, but I can tell you, I am in great hopes that inoculation will prove a success."

"It p-proves a success, you say?" *Slow down*, he barked to himself.

"*Almost*," specified Dr. Boylston, but Dr. Mather dismissed the qualification.

"M-might it be arguable, then, that it is not only lawful, but your bounden duty to make use of such a God-granted weapon?"

Dr. Boylston threw the minister a sharp look. "I will not inoculate again until I am sure that everyone I have already operated on has passed safely through the distemper."

"When will that be?"

"A few days yet, I expect. Speaking of weapons, I should like to discuss with you the possibility of publishing your transcriptions of Timonius and Pylarinus. I believe we must counter some of these spreading lies. I have seen no trace of plague, but the natural smallpox settles in more thickly every day." He looked out to sea for a moment and then turned back to Dr. Mather. "Salutation Alley has become a pit of Lamentation."

"*A voice was heard in Ramah*," said Dr. Mather with a grim smile, "*lamentation, and bitter weeping: Rachel, weeping for her children, refused to be comforted, because they were not* . . . I will consider it. How is Mrs. Esther Webb?" he asked as a parting shot. "Is she still well?"

G.D., Dr. Mather wrote later that day, quite satisfied with the foundation he had laid. *I will allow the persecuted Physician to publish my Communications from the Levant about the Small-Pox and supply him with some further Armour to conquer the Dragon.*

He would help the man. If he happened to instill in him the sense of a favor owed, well, so much the better. He had not thought this scheme up. He had not sought it out. The situation had come to him. It was the will of the Lord.

Cotton Mather rose early the next day. *G.D.* he informed his diary. *The Condition of my pious Barber and his Family calls for my particular consideration.* Edward Langdon, barber and periwigmaker, was a gallant young pillar of the Old North Church. He was also Mary Hunt's brother. That poor family, centered on their father's inn, was at the eye of a foul, spitting storm.

Dr. Mather's consideration took the form of a question that he scattered here and there through the neighborhood: *Why should Dr. Boylston hold off any longer?* That very day, the families of Salutation Alley came together to discuss the issue. Edward and his brother Josiah, and Mary and Samuel Hunt were there. The other Langdon sisters, Joanna and Elizabeth, along with their husbands, Grafton Feveryear and William Pitman. Their neighbor, Bill Larrabee. The publican, Joseph Dodge, and another neighbor, Ebenezer Thornton. Bill Merchant came, but dissented; Benjamin Bronsdon declined the invitation. But that was not a surprise; he was Mr. Cooke's brother-in-law.

The Webbs did not come, but they agreed to let the delegation know when Dr. Boylston arrived at their house.

By the time he left, a small knot of men was waiting for him at the Webbs' gate.

"We would like you to begin inoculating again," they said.

He gave a short laugh. "I already have."

Zabdiel had wrestled with himself all night long. He had not known what he would do even as he turned up the lane. But at his first stop, he had given in to Sarah's wan behest, and inoculated the Cheevers' servant lad. And then he had inoculated Esther Webb. He had put them both in the way of smallpox; he owed them some chance at deliverance. Now that he was certain it was deliverance, and not a dream.

He had not meant to reenter the fray with quite such a crowd, but he agreed to ride a few doors up the street and inoculate Mrs. Hunt, whose three children were ill, and Mr. Larrabee, whose wife and twins were sick.

It mattered a great deal to them, he told himself. But he had no more to lose: they could only hang him once.

The very next day, a Sunday, Esther Webb flushed with the first fever of smallpox. It was patent to everyone, the Webbs included, that she had taken the disease in the natural way. *While nursing her inoculated parents and grandfather,* screamed the naysayers. *He's killed her. Or just as good as.*

The word rippled out in streams of fire and anger. She was dying, she was dead, her arms and legs had rotted to bags of jelly, she had been carried off by the plague. Crowds gathered and nipped once more at Cotton Mather: scuttled through the church doors, hounded him home. *It is the Hour and Power of Darkness on this miserable Town,* he scribbled in his diary, his eyes flashing. *I need an uncommon Assistance from Above that I may not miscarry by any froward or angry Impatience or fall into any of the common Iniquities of Lying and Railing and Malice: or be weary of well-doing and of overcoming Evil with Good.*

Dr. Boylston was similarly besieged. He did not ask for help, but whenever he stirred out of doors, a Langdon or a Webb somehow seemed to be riding his direction; if it were evening, there were often two or three of them.

On Monday, a new cry blended in with the other screams and calls that crisscrossed the marketplaces: Courant! *Get your* New-England Courant *here! New England's Newest in News and Wit!*

A mere slip of a boy somehow managed to create quite a racket while staggering beneath loads of newspapers so freshly printed that they were still damp. Josiah Franklin's youngest boy, Ben. Fifteen and gawky with growth, but so enamored of a new scheme for eating a vegetable diet that he actually ate no meat: he'd made a bargain with his brother to pocket half the money that would have gone for his board and feed himself. Some said that he fed himself on less than half of it and saved the rest to buy books. Sometimes the curious thrust their noses against the windows of the printing house, just to see the wonder of a boy who ate no meat, and survived.

He'd been his brother's apprentice for three years, ever since James came home from England carting a printing press in 1717. Sometimes he thought that black-and-blue stripes on his back was all that he had to show for it, especially since business had been rocky after Mr. Musgrave had bought the *Gazette* and shifted the printing contract from James to one of his own relatives. Their odd-jobbing days looked to be over, though. Beneath his load, Ben gave such a great sigh of relief that he unbalanced himself and nearly toppled into a puddle.

A windfall had come their way, in the guise of a club of anti-inoculation physicians, mostly Scottish, who had sounded out James about setting up a new weekly paper. He had press, supplies, and skilled labor, James had said (Ben had made a face in the shadows). All he lacked was the writing, he said. And, of course, the financing.

Dr. Douglass had guaranteed both.

They had pulled it off in just over a week. The *New-England Courant* was not merely to be a list of official proclamations and a list of the comings and goings of ships, however. They dreamed grander dreams. The *Courant* was to be full of opinion and essays both humorous and educational; their model was nothing less than London's *Spectator*. Instead of the ghostly spectator who gave Addison and Steele's paper its name, the persona of this American paper was to be Jack-of-All-Trades.

So far, thought Ben, this Jack appeared to excel at only one trade—

crushing inoculation—but surely there would be others with time. Meanwhile, this one gave wide scope for virulent cleverness.

Dr. Douglass had provided the first essay: "A Continuation of the History of Inoculation in Boston by a Society of the Practitioners in Physick." To be truthful, there wasn't much in it that hadn't already appeared in the Philanthropos essay the *Boston News-Letter* had published; the sniping was nearly identical. But then, Dr. Douglass had written that piece too.

"*Infatuation,*" he concluded in the *Courant's* lead essay, "*is like to be as Epidemic a distemper of the mind as at present the smallpox is of the natural body.*"

Ben had his doubts. But he liked this new project for lightening James's temper.

Nothing about the *Courant* lightened Dr. Mather's temper. There were further hurried conferences among the clergy, deciding upon who should next take up the pen.

In fact, there was a needling flurry of feathers all over town as everyone who could wield a quill, it seemed, sat down to write somebody else in high dudgeon. The ministers, though, deemed it unseemly to answer such puppies themselves. Increase Mather solved the issue, declaring that his grandson Thomas Walter possessed just the combination of graceful wit, youth, and proper loyalty to the ministers (he was one) that was required. He would pen an *Anti-Courant*; they would hire Mr. Franklin to print it as well.

Mr. Walter was happy to oblige. So was Mr. Franklin, even as the anti-inoculators gathered at his printing house at the top of Queen Street, preparing to score their second blow.

Meanwhile, John Campbell wrote a rebuttal to the charge that his *Boston News-Letter* was stodgy. And up at the Salutation Inn, Joshua Cheever, John Helyer, and John and Joseph Webb gathered to defend Dr. Boylston: *Desperate diseases require desperate remedies,* they wrote. Mr. Musgrave snapped it up for his *Boston Gazette*.

On the eighth of August, Esther Webb's rash began erupting; by the ninth, it had thickened into the confluent smallpox. Not until the tenth did fever ripple through the rest of her fellow inoculees: just at the expected time. Dr. Mather had half hoped Dr. Boylston would begin scooping smallpox into hordes daily, but he was disappointed. Worried about Esther's fate, the doctor would not be hurried.

Nor would Sammy stop following his father with reproachful eyes. His friend Will Charnock was dying. Dr. Mather's own father didn't help;

you've lost the one boy—*my namesake*—to dancing and whoring, he said. Will you lose the other to death?

On the thirteenth, still on cue, Esther Webbs's luckier fellows erupted. Still, Dr. Boylston would not be hurried.

Over cakes and ale in Mr. Franklin's printing house in Queen Street, the anti-inoculation club concocted a delicious satire.

Dr. Boylston was to be commissioned as the major general in command of the Indian-fighting troops being gathered to crush the Abenaki up in Maine. His weapon would be inoculation, with which he would wantonly sow smallpox among the Indians. The doctors roared with laughter, as Ben kept their tankards full and passed the tobacco. It was too perfect, chortled Dr. Douglass: what better place for a doctor who insisted upon riding his rounds, rather than decently being driven about in a carriage?

Ben had even dared a suggestion or two himself, though ever so quietly, in the ear of one gentleman or another, when his brother wasn't listening. James did not like him to be clever. But his cleverness always found a way out. Why not arm the inoculator with something specific? A lancet and nutshell perhaps? Soon that was zipping around the circle, and had been included. Instead of a bandage box, add Pandora's box, he whispered in another ear. That, too, was incorporated.

It was Dr. Douglass, though, who proclaimed that General Inoculator and his illiterate soldiers would be allowed £10 bounty for every infected Indian who spread the disease to others; £5 would be granted for those Indians who died too soon to make themselves party to killing their fellows.

To this piece, Dr. Stewart added his first column, a filigree of horror about the plague in France.

At the time, Ben enjoyed both the fellowship and, above all, the clever argument. Delivering the paper on the fourteenth, though, he also saw confusion, distaste, and downright disgust on many readers' faces.

A tiny, prematurely wizened voice whispered in his ear that such overeagerness for argument was a bad habit. So much contradiction soured conversation—and he could already see that it also produced enmity, where there might have been friendship. Men of sense, he noted quietly to himself, seldom fell into it—except, he observed, for lawyers, university men, and men of all sorts that had been bred in Edinburgh.

On the evening of August 15, Cotton Mather sauntered north up Ship Street with his son, peering through glimmering mist and fog to look in shop windows. At the shop of Edward Langdon, barber and periwigmaker, the bow window was lined with faceless heads piled high with hair: chestnut, blond, gray, white. They paused for a desultory glance, and stepped inside.

Nothing could be more natural, nothing could be more innocent, thought Dr. Mather, than for a man and his son to duck out of a light rain into their accustomed barber shop, warm with musk-scented steam. The shelves were lined with still more wigs, along with tins of powder in various colors and scents, wig ties and ribbons, and stacks of stands and cases. Several comfortable chairs lined one wall, near a long table holding a gleaming array of basins and razors.

It was perhaps not so natural and ordinary for Mr. Langdon to whisk the two of them upstairs to the family parlor, but as no one else was in the shop, no one else was privy to that information.

Enthroned in Mr. Langdon's best armchair, Increase Mather was impatiently tapping his fingers together in a pyramid in front of his nose. He inclined his head slightly in greeting and beckoned all three of them to his chair. Dr. Mather, Sammy Mather, and Edward Langdon gathered in a tight circle around him, joining their hands in prayer.

They broke up with a hasty amen as they heard Dr. Boylston greet the servant at the door and make his way up the stairs. Increase pointed his grandson to a chair, though Sammy could hardly sit still; Cotton stalked solemnly about the room. Mr. Langdon stood by the window, as if the room had suddenly become suffocating.

Dr. Boylston registered a flash of curiosity when he walked in, but not yet suspicion. Even for a doctor accustomed to working with ministers, thought Cotton anxiously, three generations of Mathers might seem overkill for anything less than a governor's deathbed. The doctor made no comment, however, inoculating Mr. Langdon so quickly and deftly that Sammy barely had time to pale as he watched.

Dr. Boylston had already tucked his vial of poison back into his shirt and was packing up the rest of his instruments when Sammy darted out of his seat. Snatching Dr. Boylston's arm, he blurted, "Wait, sir, please."

Dr. Boylston froze; so did everyone else. Cotton did not dare glance at his father, who was no doubt pinched with displeasure at the boy's interference.

"Please, sir," said Sammy, "inoculate me."

Dr. Boylston looked to Cotton and Increase. "What do your father and grandfather say?"

Cotton began to reply, but his father cut through his stammer. "I have been hoping sir, that such an opportunity might present itself," said Increase. "There is not a moment to be lost."

Dr. Boylston's whole face radiated with sudden pleasure. He bowed. "I am honored, Reverend, by your trust. And I cannot tell you what a relief your support will be, to me and to all those who have braved the operation, and who are considering it."

His words fell like pebbles into a deep well of silence.

Mr. Langdon cleared his throat. "The Mathers, Doctor, are in an unusual position, due to their ministry. I am sure you will understand that they require an unusual degree of discretion."

Surprise blanked Dr. Boylston's face, followed by consternation and a flash of anger, quickly controlled. "Surely you cannot mean that you wish me to inoculate the boy in secret?"

Anxiety knotted around Cotton Mather's heart. Again he opened his mouth, and again his father stole the speech from his throat.

"Discretion, sir, is paramount," the elder minister pronounced.

Dr. Boylston resumed putting his things away. "I do not operate in the dark," he said. "For anyone."

Sammy dropped to his knees; his eyes were huge and dark. "Please, sir." His voice sank to a harsh whisper. "My best friend died this morning."

Dr. Boylston glared down at the boy. Cotton Mather started forward, but his father held up a hand, and he stopped.

After a long moment, Dr. Boylston looked back up, not at Increase, but at Cotton. "I will do it for the boy's sake, Reverend. As I did with my son, you must put him at grave risk daily by your visiting so many rooms thick with the contagion's poison." He shifted his eyes to Increase. "Do not ask this of me again."

Increase nodded, and Dr. Boylston drew the poison out once more, and wiped his lancet clean.

For all his desire, Sammy was not a good patient. At the first scratch of the skin, he went white and began to tremble. Watching his son, Dr. Mather, too, began to quiver. Dr. Boylston worked fast, but not fast enough. Just after he had bound up the wound on Sammy's arm, the boy fainted dead away, and his father staggered back into a chair.

"He is a delicate child," said Increase as Dr. Boylston and Mr. Langdon lifted his grandson onto the sofa. "One cut will do."

"I cannot answer for that," said Dr. Boylston tersely, waving smelling salts under the boy's nose. "If you will not follow the procedure properly, I cannot say it will work."

"It is enough," declared the elder Mather as the boy came to, moaning.

Dr. Boylston bowed. "I will send my bill in the morning," he said as he gathered up his things and took his leave; Mr. Langdon showed him out.

The two elder Mathers pretended they did not hear the voices raised in the passage as the doctor told his host exactly what he thought of that evening's subterfuge.

G.D. Cotton Mather wrote later that night. *My dear Sammy is now under the Operation of receiving the Small-Pox in the way of Transplantation. The Success of the Experiment among my Neighbours as well as abroad in the World and the urgent Calls of his Grandfather for it have made me think that I could not answer it unto God if I neglected it. At this critical Time, how much is all Piety to be press'd upon the Child!*

And it may be hoped with the more Efficacy because his dearest Companion (and his Chamber-fellow at the College) dies this Day of the Small-Pox taken in the common Way.

If only Dr. Clark would allow him to bring Lizzy into this fellowship of safety, he would rest easy. But Dr. Clark had made it clear that she would suffer no such operation while living under his roof. And with Lydia's glittering eyes following his every move, Dr. Mather knew he could not have his daughter back in the house. Lydia would not dare to touch Sammy, but the girls she would torment night and day.

Dr. Douglass conferred with Dr. Clark, and Dr. Clark conferred with his brother and the rest of the selectmen. After being threatened with a felony indictment, Dr. Boylston had now tested them not once but twice. They would be a laughingstock if he walked away from such threats unscathed.

"We will get an indictment," said Mr. Cooke. "And then we will get a conviction."

For the first few days, as the disease burrowed into Sammy, Dr. Mather hovered at his door, full of generosity and nervous energy. He would press his many terrified kinsmen to undertake the wonderful operation, he thought. For the sake of the world at large, he would write a treatise for the London press—especially apropos, now that he could lay claim to notable experience. For the sake of his own humble corner of the world, he would recommend the insertion of some edifying passages into Mr. Campbell's *News-Letter*.

The twentieth—the sixth day, the usual time for the first fever to bloom in inoculated smallpox—came and went, leaving Sammy cool. The next day, the tiresome *Courant* struck again: and again, the lead column was anonymous but obviously by Dr. Douglass. At the Mather house, the day crawled by, and both father and son began to fret. Dr. Boylston promised a blooding on the eighth day, if no fever appeared.

The morning of August 22 hunched into the afternoon. Minutes before the doctor arrived, headache hammered through Sammy's skull; his skin was soon clammy with sweat. Obadiah must have given Dr. Boylston the news out in the yard, thought Dr. Mather; the doctor was humming as he stomped up the stairs.

"You are cheerful today," he said acidly, as the doctor was shown into Sammy's chamber.

"You will never guess who I inoculated this morning," answered Dr. Boylston.

Dr. Mather gave up with a quick frown. He did not care; he cared only about Sammy.

"Samuel Valentine," crowed Dr. Boylston.

Dr. Mather's heart rose in his throat, spilling over with sweet relief and not a little sour-green envy. For he knew as well as anyone what that meant.

"Bloody hell!" swore Elisha Cooke when Dr. Clark delivered that same news to the select men in their customary room upstairs at the Bunch of Grapes Tavern. "Bloody hell," he said again, as it sunk in. The news was surely worth two such epithets, possibly more: for young Valentine's father was John Valentine—no inconsequential ally of the governor's, but His Majesty's advocate general for the provinces of the Massachusetts Bay and New Hampshire, and the colony of Rhode Island. He was, in short, the crown's chief lawyer in New England. To make matters worse—as if they needed to be made worse—the boy's mother was Mary Lynde, daughter of old Judge Samuel Lynde, and niece of the present judge and councilor Benjamin Lynde.

With Mr. Valentine party to the operation, there would be no indictment on a charge of felony murder, or felony anything else for that matter. The governor, Council, and all the highest legal apparatus of the province might as well have sent trumpeters on white horses clanging through the streets, proclaiming inoculation to be right, good, and necessary.

"Dr. Boylston must be stopped," insisted Dr. Clark.

"Oh, he will be stopped," said Mr. Cooke. "They will all be stopped."

The next day, Dr. Boylston inoculated his own eldest son and namesake, Zabdiel junior, who rushed home after finding that he had lain in an infected chamber two nights running. One of the college friends he had been bunking with for the summer break had broken into the dread fever just that morning. That same day, Dr. Boylston inoculated three more Langdons: Edward's much younger brother and sister, Nathaniel and Margaret, and his niece Joanna Syms along with Ebenezer Thornton's new bride, Elizabeth, just nineteen. A neighbor of the Langdons, Mr. Thornton was one of the wealthiest men in the North End.

At the opposite end of Boston's world, out on the Neck at the Roxbury line, the General Court descended upon the George Inn. The country men had absolutely refused to set foot in the cloud of contagion that enveloped the city. Even the governor had recognized that to demand a meeting in the Town House was futile.

Owned by Jerusha Boylston's uncle, Stephen Minot, the rambling old inn was known far and wide as a jolly place to break the long ride—and even longer walk—between Boston and Roxbury. With the entire General Court squeezed inside, not to mention regular wanderers and a small army of serving girls handing out beer, strong Madeira wine, rum punch, and gin, though, the huge open common room that took up almost the entire ground floor no longer seemed so spacious. In fact, it seemed hair-raisingly cramped and fetid. It was impossible not to draw breath that reeked of having already been breathed by someone else in the midst of drinking and smoking. Hoping to bake, sting, or drown the invisible contagion and render it harmless, most of the men smoked and drank all the harder. Now and again, they looked at each other askance, and went silent or stepped outside for a breath of the hot, humid air of late summer. In such a crowd, thought Dr. Clark as he gazed around the room, the angel of death had only to hover over one man and breathe through his breath to spew death over a multitude.

Mr. Cooke began agitating for a move to Cambridge. The urgency of that move, however, was soon lost as the House began squabbling with the governor and council upstairs over who had the right to send what kind of messages to whom and when. The minutes ticked away.

In town, word of Sammy Mather's inoculation leaked out; crowds now followed Dr. Mather everywhere. He had forgotten his promise to help Dr. Boylston. The following day, however, the twenty-fifth of August, the doctor gently recalled it for him as they stood together, watching the rash that had at last begun to flow across his son.

G.D., Dr. Mather wrote after the doctor had departed. *I will assist my Physician in giving to the Public some Accounts about relieving the Small-Pox in the way of Transplantation, which may be of great Consequence!* Odd, he thought, how quickly Dr. Boylston has become "my" physician. He skimmed a few pages back: yes, only a few weeks ago, he was a stranger: "the" physician. Dr. Mather bit the inside of his lip and hoped tightly that the shift would turn out to have been a good one. Sammy's fever had not gone off as he thought it should. Dr. Boylston, however, was not at all properly distressed. Indeed, the doctor went so far as to look pleased. *Pleased!* No matter how hard Dr. Mather suggested that his son's case surely ought to be declared hazardous, Dr. Boylston remained implacably and most irritatingly sanguine.

Dr. Mather turned with renewed zeal to supplying his son with instructions for suitable prayers, cries, and offerings to heaven. The boy would have to make quite a noise, he grumbled to himself, to counteract the clamor in the street.

Out on the Neck, the House posted guards at the doors to the inn to keep strangers out of their chambers. Inside, they went on bickering with the governor.

Up in Salutation Alley, Esther Webb was recovering from a fearsome bout with confluent smallpox; her cousin Abigail, John's daughter—also uninoculated—was dying. On the twenty-eighth, the *Courant* appeared yet again, though notably mutilated. A delegation from the governor had represented to Mr. Franklin exactly how much trouble he might get into if such libel continued; his own father had been less polite.

He had at last canceled Dr. Douglass's column, though he left a whole page blank, in expensive if quietly eloquent protest. A waste of spirit in an expense of paper, someone had quipped.

Still, what was left was bad enough. The lead column written by a minister, no less. Even if it was that Anglican prig Henry Harris of King's, and it was in tone quite different—being at least rational and void of personal insult—still, such public mixing of journalism and divinity was shameful.

> *G.D. This miserable Town is a dismal Picture and Emblem of Hell; Fire with Darkness filling of it, and a lying Spirit reigning there; many members of our Churches have had a fearful Share in the false Reports and blasphemous Speeches and murderous Wishes in which the Town is become very guilty before the Lord.*

Again and again, he warned his flock to repent, lest they provoke the Lord to terrible vengeance, even in His holy places.

On August 29, as Sammy's pocks were maturing into full pustules, the fever veered around and came roaring back. Dr. Mather spent hours in solitary prayer, summoning the strength to offer up his son as a sacrifice to the Lord. Dr. Boylston, however, still refused to take proper alarm, scribbling in his case notes only that the boy had a "brisk" fever. His own son, he said, had suffered much worse. It outraged Dr. Mather: no matter how high Tommy Boylston's fever had spiked, it had all been within the bounds of the first fever. His son's warmth, surely, was a harbinger of the dreaded secondary fever. He stomped angrily up to his study.

> *G.D. the Condition of my Son Samuel is very singular. The Inoculation was very imperfectly performed, and scarce any more than attempted upon him; And yet for ought I know, it might be so much as to prove a Benefit unto him. He is, however, endangered by the ungoverned Fever that attends him. And in this Distress I know not what to do; but O Lord, my Eyes are unto thee!*

If only Providence would reveal some sign that he was Doing Good.

Sometimes, Providence required to be provided with a slate. Reaching across the clutter of his desk, Dr. Mather slid his Bible toward him. Holding the book gently in one hand, resting its spine against the desk, he shut his eyes, said a quick prayer, and released his hand. With a small thud, the book fell open.

He opened his eyes, letting the black and white resolve into a single verse:

Go thy Way, thy Son liveth.

Tears sprang to his eyes. It was the very passage he had been hoping beyond hope to read: Jesus healing the son of a nobleman at Capernaum. Even as this thought slid through his mind, though, suspicion slithered in its wake. It was too perfect; he had somehow caused the book to open just at this point.

He had *not* influenced the outcome, he told himself; he had not. Look: hadn't a paper lodged just behind the page in question put the book at some disadvantage for opening at this longed-for place? That the Bible had fallen open here anyway was surely the very sign and wonder for which he had pleaded. Providence had not merely spoken, but shouted the righteousness of his ways.

Dr. Mather's heart lifted, and he sped downstairs to see his son.

❧ 6 ❧

NEWGATE

To:
Sir Hans Sloane
In his house in Russell Street
Bloomsbury Square, London
Tuesday, August 8, 1721

Honoured Sir:
*   This comes to give you Notice that the Operation of Inoculating the*
Small Pox on the Prisoners in Newgate is to be performed to Morrow
morning about Nine o'clock; At which time Your Presence there will be
very Acceptable to

     Honoured Sir,
       Your most obedient humble Servant,
       Charles Maitland

THE following morning at nine sharp Mr. Maitland, the king's physicians, Sir Hans Sloane and Dr. Steigerthal, and the Prince and Princess of Wales's apothecary, Mr. Lilly, entered the hall where the prisoners had first been chosen, and where they had been gathered again. Twenty-five more physicians, surgeons, and apothecaries jostled through the door behind them, including Dr. Harris and Dr. Keith. Many were members of the Royal College of Physicians and the Royal Society; a few were ambitious young doctors from the Continent. To their noses, they held clove-studded oranges or handkerchiefs drenched in perfume.

A barrier like a knee-high fence had been run across the middle of the room, parting the prisoners from the spectators. On the prisoners' side, there were six high-backed chairs and a table. On the spectators side, the armchairs had been pushed to the back and a row of benches installed. The men shoved the benches aside and crowded forward in a huddle.

On the other side, the prisoners sat pale and staring, as Sir Hans Sloane stood to the fore, welcomed the company, and launched into a brief lecture describing the operation as performed by Drs. Timonius and Pylarinus in the Levant, and now, in their own city of London, by Mr. Maitland. Here he stopped to bow gracefully to the surgeon; the surgeon bowed in turn, first to Sir Hans, and then to the gathered assembly. In a ripple of heads, all the men bowed back, save Dr. Wagstaffe and Dr. Freind, who stood with defiantly straight backs, their faces pinched with contempt.

Sir Hans ignored them. "In order to demonstrate the operation's power in itself, it has been determined that no art or medicine shall be used to promote the eruptions—not even so much as obliging the patients to keep to their beds. The whole process is to be left to nature—"

"Nothing about it is natural," came a call from the back.

Sir Hans rolled smoothly on: "—assisted only by a strict and regular diet. Furthermore, there has not been the least encouraging or favorable circumstance attending any of the prisoners before the operation."

This roused gruff laughter: it was hard to imagine circumstances less encouraging than awaiting the gallows in Newgate. But the point was taken. *Applebee's*—London's gadfly of a Tory paper—had been shouting that the prisoners were being prepared for a dubious smallpox experiment by means of purges. *As if purges might somehow corrupt the outcome*, snorted Mr. Maitland to himself.

Sir Hans gave the nod for Mr. Maitland to proceed.

He opened the little gate in the barrier and crossed into the prisoners' side of the room. As Sir Hans put to rest the theory that a needle must be used—much less Dr. Pylarinus's golden needle—and extolled the praises of a modern lancet, Mr. Maitland drew out his own and stepped into a long, slanting stream of light from a high window. He wanted the clearest view possible of what he was about to do.

With pardons dangled before their noses, the prisoners had all agreed to participate, but now, with that blade flashing in the sun and so many gentlemen peering over the rail like fiends, all six shuddered and recoiled. Mary North gasped aloud and gripped Lizzy's hand.

Was there not a basin on the table? It was just as their tormenters had foreboded: the glittering gentlemen with their wolfish faces would fill it with blood and pass it around like a communion cup.

"Who's to be first?" asked Mr. Maitland.

A short, sharp wail rose over the table, though none of the six could have said who voiced it. Lizzy took a deep breath and tried to recall the vision of Mr. Maitland's kind eyes. However, if it was to be bad, best get it over with. She untangled her hand from Mrs. North's grasp, patted her arm once, and pushed back her chair. "I'll do it, sir," she said.

Every eye in the room swiveled to watch as she stood.

"Oh, Lizzy," whispered Mrs. North, *"no."*

Lizzy tottered and gripped the edge of the table as a hot black wave rolled through her. Somehow, she forced her feet forward to Mr. Maitland.

Necks before and behind her craned to see as she rolled up both sleeves at Mr. Maitland's request. The hands plucking at her looked like her own, but she could not feel them. Surely they were someone else's.

"The operation," said Sir Hans, "is performed by making a very slight shallow incision in the skin, about an inch long."

Lizzy shut her eyes. If the cut was to come at her throat, she didn't want to see it. For a long hot moment, she felt nothing. Then she heard a gasp from her fellows, and a cold line drew down her right arm—and stopped. Two footsteps, and another stroke down her left arm.

"Now your leg, please," said Mr. Maitland's voice, and she hitched up her skirts.

Another couple of footsteps, and the same cold line drew down her right thigh.

"Good girl, Lizzy," Mr. Maitland said quietly in her ear. "You can open your eyes now."

The room was filled with eyes. She glanced down at both arms. A few droplets of blood had beaded on the surface of each cut. That was all. Her throat was untouched.

"Great care should be had in making the incision," said Sir Hans, "to go just deep enough to draw blood, but not all the way through the skin, for in that instance it may be attended with very troublesome consequences."

Fear flooded down and away, and for a moment, Lizzy thought she might have peed where she stood. She had not, but her cheeks flushed crimson, shamed by the thought.

"After the incisions are made," Sir Hans continued, "a cotton is dipped in the ripe matter of a favorable kind of the small-pox."

Mr. Maitland wrapped a bit of cotton around the end of a toothpick, dipped the stick into a vial, and stepped back toward Lizzy.

She shut her eyes again. Perhaps it was poison; perhaps it would set her blood afire, shooting flames through her veins. In the end, all she felt was a gentle touch as Mr. Maitland smeared each cut once.

"The matter is put into the wound," said Sir Hans, "and covered by a plaster for twenty-four hours, after which it is removed."

Applause scattered like dry leaves between the stone walls, punctuated by the thumping of walking sticks on the floor and a few calls of "Bravo!" and "Well done!"

"Preposterous," announced Dr. Wagstaffe. "You cannot pass on the smallpox through the skin; it must be taken into the lungs or the gut."

"That is all, Mrs. Harrison," said Mr. Maitland with a smile, as he finished fixing the third bandage in place. "You may sit down now, and send up someone else."

She turned and saw her fellows as intent upon her as the gentlemen were. "It don't hurt a mite," she murmured as she resumed her place at the table. Cawthery and Alcock jumped up: now that it was safe, they wanted it over with. Mrs. Tompion took her turn, and then Lizzy pulled Mrs. North up by the hand and propelled her forward.

After Lizzy's return, Evans had lounged back in his chair, sneering. When it came time for him, he swaggered up and stood feet apart, hands folded in front him, as if to say, *Do yer best, you bloodsucking butchers. You can't touch me, an' we all know it.*

But he had been just as afraid as the rest of them, when it began. It was the first emotion Lizzy had seen in his chilly eyes.

For the next two days, little happened. All six prisoners slept well and woke refreshed: for a few blinking moments Lizzy had trouble remembering whether the operation had already been done, or whether she had dreamed it.

They dressed, walked about, and ate hungrily—at the king's expense, who wouldn't? The only unpleasantness was being on display all day, visitors coming and going, sitting on the benches and gawping at them, as they whiled away the hours. Sometimes Mrs. Tompion read from the newspapers that the gentlemen left behind, which Lizzy liked; she had not known the world had so many doings in it. Sometimes they gambled. But mostly they just talked and drank.

Mr. Maitland was the only gentleman who crossed the boundary. Their pulses were fast, he noted, scratching his chin, but he could not detect any sensible cause.

"You mean like fear of catching the smallpox?" sneered Evans.

Mr. Maitland's worries were twofold: He had to steer this experiment between the two dangers of death and nothingness: between serious smallpox and a distemper so light that it might not be smallpox at all—or not small-pox enough to produce a survivor's protection.

On the morning of Saturday, August 12, the fourth day of the experiment, the incisions were still not inflamed. Dr. Wagstaffe smugly noted in his diary that all six prisoners were "very well." The prisoners and even the supporting physicians, on the other hand, began to get restless.

Mr. Maitland knew it was early, he knew he should have patience, but he felt a growing dread all the same. Perhaps the matter he used had been defective; he had been obliged to collect it the day before the operation and let it sit in its cold little vial in his surgical kit for at least fifteen or sixteen hours—for the very good reason that they had chosen a donor far from the prisons and stews of London, a boy who lived an otherwise healthy life in the country. But perhaps they had let their concern for a clean subject outweigh the need for fresh matter.

At Sir Hans's urging, he went in quest of likely matter to be had closer by, and found it at last in Christ's Hospital, just down the street. At about six o'clock that night, he cut new incisions in his patients' arms. This time, he swabbed them with the new matter in grim abundance, swirling the cotton deep in the cuts.

Unfortunately, he used his new supply with such abandon that he ran out by the time he got through John Alcock's right arm; Alcock's left arm had to go without. Evans got no new matter at all: but that was little matter, Mr. Maitland remarked jovially, as Evans had already had enough to last him a lifetime.

Mr. Evans scowled and spat.

Really, thought Mr. Maitland, *he's a right nippit blackguard*.

Watching the disapproval in Mr. Maitland's eyes, Lizzy agreed: Evans followed her, as many men did, with his eyes. But where other men undressed her, she had the feeling that Evans was peeling her, slitting her to bits, and laughing. She did her best to keep Cawthery between her and him. Given time, Evans might think Cawthery into a corner; on the other hand, Cawthery could knock Evans's brains out in one smack. When Cawthery was around, he kept his eyes down.

"Listen to this," said Mrs. Tompion. In a surprisingly good imitation of Dr. Wagstaffe, she read a snippet from *Applebee's*. Felons in fear of death, no doubt, were duping the doctors "by pretending that they have never had the smallpox, when perhaps they have had them." She looked sharply at Evans. "I think they mean you, ducky." He shrugged and tossed down a card, winning the hand he was playing.

Mr. Maitland sighed. No doubt Evans was capable of cruel falsehoods, but in this instance, he had not lied: he had had the smallpox in jail last September. They had included him precisely because they *knew* he'd had it. But the story was easily twistable, and *Applebee's* seemed to relish the twisting. But then, *Applebee's* was firmly committed to ravaging any project the king and his Whiggery-jiggery might endorse. Not that the Tories could quite say that, of course, at least not in print. They contented themselves with taking potshots at the prisoners, the procedure, and the foreigners, Jews, and women who had dreamed up such quackery to begin with.

"Do you think Dr. Droop-staff and his Friend leave this place and run straight to the paper to wag tongues over everything they'd like to think they've seen here?" asked Mrs. Tompion, to no one in particular. It did not bother her in the least that Dr. Wagstaffe was in the room, right up next to the railing. She gave him a slow, wicked smile, and he stalked from the room, to the sound of her laughter.

The following morning, the five who had been reinoculated all woke to the throb of their arms. Unwrapping their dressings, Mr. Maitland was pleased to find all the incisions inflamed and festering. His patients' pulses were noticeably quicker, and their urine cloudy. Except for their sore arms, though, none of them felt sick.

Lizzy went for a walk with Mrs. North in "the garden," though it was little more than a stone passage between the prison and its high outer wall. Still, thought Lizzy, you could see a long wide ribbon of sky. Once, she saw a bird flying high overhead.

Though the Princess of Wales stood by her unquailing, Lady Mary grew weary of the curiosity and thinly veiled disgust of the crowd that went on swelling at her door, as the news of her experiment rumbled through town. She retired to her country house in Twickenham. The soprano Mrs. Anastasia Robinson, the composer Giovanni Buononcini, and the castrato Senesino had retreated there as well; Lady Mary wrote to her sister in Paris that she was melting her time away in perpetual concerts.

She did not bother to mention that she was running from the inoculation controversy; she did not bother to mention the word *smallpox* at all. Her poor sister, after all, was fighting off madness in exile and alone. So Lady Mary chattered instead about Molly Skerrett, a little thread-satin beauty who deserved better connections than she'd been born with. She'd welcomed Molly into her house as her companion, wrote Lady Mary; their long talks made her think of those she had enjoyed long ago with Frances, walking arm in arm through the grounds of Thoresby. And would Frances please not forget the fine silk she had promised for young mistress Mary? She was growing quite the little woman, and was almost as much fun to decorate as a new house; Lady Mary and Molly played with her every day.

When the music stopped and the child was whisked off to eat or sleep or be coaxed out of tiresomeness by her nurse—now quite well, and what a relief—Lady Mary peppered Mr. Maitland with notes of advice, in an entirely different tone.

With Mr. Maitland's experiment well under way, Dr. Richard Mead began his own, on a seventh prisoner, a young girl of eighteen. Sir Hans had somehow managed to take charge of the Turkish inoculation—though really, thought Dr. Mead, it was by rights his; he had known Lady Mary since girlhood, and that ought to have counted for something. Instead, he had had to settle for a slightly different experiment. Nonetheless, Dr. Mead had high hopes for this other method, from China. It did not require cutting.

Which wasn't to say that it did not have its unpleasant moments, he thought. *If only the girl would lie still!* He picked up a small bit of cotton and dipped it in matter he taken from ripe pocks that morning. Laying one hand firmly on her head, lest she wriggle, he proceeded to pack her nostrils with the pocky cotton.

The papers, quite shamefully, claimed it had been done while the girl was asleep.

Right on cue, the eagerly awaited rashes bloomed across Mr. Maitland's patients on Monday morning, the sixth day after their inoculation. Red spots and flushings had appeared on all the five, but the marks were clearest on Mary North, especially about her face, neck, and breast. "The engrafting has taken root," he observed with satisfaction.

"Mary, Mary, quite contrary, how does your garden grow?" quipped Mrs. Tompion, though her symptoms were quite similar.

They were still all without any nausea, headache, or thirst, though when pressed, they agreed that they might have been a little hot in the night. All of them, that is, except Evans. He had suffered no twinge whatsoever, and made no effort to satisfy the doctor on that point. By evening, his incisions had dried up entirely.

The next day, Mr. Maitland found them all much the same, though by nightfall, the spots were darkening and then paling in the center as they swelled into blisters.

The rash was a relief, but the lack of sickness was beginning to make Mr. Maitland irritable. He had not wanted any part of this—had done his best to refuse, but Sir Hans and the Princess of Wales would have none of it. And behind them had loomed the long shadow of the king. So here he was. But the last thing he needed was a failure, what with the entire Royal College of Physicians and Royal Society staring over his shoulders. The Princess of Wales and the king himself, too, if you counted their eyes by proxy.

It didn't help that Dr. Mead's poor girl suffered much more than all Mr. Maitland's six patient put together. Not that he'd wish her torments on anybody. Sharp pains had begun to knife through her head her soon after Dr. Mead had packed her nostrils; her fever had spiked the same day and had never left her till this very morning, when her eruption, too, had begun. Lizzy had stayed with her night and day, he saw, doing her best to cool the girl down with damp rags.

"It does not as yet look the least bit like the smallpox," sniffed Dr. Wagstaffe, over his shoulder.

"No," said Mr. Maitland. "If we are lucky, it never will. It looks, instead, like inoculation for the smallpox." He turned to face Dr. Wagstaffe. "Otherwise, there would be little point in inoculating, would there?"

On Wednesday, August 16, though, he breathed a sigh of relief. The rashes continued developing well, and at last his patients' incisions began to discharge a thick, purulent matter. At the bend of her thigh, near the incision on her leg, Ann Tompion had produced a satisfyingly large yellow pustule. Alcock had even suffered a slight fever in the night; his urine was notably cloudy, and he had more fresh pustules appearing on his face and arms. Cawthery had a large yellow pustule on his left cheek, and several small ones on his face.

By Thursday, Alcock's pustules were ripe with yellow matter, ringed with red. Of the five patients with pocks, he had by far the greatest number: no less than sixty. Though she had fewer, Mrs. Tompion pocks looked similar, especially on her right arm and thigh. A few other fresh ones were scattered about her chin and mouth. Lizzy had the fewest; she could hardly count ten. But at least she had some. At last, Mr. Maitland was happy to say, his chickens were properly speckled with pocks you might find on any natural smallpox patient.

"I will concede that the prisoners' appearances are similar to each other," said Dr. Wagstaffe. "But they bear no resemblance whatsoever to the smallpox. Look at that woman's arm." He pointed at Mrs. Tompion. "A boil with a bit of matter in it, I give you that. But it has not altered a whit from the first day of eruption, which is contrary to the progress of the true smallpox," he snorted.

"It has not altered since the first time you saw it, perhaps," replied Mr.

Maitland icily. "But I assure you, it began as a red pinpoint fleck, and has developed through the stages of a true pock, though more quickly than in natural smallpox. There are those, sir, who regard the speed of inoculation as one of its blessings, not one of its failings. Furthermore, it has not quite remained unchanged. It has grown."

"It's a pimple with matter in it!" cried Dr. Wagstaffe.

"If it has matter in it," retorted Mr. Maitland, "why may it not be a pock?"

"Because there is *one* of them," said Dr. Wagstaffe. "Whoever heard of one pock?" He turned and walked out of the room as if trailed by robes of victory.

"Don't you worry sir," said Lizzy. "We'd all much rather have one small pock, than the smallpox."

Mr. Maitland was gratified to hear someone from the other side of the barrier agree. "Man's a sanctimonious bag of vapors," said a clear, light voice from the back corner. "I've seen inoculations in the East, and now I've seen 'em here, and I'll tell anyone you please that your incisions and eruptions are the very same as those I've observed in Constantinople."

The whole room turned to look at the speaker. Lizzy and Mary stood up so as to be able to see; after a moment, even Mrs. Tompion joined them. He was a slight fellow with a black mustache, leaning casually back in an armchair by the fire. He had affected, as some of London's eastern merchants and travelers did, the clothing of the East: a glimmering caftan that seemed to have been made of gold softened until it flowed like water, a red velvet turban, and a jewel in one ear. But the voice was honeyed English. "And that is not a few, you can be sure. For my money, sir, you can also be sure that none of your patients will ever again be infected with the smallpox."

"Much obliged for your kind words of support, sir," said Mr. Maitland, making his way through the crowd. "Might I beg the pleasure of your acquaintance?"

The man stood and thrust out his hand. "Mr. Cook, sir. Turkey merchant. Pleasure is all mine."

"Not at all," said Mr. Maitland. "Might I offer you some refreshment in a more auspicious environment, sir, where we may discuss the matter further?"

Lizzy sighed as Mr. Maitland led Mr. Turkey-Cook away. She would dearly like to have heard their conversation.

In the carriage at the front gate, the man sat back and watched Mr. Maitland with bright dark eyes. "Where shall we go?"

"Child's Coffeehouse, I think. Much the best in the vicinity for intellectual discussion. Unless you have another preference, *my lady?*"

"Damn," said Lady Mary.

The surgeon raised a brow, but she waved him off. "As long as I am dressed like a man, I will talk like one. How long have you known?"

"You may swear like a sailor, my lady, and I would still know your voice. How long have you been growing that mustache?"

"As long as I have been feeding my girl's ridiculous rat of a dog—never did like small dogs, but this one has at last proved its worth," she said, patting the black fuzz carefully glued to her lip. "Except that it does rather make me want to sneeze."

"Everyone sneezes in Child's. Great deal of snuff. And Turkish tobacco too."

"Then we are still going?" She sounded like a young girl being granted permission to attend her first ball.

He shrugged. "It is your lark, my lady. So long as you allow me to maintain my ignorance, I will maintain your disguise. For a price."

"Which is?" she said sharply. Through the carriage windows, the dome of St. Paul's loomed large and close overhead, and then disappeared altogether as they rolled into the churchyard and drew up at the door of Child's.

"Just regale the company with lovely stories of successful inoculation."

For two hours, "Mr. Cook" happily drew a smoking, sneezing circle of men—clergy, proud university wits, poets, and booksellers—close around her as she spun tale after salacious Turkish tale, until the men supposed they had stumbled into Aladdin's cave rather than Child's Coffee house. They ended with a carousing toast to the undoubted success of the Newgate experiment.

"Who is that ferret-faced fellow glowering in the corner?" she asked as they were leaving. "He looks even more like a rat than Mary's dog."

Mr. Maitland glanced over and groaned. "Isaac Massey. Apothecary at Christ's, and therefore my esteemed colleague."

Mr. Massey began to rise, as if he might step over to speak to them. One glance at the Machiavellian smile on Lady Mary's face made Mr. Maitland take her elbow and firmly steer her out the door and into his coach.

"As it is, Dr. Wagstaffe will already know everything we've said before we even reach your door," he said to her protest, "and will be sharpening his knives. He already feels he needs to discredit me. I would prefer he didn't feel the need to flay me alive as well."

* * *

The next day, Friday the eighteenth, Alcock's pocks looked the same as the day before, though fuller and larger. Unfortunately, his fever had soared, which had nothing to do with the smallpox. He had jail fever.

Mr. Maitland instantly quarantined him from the others. Lizzy begged to be allowed to nurse him, but Mr. Maitland adamantly refused. "I have no protection to offer you from jail fever, my dear, but distance. It is a highy contagious and malignant fever, and I cannot risk losing you. It was a fine offer, however," he said as her face fell. "Take care of the others," he suggested.

She did, though they didn't much need it. Their only real discomfort came from their incisions, which bloomed larger by the day and ran copiously.

"Haven't we grown nice?" said Mrs. Tompion with a yawn. "Too particular to abide so much as a smear of dirt on our sleeves."

Wiping her arms and her leg yet again, Lizzy looked curiously at the thick yellow pus oozing out of her. Dirt was not really what she would have called it. It looked more like rancid butter, though it smelled considerably worse.

On Saturday morning, Mr. Maitland stopped in to see Alcock first, and emerged in a rage. "Do you know what that Alcock has done in the night?" he roared. "He has taken a pin and pricked every last pustule he could come at."

Lizzy felt giggles rising and quickly looked at her feet and coughed.

"Yes, Alcock was feverish. Yes, he was possibly delirious," Mr. Maitland reprimanded the staff. "But you are being paid to *watch* him, not to watch him make a hash of himself and the experiment, all at once."

The remains of Alcock's pustules were already crusting; a few had already scraped off. Most were still ringed by red: but as far as watching the development of inoculated pocks, Alcock's were ruined. With perverse solidarity, his incisions stopped running too.

Across the next two days, the others' pocks also began to dry up, though their incisions still ran. Then even those slowed and began to dry up.

Applebee's, read Mrs. Tompion, was now grumbling that "any Person that expects to be hang'd may make Use of it, if they please," to get off scot free. Mr. Maitland was inclined to interpret this as an inside-out compliment. "They smell defeat," he said with a smile.

Neither Dr. Wagstaffe nor Dr. Freind proved ready to surrender, however. "It is no true smallpox," they insisted as invited doctors assembled for a final consultation. "There has been no regular rash," Dr. Wagstaffe said with contempt, "except in Alcock and that girl who had it stuffed up her nose. In the others, it is more likely to have been the chicken pox, and therefore cannot possibly have made the prisoners proof against future infection."

"The prisoners did not have many pocks," conceded Sir Hans. "However, the second incisions, by which such a vast discharge has been made, may have been a mistake. They seem to have impeded the eruption, rather than contributing toward it. Perhaps they drained too much of the poison."

"First you had it that the second incisions were the solution," objected Dr. Wagstaffe. "Now you point to them as the problem."

"Furthermore," proclaimed Sir Hans, "the prisoners' experience of the practice answers the Turkish descriptions exactly. The pocks that did ripen have followed the development of natural pocks, though with more speed and less fullness. In conclusion, we firmly believe the prisoners to be, in all respects, safe from any future infection."

"Preposterous," said Dr. Wagstaffe over the applause, in exactly the same tones he had said it the very first day. "And premature, as well," he added.

Later, as Sir Hans and Dr. Steigerthal were taking their leave of Mr. Maitland, Sir Hans shook his head and said, "Odious as Dr. Wagstaffe is, I am sorry to say, he has a point. I fear we must devise another test, somehow, to demonstrate the protection."

"No," said Mr. Maitland. "No more tests."

"Think on it," said Sir Hans.

On August 24, Mr. Maitland purged Alcock and Cawthery, to clear their systems of the last remaining poison. He did not bother with Evans. *Purge all his poison, and there'd be nothing left*, he thought.

He had ordered drafts for the three women as well, but when they were brought in to the women, they refused to drink. "It's not the right time of the month for a purge, sir," said Lizzy uncomfortably. "Not for all three of us, as of this morning."

He checked with the laundresses, just to be certain, but they assured him it was just as Lizzy said: all three women had begun menstruating within fifteen minutes of each other.

He sighed. The proclamation of victory would have to be postponed.

Four days later, Mary North unaccountably washed in cold water. Even more unaccountably, the wardens let her. She went down with a violent colic, which lasted near two days and gave all the doctors a fright. All they needed now was to have her die of stupidity within sight of triumph. The opposition would not allow it to be a cold; they would have it that it was the inoculation.

Sir Hans read a stern lecture to the staff. Mr. Maitland, for the second time, lost his temper, this time with his patients.

"After all that risk, and in sight of pardon, must you come close to killing yourselves through idiocy?" he said irritably, pacing back and forth in the women's chamber.

"I could not stand the smell," whimpered Mrs. North. "Not one minute longer, I couldn't." And then she doubled up in pain again.

Lizzy looked at Mr. Maitland reproachfully, and he stomped out of the room.

He was tempted, on the way home, to wonder whether Lady Mary's suspicions of knavish physicians were not so far off after all. Perhaps Dr. Wagstaffe—*No. He would not go there. Not without evidence.*

Two days later, on Wednesday, August 30, Mrs. North was still griping, but the pains had weakened to nips. Pushed by Sir Hans and Dr. Steigerthal, Mr. Maitland refused to wait any longer. Served up purges again, all three women drank them down. Along with everything else in their bellies, the potions carried off the last of Mary North's colic pains.

The next day, the men took their second purge; and on the first of September, the women swallowed theirs.

For all intents and purposes—save the all important papers of pardon—the experiment was over.

That evening at home, Mr. Maitland sat down to draft the report that Sir Hans Sloane would take to the Princess of Wales, and then to the king himself. The papers, at any rate, had said the king had demanded an accounting.

The experiment has perfectly answered Dr. Timonius's account of this practice, and also the experience of all who have seen it in Turkey, he wrote. A doodle grew into a turkey cock; he shook his head and scratched it out. He had to focus on the here and now. On London, not Constantinople. On Newgate. He began again. *Considering the subjects' age, habit of body, and circumstances* . . . He stopped again. He had to be precise, but he did not like sounding so ichie nor ochie. Wavery-quavery, Lady Mary would have said. He especially did not like Sir Hans frittering on about still more tests.

He threw down the pen and sat back in his chair. After a few moments, he drove himself forward to the edge of his seat. He dipped the pen firmly in the ink. At the bottom of the page, he dashed off one more sentence in uncharacteristically large letters, sweeping back beneath it in a flourishing underline:

It has been successful far beyond my expectation.

⁎ 7 ⁎

AN HOUR OF MOURNING

Dock Square, Boston
Wednesday, August 30, 1721

ZABDIEL unwrapped the unbound proof sheets of his new book—
his book!—and looked at them lying heavy and solid on the parlor
table with a curious satisfaction and a pride that startled him. He had hurried that morning, inoculating Reverend Mr. Colman's nephew as promised and visiting all his other patients, both natural and inoculated, in time
to snatch one hour for dinner—and savor the new wonder of authorship.
He was lifting the sheets from their wrapping when he heard a high-
pitched bellowing below. He glanced out the window and saw Mary
Dixwell puffing up the street, wailing and blubbering. He stepped quickly
back, but it wouldn't have mattered. Without bothering to look up, she
rushed right up to the shop door and began rapping in desperation, pausing only to press her nose against the curving glass of his bay window.
Surely she could see that the shop was shut up for the dinner hour?

She began rapping again, her wails rising in intensity. Zabdiel sighed,
laid the book back down, and made his way downstairs, nodding to Jack to
let Mary in.

She nearly tumbled inside as the door opened. He helped her, heaving
and out of breath, to a seat. She was a big boned and pleasantly fat woman
who looked strong as an ox, but for all her bulk she had the delicate constitution of a consumptive. "Now, Mrs. Dixwell," he said, "what's the matter?"

"Oh, Dr. Boylston," she moaned, fanning herself, her chest heaving so
that the gold chains around her neck glinted in the afternoon sun, "I've
had such a fright, you don't know."

She was certainly trembling all over. "Have the children taken a turn for the worse?" he asked quickly. All four of them were down with smallpox. At his recommendation, Mary had turned their care over to a nurse, but she had balked at either sending them away or removing herself. She had merely confined them to the upper floor, where she could at least hear her babies, and they could hear her, singing them lullabies.

"*No.*" She shook her head and took a deep shuddering breath. "No. It's old Mr. Johnson, two doors down from our house. I pass his place every day. He's a bit of an invalid, you know, and we hadn't seen him for a week, so Mrs. Franklin and I, we put together a basket and went to check that he was all right. We knocked but heard no answer, none at all, so we opened the door." She clutched at Zabdiel. "Oh, Dr. Boylston," she whispered, "he rolled right out atop us, though we leapt back, you can be sure. . . . Dead at least a week, and halfway rotted before that with the confluent pox. He looked to have died trying to crawl out his own door. The stench was loathsome." Her throat moved convulsively, and she was turning green.

Jack handed her a glass of water. She gave him a grateful look and took one sip, but then stopped. A sob welled up from deep within. "There—there were—there were maggots." The last word rose and twisted into a shapeless wail.

He sat down by her and took her hand. "Mary, hush now."

"No, no, no," she shrilled. "*Inoculate me.*"

"I cannot recommend that, my dear," he said with a firm calm that reached her more clearly than his words. "You have had a great fright, and you know you are not strong. The Turkish doctors recommend a preparation of a thin, cool diet and a calm mind."

She tightened her grip on his arm. "Today. *Now.*"

Hysteria rippled through her in waves. This time Jack brought a glass of wine. Zabdiel stirred in a good strong dose of laudanum and sent Jack for Mr. Dixwell.

Mrs. Dixwell's husband John was a puzzle. A sternly ascetic Puritan with regard to himself, he was also a goldsmith who had grown rich spinning gold into jeweled treasures that would have delighted the Queen of Sheba; he prized his wife as an obedient, pious, and decorative pet. Surprisingly, he sided with her in the matter of inoculation, even after having the dangers of her agitation pointed out. "There are those," he said, "who argue that inoculation trespasses on the prerogative of Providence. But sometimes one must surely marshal the world into place, to make way for Providence."

"You have been listening to Reverend Webb," said Zabdiel, as he cleaned his lancet with a sinking heart. Desperately embracing inoculation was no more rational than despising it unseen, and possibly far more dangerous: but how could he say no to those who knew the risks? Who weighed them against a real and known threat of smallpox, and begged for a chance for deliverance?

Mr. Dixwell, a ruling elder of Mr. Webb's New North Church, nodded. "I have. And no doubt the minister would agree, though too late, it would seem, for his own family—his wife, I have heard, has been taken sorely ill with the distemper."

Zabdiel knew that—he had seen Fanny Webb just that morning, after visiting her husband's cousin Esther, who was slowly recovering, and her sister-in-law Abigail Webb, old John's daughter, who was not. Abigail had chosen not to be inoculated, and now hovered very near death. But he said nothing.

Mr. Dixwell paused only briefly; when it became apparent that Dr. Boylston was not going to discuss the Webbs, he pressed on. "That particular lesson, though, is a teaching from my father."

A formidable family, thought Zabdiel. Proud enough to make the marshaling of Providence an earth-shaking habit: John Dixwell's father, of the same name, had been one of the fifty-nine men who'd signed the death warrant of King Charles I at the end of the Civil War. For a while, he had been hailed as a hero. But when England's experiment as a kingless republic had foundered, the Restoration of King Charles II transformed him from hero to assassin. *Regicide*, hissed cruel shadows at his heels, and the whole family had slipped into hiding in America, under the name of Davis. John Davis's son, however, was not a man to hide from man, law, or God; he seemed never to have tasted either fear or doubt, thought Zabdiel, uncorking his vial of smallpox. As an adult, Mr. Dixwell had moved to Boston and resumed his father's rightful name.

"Whenever you are ready," said Zabdiel. The Dixwells clasped hands and prayed for an outcome pleasing to the Lord, and then Mary Dixwell rolled up her sleeves, and took the infection into her blood.

Dr. Mather stopped himself just outside the door to his son's chamber. He said a brief prayer to calm himself, and then he pushed open the door.

Sammy was shivering with a fever as high as ever. "Let me be bled, Father," he said through chattering teeth.

Where God does not appoint a clear path, men must struggle as best they can through the darkness, Dr. Mather told himself. Aloud, he sent a maid running for Dr. Boylston.

Dr. Mather crowded so close behind Obadiah as he opened the door that Zabdiel had a brief image of a two-headed footman, one head black and close cropped and one white with towering, feathery hair. Dr. Mather reached around to fairly pull Zabdiel inside. "Sammy has fallen into an un-pacifiable Passion to have a Vein breathed," he said, dispensing with the niceties of greeting.

Where did the man get such phrases? Why, if you had to fight a stammer, would you put yourself through such hoops?

"Qu-quite unpacifiable," Dr. Mather continued. "I beg, Doctor, that you will gratify him."

Zabdiel ran lightly up the stairs three at a time. He liked to at least glimpse the boy before the father smothered all possibility of an objective interview. Just that morning, the boy's fever had been brisk, as it had been for two days, but unless something drastic had changed, it was moderate. By no means dangerous, and certainly not the worst-ever smallpox fever—not even the worst-ever inoculation fever, as Dr. Mather, in his proud need for his family always to be best or most, had hinted he wanted Zabdiel to say. On the days he came to the Mathers from Esther Webb's bedside, Zabdiel had sometimes found it difficult to keep his temper in the face of Dr. Mather's tangle of morbid fears and desires.

Now, striding into Sammy's chamber, Zabdiel shook his head. For once, it was worse than the boy's father had said. Sammy was curled in a corner of his bed, weeping and shaking, plucking at the bedclothes and muttering. The moment he saw Dr. Boylston, he scrabbled toward him, crying, "I am burning up, I am burning to death. Let me be bled, oh, let me be bled!"

What the boy has fallen into is hysterics, thought Zabdiel. *Maybe that will be our next epidemic.* He took hold of the boy's wrist with one hand and felt his forehead with the other. The fever remained brisk, but it was not appreciably different from before. His pulse, though, was rapid and jittery. What was starkly different was his fear.

Dr. Mather arrived huffing behind Zabdiel. "An impression of such violence, you see, as if it came from some superior Original, I am sure of it."

Zabdiel threw a sharp look over his shoulder. The last thing he needed was for Dr. Mather to be divining medical directions from angels. It was the last thing Sammy needed too. Zabdiel did not like to be overly skeptical on the subject of the heavenly host; angels no doubt abounded. He hoped there might be several breathing the light of God into the room right at this moment. But really, on the subject of divining superior but invisible forces, Dr. Mather had been misled badly in the past.

On the other hand, a light bleeding could do no harm to the boy at this point, since the eruption was well out. And it might do some good.

He let a few ounces and added to the boys' self-prescription another small glass of wine laced with laudanum. Soon afterward, the boy slid into a sweet sleep.

"And now, sir," said Zabdiel, as they left him, "if you have a moment, I should like to show you the fruits of our labor." They went upstairs to Dr. Mather's library, and Zabdiel pulled his book from a pocket and opened it to the title page:

Some ACCOUNT
of what is said of
Innoculating or Transplanting
THE
Small Pox.
By the Learned
Dr. *Emanuel Timonius,*
AND
Jacobus Pylarinus.
With some Remarks thereon.
To which are added,
A Few *Queries* in Answer to the *Scruples*
of many about the *Lawfulness of this Method.*

Published
By Dr. ZABDIEL BOYLSTON.

BOSTON: Sold by S. GERRISH
at his Shop in Corn-Hill. 1721.

They celebrated over their own glasses of wine, minus the laudanum. For it was the work of both men, though Dr. Mather had withheld his name: it set forth his transcriptions of the Royal Society's inoculation papers, followed by Zabdiel's carefully polished rebuttals of Dr. Douglass's and Dr. Dalhonde's arguments against the operation, as well as forthright rejection of the *Courant's* nattering. It finished with a few of Dr. Mather's learned musings on inoculation's lawfulness with respect to piety and Providence.

"A trifle, a trifle," said Dr. Mather with a bow, as Zabdiel thanked him for his help. But the minister was obviously gratified. "Let us hope it may move men to consider the subject rationally."

At dawn a few days later, Zabdiel saddled up Prince for a long morning ride. Except for the weather, which was miserably wet to the point of threatening to rot the crops in the fields, he dared to hope that things were looking up as they trotted out of town and the stallion stretched into a canter. Esther Webb had survived, and all the people who really mattered—herself and her parents, most of all—believed strongly that her case of confluent smallpox had not been caused by the inoculation, but by nursing her parents while they were under inoculation.

It did not, by any means, lessen Zabdiel's guilt for his part in causing her suffering and her ruined face, but it did both exonerate and implicate inoculation quite usefully. Inoculation had not produced any more than a light case of distinct pocks in any of the patients who undertook it. On the other hand, those who would argue that their cases were so light as to not count as smallpox at all were handily contradicted by Esther's experience. For if her parents' inoculated pocks were not true smallpox, then how did Esther come to catch it from nursing them?

Then there was the issue of trust. The morning after he'd inoculated Mrs. Dixwell and bled Sammy Mather, Mr. Samuel Jones had asked him to stop by his smithy and inoculate him—a family man, in the prime of his life—and a blacksmith too. Not likely that he'd calmly take such a step if he thought he might die—or that ulcers would rot his arms to the core, laming him for life. Most importantly for Zabdiel, Mr. Jones had married into the tight-knit Webb-Adams clan. He was an emissary of sorts; his inoculation served as a quiet shout to the world: *We believe in Dr. Boylston.*

His own son Zabby had erupted, and looked to do well. All his other patients were doing well too. They were growing in numbers, at any rate. And in desperation: Take the twenty-year-old daughter of Joe Dodge, the Salutation Inn's publican. She had been determined to be as brave as her friend Esther Webb at first; she had undertaken to nurse her own sister, though she herself had never had the disease. By the seventh day, though, she was terrified by the bubbling and bloated monster that lay in the bed where her sister had been; she and her mother fled to him in tears, begging for his help.

Best of all, since the inoculation of Samuel Valentine, the cloud of a murder charge had lifted.

He rode through the gate and out onto the Neck, forcing himself to veer close by the gallows once again. But Joseph Hanno was gone and so was his scent, both in reality and in Zabdiel's head. All that was left was clean: the sky and the sea and, far out in the marshes, a million birds wheeling and dancing through a rain-washed dawn.

Back at home, he wrote to Jerusha. Just two words, but they gleamed beckoning and beautiful on the paper: *Come home.*

At the bottom of the page, he had added one more: *Please.*

* * *

When he visited young Samuel Valentine on September 5, the boy's uncle, Judge Benjamin Lynde, was there. "Miraculous," he said, rising from a chair next to the boy's as Zabdiel entered. "I would bare my own arm this instant in support, sir, would it do you any good."

He did the next best thing. He had Zabdiel inoculate his seventeen-year-old black slave. "Fine fellow," said the judge. "Spent the last two years training him as footman, you know. Don't wish to lose him now."

Things were definitely looking up, thought Zabdiel.

On Wednesday, September 6, there was a break in the clouds, one brief shiny day streaming with the slanted light of autumn. That afternoon, a carriage rolled up and deposited Jerusha and the girls on the front step. She went straight into Zabdiel's arms and stayed there. The girls ran through the hall, fluttered through the kitchen, and burst into the garden to show Tommy and John and Jackey their treasures from Roxbury.

Presently, Zabdiel led Jerusha up the stairs to the parlor and opened the door, as if ushering her into a king's treasure house. Zabdiel junior was lying in state on the sofa with a book—a sight that made her fairly gasp. She inspected his thirty or so pocks, which were already scabbing nicely, and felt his cool forehead. And then she smothered him with mother's kisses that made them both laugh, and made Jerusha cry too.

Not half an hour later, the three girls in turn sat bravely on Zabby's lap while they had the operation. He had promised them each a ginger candy if they could watch the whole thing and yet not squeal, and all three of them worked hard to earn their prizes. Jerusha said they must not actually eat the amber sweets until after dinner, though, so they made a centerpiece of them. For the girls' sake and Zabby's the meal had to be meatless, but Moll had made it festive as possible: fried eels with parsley and lemon—*eel season, already!*—a salad of purslane, spinach, capers, and raisins in an oil-and-vinegar dressing, and apple pie.

If there was any jolt of unhappiness in the day, it had been Tommy's that morning as he dismantled the pirate ship. Tomorrow, it would be back to the Indian game.

"Those girls won't be playing Indians in this rain, with them pocks raised on 'em, I can tell you that," said Moll, one eye on the sky, the other on Tommy's moping face. "I bet those girls'd love to play pirates. You ever asked 'em?"

"It won't be the same," grumped Tommy.

"No, but it won't be the same old Indian game either. You just sail that ol' ship right on upstairs, and see what happens." She demanded the sacrifice of his mother's best sheets, though, as the price for Captain Roberts's liberty. "That's a pirates' world," she said, handing him an old gray blanket instead. "Win some, lose some. 'Sides, you need a set of dark sails."

On Friday, Moses Pierce stepped up from his glass workshop next door to Tom Boylston's shop and warehouse on the Town Dock and begged Zabdiel's attendance on his little family; all three children were ill. His wife, Elizabeth, would not leave them, though, so they had decided that she should undergo inoculation. "I can't try it myself," he said anxiously, twisting big hands scarred with fire and glass, as if he were confessing a crime. "I had it back in '02."

"Me too," said Zabdiel, and the man broke into a relieved smile.

That evening, Zabdiel rode home with Mr. Pierce to North Square, into the very shadow of Selectman William Clark's grand mansion, with its three brick stories and twenty-six rooms—and a king's ransom in windows, said Mr. Pierce. "Not as what I'll be called upon to replace them in the future, when he finds what I've inoculated Elizabeth right under his nose."

Across the street, the Clark house brooded silently, but Zabdiel felt the prickle of watching eyes.

On the way home, he stopped in to see Mrs. Dixwell in Union Street. She was a little jittery, but he showed her her own forearm, peppered with a light scattering of red flecks, and coaxed her back into calm. On the uppermost floor, three of her children were doing well, but ten-month-old Mary, her newest darling and her namesake, was in grave danger. In low, urgent tones in the stairwell, Zabdiel urged Mr. Dixwell to keep the news from her.

"*Thou shalt not lie*, I am commanded," said Mr. Dixwell gruffly, his face gaunt with sleeplessness, "and I shall not. Nor will I tolerate lying in the servants."

"Do not lie, then," said Zabdiel, very close to exasperation, "but try to keep the truth from her. It is paramount that she remain calm and cheerful. We do not want her blood or her spirits troubled any more than they are."

On Saturday, he inoculated his brother. Jerusha shamed Tom into it, telling him that out in Roxbury, Sarah was fretting over his safety, to the point of harming the unborn child. "A boy," she added, "by the way she's carrying him. And a feisty one too. He kicks from noon to night."

Later that day, yet another Webb—Bethiah Nichols, old John's thirty-year-old daughter—rushed in and begged to go under his poisoned knife. Her youngest sister, Abigail, had died the week before; her sister-in-law

Fanny Webb, the reverend's wife, lay so sick that she was swollen beyond recognition. What with her father and her aunt and uncle inoculated, with Esther, Abigail, and Fanny so ill, and now with her own children sick, Mrs. Nichols wept that she had lived in the way of infection for over a month, haunted by inoculation day by day. Time and again, she had dithered and drawn back just as she told herself she was ready. Now, in hope and fear, she had made herself stay with Esther until he came. Even then, she had come close to fleeing the back way out the house as he entered at the front.

With his soothing encouragement, she undertook the operation. He left her sitting by Esther's side with a teary smile on her face.

On Monday, things began to slip and crack. In Union Street, Mary Dixwell's rash went on thickening; if it did not stop soon, he would have to concede that the inoculation had failed. *No*, he told himself. *Not failed:* she had caught smallpox in the natural way, before the operation.

Worse was the news that Bethiah Nichols was already feverish. His heart sank. It was only the third day of her inoculation. In her case, there could be little doubt: the operation had come too late. *Why the Webbs again, Lord? Why the Webbs?*

It wasn't, of course, only the Webbs. Funerals had become so frequent that the bells filled the air from morning to night with deep, booming carillons of death. Following a recent resolve passed by the General Court, the selectmen (who had pushed that resolve through the court in the first place) met to regulate funerals. No funeral should toll more than one bell—no more of the full pealing tangles of sound, they decided. And no person should have the chosen bell toll more than twice—or, in the case of Indians, Negroes, and mulattoes, more than once. Furthermore, funerals were to be kept to one hour of mourning, between five and six in the afternoon. It sounded draconian, they told the dubious ministers, but really, how could the doctors urge their patients into cheer when death was sounding incessantly around them?

On Tuesday, the Reverend Mr. Colman had Zabdiel inoculate his daughter Jane. Mr. Melville, keeper of the prison, and his wife, Mary, scion of the vast Willard clan of the Old South Church, put their son and daughter under the operation. As if the Salutation crowd did not want either the world or Zabdiel himself to doubt their faith in the face of tribulation, still another put himself under the operation: this time it was the baker Grafton Feveryear, another of Edward Langdon's brothers-in-law.

That evening the Boylston girls sparked into their fevers. For a few hours Zabdiel and Jerusha held their breath, but unlike Tommy's, the girls' fevers were mild.

On Wednesday morning, September 13, a black servant in silver-lace livery strutted up to the door with a message he stressed was urgent: Would Dr. Boylston be so kind as to attend Mrs. Margaret Salter?

He very nearly was not. At thirty, she was a weakly hysterical woman who was ill every other day—a perfect physician's nightmare. Though, to be honest, she was also a physician's gold mine. Her real attraction at the moment, though, was that she was the niece of Selectman John Marion. By marriage, admittedly—but still, she was family. It might—just might—be a way to force one of the selectmen to witness inoculation, willy-nilly. Unless Mr. Marion planned never again to lay eyes on his niece.

Stilling a tiny voice of warning, Zabdiel agreed.

That evening, he somehow found the time to slide into the Salutation to meet Cheever over a pint.

"Mrs. Dixwell's pocks fluxed in her face this morning, and Mrs. Nichols's pocks sprouted in hordes this afternoon," said Zabdiel. "On only the fifth day. None of her cohort of inoculees have yet felt so much as a feverish twinge."

"What do the Webbs say? What does Bill Nichols say?"

"Good men," said Zabdiel. "Sat there patiently while I explained the different numbering of days between inoculated and natural smallpox. On top of that, they grasped the point before I explained."

"There's no doubt Bethiah's is natural?"

Zabdiel shook his head. "None. Not with her." He sighed. "Though there are plenty out there who'll be more than happy to doubt it."

"In French and Scottish?" asked Cheever, but got no reply. Behind the house, a horse screamed in terror, the high twisting sound nipped by the deeper shouts of men and the clash of shod hooves kicking against walls. With everyone else, they rushed into the stable yard.

Someone had tossed hot tar on the horse's saddle, followed by a scattering of feathers. Some of the tar had dripped down on the horse's back and belly and no doubt burned it; it was wild with panic that was shaking hot drops of the stuff all over the yard.

The poor man who owned the horse was nearly as frantic as the animal was, running about, yelling and clutching his hair. After watching him for two minutes, Zabdiel told Cheever to haul the man inside for a drink and had the Langdons clear everyone else out of the yard. Then he and Jack went to work.

Fifteen minutes later, they had the horse calmed down to a shivering stand, long enough to get the saddle off. After another fifteen minutes of jittery walking, the gelding allowed himself to be led into a stall, trusting them enough to let them put some ointment on its burns. They weren't bad; thankfully, the poor beast had been more frightened than hurt. Zabdiel left Jack working the rest of the tar out, and keeping an eye on the other horses too.

When he reentered the pub, Cheever was alone by the big fire.

Zabdiel looked about for the horse's owner.

"Lightweight," said Cheever, blowing a large ring of smoke. "Two glasses of rum punch and his forehead did a double bounce on the table. Langdon's treated him to a bed upstairs." He still had a small row of full glasses lined up in front of him. He slid one across the table at Zabdiel. "He's a visitor. Says he knows no one in town; he's just stopped here on his way up to see cousins in Cambridge. So, he asks, why would someone tar and feather his horse?"

"Why would a man like a mouse have a horse like that?" snorted Zabdiel, tossing the rum down his throat. "That's a better question. Or at least one with a less obvious answer." He fixed Cheever's eye. "Did you get a good look at him?"

"Two rums' worth."

"No, the horse."

"In the dark? With him thrashed about like hurricane?" He slid another rum toward Zabdiel.

Zabdiel sipped at it. "He looks just like Prince. I might have mistaken him myself. Except, of course, that his pockets have been picked." He threw back the rest of the rum, and then started to chuckle. "Meant for me, of course. Only, my foe in the dark can't tell the difference between a horse who's been castrated and one who has not." His snickering broke into laughter, and soon he and Cheever were roaring till they cried.

Eventually, the laughter petered out. "You watch your back," said Cheever. "Bastard who did that'll try anything."

"I'll be fine," said Zabdiel.

Nonetheless, the Salutation Alley men tightened their knot around him. They gave up all pretense of happening to be riding the same direction; two of them began accompanying him wherever he went.

"I am not a virgin in distress," he once said testily to Cheever. "I do not need to have my hand held."

"Glad to hear it," said Cheever. "I don't think we could manage an escort of eight, plus a chaperone for hand holding."

On Thursday the fourteenth of September, Zabdiel's brother edged into the fever even as his own girls left theirs behind, and headed into the rash. Up in Salutation Alley, Fanny Webb gave her husband one last look of longing and regret, and let go of life.

Grieving for her, and even more for poor John, who looked pithed for all that he was a minister and must urge proper Christian fortitude in the face of sorrow and death, Jerusha gripped Zabdiel's hand and held her breath as she watched the rash sow its way over her girls. Before she had even dared to hope, it slowed and ran out of seed. Young Jerusha had no more than forty or fifty quickly ripening flecks; Mary and Lizzy had more than she did on their faces, but they skated lightly on the surface of the skin: they would leave no scars.

On Saturday afternoon, high thin clouds scudded overhead as the New North Church filled with every Webb and Adams in town for John's sake, and every Bromfield for Fanny's. Behind them came the ruling elders and deacons of the New North, out of respect for her husband, their pastor, and all the province's councilors and judges as well as the governor and the lieutenant governor, out of respect for her father, Councilor Edward Bromfield. Behind that streamed the regular congregation and the Webbs' friends and neighbors. Every house in Salutation Alley emptied into the church, which soon began spilling people back into the streets. The minister's young wife had held many a pock-ridden hand in the neighborhood when no one else could or would, without a thought for herself. Her husband and father were respected; she had been loved.

Like a long-legged bird of doom, the Reverend Dr. Cotton Mather stalked into the pulpit to deliver her funeral sermon. But even as he intoned, *This brave and beloved servant of God*, Zabdiel's mind wandered. Fanny was beyond help, but he said his own silent prayers for John, who would be lost without her. And for John's sister Bethiah Nichols, who might yet be saved, Lord willing. But no longer, he thought, in the absence of the Lord's concerted help. Zabdiel had visited her on his way to the church; she was full of small, depressed pocks that were already confluent, and still they were spreading. Her throat was dry and sore, and she was racked with a dry cough. Her progress did not look good. In fact, it looked damned poor—He caught himself and glanced about, as if someone might have heard the rough urgency of his thought. Still, she might yet be saved. Where better to hope for that than in a house of God?

Afterward, as the bearers carried the coffin from the church at a slow march and set it on the hearse, the funeral bell found its bronze voice. It tolled, once and then a second time, fulfilling the legal limit of mourning. But the shipwright and anchorsmith pulling the bell rope with arms thick as oaks cared nothing for the selectmen and their decrees of how many times a bell might be tolled, and when; they grieved for the young woman who had cradled their dying children at the stinking worst of the distemper, when no one else would come near, least of all the selectmen. The bell boomed out again. A murmur of surprise and satisfaction rose and died away, and still the bell tolled.

"It is expressly flouting the law," muttered Mr. Cook in a tone he knew would carry to Chief Justice Samuel Sewall, three feet ahead. "Twice only, and once for Negroes."

"It is the first public funeral I have seen without the ostentation of scarves and rings," remarked the judge to his son in clarion tones. "It has a very good character."

Mr. Cook scowled, but fell silent. The bell tolled twenty-eight times, once for each year of her too-short life, as Frances Bromfield Webb's funeral procession wound west up Snow Hill to the burial ground and laid her in ground so sodden that the earth itself seemed to be weeping.

Later that evening, a carriage drew up at the Boylstons' door, and a small party of Reverend Webbs's Adams cousins descended. Mr. Jones had been inoculated two weeks before and had done well; only a few scabs still clung to his skin. Now he and his wife—one of the Adams clan—wanted their five-year-old daughter Mary inoculated. With them was Mrs. Jones's eldest brother, Samuel, along with his wife and four-year-old daughter, both also named Mary.

The Adamses had already lost two children to other childhood disasters. "I cannot bear even to think of losing my last little lamb too," said Mrs. Adams, holding the child tight, as if some dark wind might snatch her away. "But it was hard not to fear it this morning." She had decided in the midst of the funeral, she said, that she and little Mary should be inoculated without delay. Samuel had agreed so heartily with her scheme that he had driven straight here on the way home, without so much as looking left or right.

Rolling a hoop with a stick, Tommy went sprinting by the bay window facing the street, and John ran yelling after him. Wild laughter could be heard around the side of the house.

"Whenever you're ready," said Zabdiel, picking up his lancet.

On the seventeenth, Zabdiel's brother's pocks came out; Mrs. Nichols's rash went on thickening.

On Monday, September 18, Mrs. Dixwell's pocks at last began to scab, though her face, more truthfully, could no longer be described as having pocks. It was one vast swollen boil. Her throat was raw and her breathing ragged.

In her big house in Marlborough Street, surrounded by servants, Mrs.

Salter detected a fever. She detected a headache. She demanded laudanum.

Zabdiel detected impatience, but did his best to quell it.

In a move of unforgivable pride, Governor Shute proclaimed a Day of Thanksgiving in October, provoking dark muttering all over town. Not that anyone was opposed to giving thanks, when it was merited. But just then, with the epidemic's furor still rising around them, it seemed dangerously imperious, as if setting a date by which the Almighty must behave. Almost as dangerous a temptation of the wrath of God, muttered some, as inoculation.

The next morning, the advocate general of the province responded by having his daughter, Elizabeth Valentine, inoculated.

By Wednesday evening, Mrs. Dixwell's face had scabbed over completely; bloody pus seeped through cracks in the thick crust. The next day, the scabs on her body began to slough off, and her incisions opened wide, disgorging rivers of poison. Both John Dixwell and Zabdiel clung to hope. She was feeling more comfortable; her breathing had eased, and her fever was still moderate. Maybe the scabs and the incisions would eject the poison from her body.

That afternoon, Zabdiel allowed Mr. Dixwell to bring their two eldest children—ten-year-old Basil and six-year-old Elizabeth—in for a visit, which gave her great joy and, as they were recovering nicely from their own bouts with smallpox, put them at no danger. John, only three, they kept in the nursery, fearing that he would scream in terror at the figure on the bed, who was not, could not, be the big, warm, cinnamon-scented mother he missed. Surely, such a scene would only upset them both.

Basil and Elizabeth were charged not to mention their little sister Mary at all; Zabdiel still thought it too dangerous for Mrs. Dixwell to know that her littlest now lay in the earth.

In the midst of this visit, Zabdiel was called away to see Mrs. Margaret Salter, who had taken a sharp turn for the worse.

When he saw her, she pointed to three flecks—two on her face, and one on her arm—and wailed. He was inexcusably short with her, he thought glumly afterward. After explaining for the tenth time that the appearance of *some* rash was to be expected, he abruptly took his leave and returned to Mrs. Dixwell.

As he rode back to Union Street, the funeral bells began to toll all across the city; it was the mourning hour. Five o'clock.

Mrs. Dixwell's windows were all wide open and the air in the room was crisp and cold, cut with the scent of burning leaves outside and cinnamon oil within, though neither masked the thick miasma of her pocks. The children had gone, and she was shaking with hysteria. "My baby," she wailed, as he walked in. "My Mary, my baby, my Mary." She could hear her baby's sweet voice, she said, calling her to heaven. She would die in the night and be eaten by worms.

"She asked," said John stonily to Zabdiel's silent question. "Point-blank."

Zabdiel sighed. He dosed Mrs. Dixwell with laudanum and sat with her until the crying and shivering went off, and she drifted into heavy purple dreams.

The next day, he visited early in the morning. She was groggy, but seemed refreshed and calmer.

That afternoon he slipped away to see other patients. Mrs. Nichols, thankfully, had held steady for about a week: she hadn't improved appreciably, but she hadn't worsened, either, and that, at this point, seemed a gift of grace.

Mrs. Salter was lying back on her pillows, a looking glass lying hopelessly in her hand. She had several pink bumps already filling with clear liquid; about two dozen, he estimated. "Twenty-five," she snapped. He assured her this was a fine sparse number, but she would have none of it: she had a splitting headache, vapors, and she was dying, she announced.

He returned to Mrs. Dixwell. She had done well all day, but as the bells boomed out again at five o'clock, she began to shake and wail afresh. Ominously, her fever rose with her hysteria. Zabdiel bled and blistered her, but to no avail; the fever soared higher and higher.

The next morning, Saturday, September 23, the fever stopped rising, but it clamped around her like a vise, inside which she shivered uncontrollably. Zabdiel drew John aside, and began to prepare him for the worst.

Later, among the stately houses of the South End, he inoculated the only son and heir of Councilor Thomas Fitch; the powers that be, it seemed, were slowly coming around to inoculation, even as his own faith began to waver.

In the Town House, the selectmen met to discuss the problem of firewood: supplies were already dangerously low, and there hadn't even been a cold snap yet, not a real one. But the sloopmen who sailed it down from the forests of the north had no wish to touch at Boston. Dr. Mather had sent them a suggestion, and this time, they admitted it was a good one. The selectmen let it be known that if the sloopmen would moor their sloops at the Castle, the town would bear the cost of hiring crews to run the boats over from the Castle to the Long Wharf, unload them, and return them empty and aired.

They could not face a smallpox winter without fuel for cooking and for heat.

* * *

On Sunday morning, September 24, Jerusha shepherded Zabdiel and the children to church: it was to be a familial day of Thanksgiving, for the girls had shed the last of their scabs. Everyone in their little family was safe.

The children, she knew, had decided in hushed conference among themselves that they would pray hard for the souls of their papa's sick people. Jerusha smiled, anticipating their little faces screwed up tight as they pressed their prayers toward heaven. Perhaps those prayers would help; she certainly hoped they might, though she silently asked pardon for her entirely selfish reasons. If Mrs. Dixwell were to die, the simmering mob that trailed her husband night and day might explode. But the mob was not half as harsh as Zabdiel would be on himself.

She shook off her gloom. Misery might always come tomorrow; it was her duty to the Lord to celebrate His glories as they came. And what glories they were: six fine children, hard pressed to keep from skipping to church, safe once and for all from the smallpox. The angel of death had passed over their door.

She knew she must look grave, she knew she must join the congregation in begging for mercy for all of Boston. But exaltation and praise bloomed bright in her heart. She was looking forward to the singing.

For his part, Zabdiel had promised Jerusha that he would focus this morning on thanksgiving, so he had thrust Mrs. Dixwell to the back of his mind. As they crossed the street, he clung to the successes for which he could give thanks: his family's safe passage through inoculation, Jerusha's return. Cheever. Helyer. Dr. Mather's support, however strange and sly it might be. Across town, Mr. Adams and his little girl Mary had begun to erupt and looked to do well. Mrs. Adams was a bit of a concern—she had not yet felt so much as a single flash of fever. But too little sickness was a much nicer problem than too much. Young Mary Jones, too, inoculated the same day as her Adams cousins, had a fine sparse rash of pocks creeping across her.

And then there was Mrs. Salter. Her pocks had ripened to pustules; though she refused to believe it, she would soon be fine. The sooner, the better.

Just before they entered the church, someone plucked at his sleeve. He turned, and a black man he did not recognize leaned forward and whispered in his ear the words he had been half dreading all morning. "It's the missus. I am to beg you to come at once."

He turned to Jerusha, but she had heard. Her pale eyes wide, she gave him a quick smile of encouragement and said, "Go. We will pray for you."

Zabdiel sighed, though whether it was more relief at being released from false thanksgiving or regret for the summons he had known must come, even he could not say. Jack materialized, behind him, and they headed back for the barn, the other black man in tow. Five minutes later, they were trotting north.

At Mr. Dixwell's shop, where Union Street ran into Hanover, Zabdiel was dismounting, when the servant ran up behind and puffed, "Pardon, sir, but may I ask why we are stopping here? I was to beg you, sir, to come straightaway."

"Isn't your mistress Mrs. Dixwell?"

"No, sir. Mrs. Nichols. She's begun to bleed. Before her time, if you get my drift."

"*Mrs. Nichols.*" Zabdiel blinked twice, and then tossed himself back in the saddle and leapt into a canter north up Hanover Street, toward Wakefield Alley.

Bethiah Nichols was weepy, but Zabdiel had no time to coax her out of it. "You told me you were not with child," he said, a little sharply. "Are you sure?"

She sniffled and looked away, and presently she nodded and whispered, "Eight or nine weeks gone. I was afraid you would not agree to the operation."

Zabdiel's heart turned over inside him, and pity came back. He took her hand. "I would not have. I am afraid you are losing this baby, my dear," he said.

She sobbed in silence, and he let her cry. There was nothing else he could do.

He stepped out for a breath of air; Jack ducked out with him into the empty streets. "I'll be fine," said Zabdiel impatiently. "The good folk of Boston are in church."

"Ain't the good folk I'm worried about," said Jack.

On their way home, they stopped in at the Dixwells'. Mary Dixwell's fever had wrapped her ever tighter in suffocating heat; she was shaking so constantly now that it was hard to tell when the feverish shivering stopped and the convulsions began. Zabdiel remained by her side all that afternoon, praying privately for a miracle, knowing he would not get one. Just before the churches were to let out from afternoon prayer, he sent Jack north to Salutation Alley. Presently he reappeared with Reverend Webb and a phalanx of Mr. Dixwell's fellow ruling elders and deacons of the New North Church.

Outside, a crowd of the already mourning, the curious, and the perpetually angry mingled around the house. Some prayed loudly for Mrs. Dixwell's deliverance; some wished just as fervently, though more quietly, for her death: as just retribution for the poor king done to death by her father-in-law all those years ago, as punishment for her own temptation of Providence. What was the difference, someone wheezed, between her death and suicide? Heads nodded, and eyes slid knowing looks at each other.

Dr. Douglass drove by in his carriage and eyed the crowd with satisfaction. *Pride goeth before a fall*, he observed to Mr. Stewart, and drove on.

Zabdiel remained by Mrs. Dixwell's side into the evening, fending misery off from her final moments with laudanum, while John Dixwell knelt by the bedside in prayer. Mr. Webb and the men of the New North surrounded him, their voices blending into a strong, deep, comforting river of sound. Through the old-fashioned diamond panes of the windows, the trees smoldered with the fires of autumn, their edges curling gold, bronze, red, orange, peach, mahogany, and yellow. As the sun touched the tip of the three-peaked mountain to the west, the whole world briefly flamed bright. To the east, the tide slid whispering away from the land, and as the light quietly failed, Mrs. Dixwell's spirit sank with it into death.

❧ 8 ❧

THE KING'S PARDON

Newgate Prison, London
September 6, 1721

THE others had hauled the tapster from bed as the sun rose and were already celebrating their pardons in the taproom, but Lizzy Harrison lingered in her chamber. She ought to celebrate—she ought to—she knew it as well as anybody, but she felt more like crying.

The gates were to open to them later that morning; king's pardon in hand, she would be free.

Lizzy looked about at the empty room with its three rough beds, mismatched chairs, and tipsy tables, its walls decorated with scrawls of charcoal. It was the finest room she had ever lived in. Against all expectation, she had been happy here too. Had felt useful. But as of nine o'clock, she had earned the right to be turned out from it.

To go where?

She stared at a small patch of sun sliding across the table, as if she could burn it into her vision. No other room she was ever likely to inhabit would be pierced by so much as one window: London's tax on windows ensured that. Here she had two. So what if they were barred? So what if she could not read the scrawls on the walls? Hadn't Mrs. Tompion read most of them to her?

A jangling of keys shattered her reverie. "As is one of them medical gentlemen wishes a word with you, Lizzy 'Arrison," leered the jailer, as if to say, *And don't I know exactly what word it is he wants, my Lady Lie-back*. He smelled of onions, bad teeth, and gin. "In the small parlor. Doubletime."

Her already sinking spirits dropped into the dungeons. She was no green girl, she told herself tightly, as she had so many times before, but now it sounded hollow and sad. The old London was already pulling her back to the old expectation of all she was good for. With one of the doctors, no less.

She was too proud, though, to let the jailer see her distress. She rose as haughtily as she imagined the Princess of Wales herself might, and sailed out of the room without so much as a glance at the man.

The parlor looked empty. Perhaps the man, whoever it was, had thought better of himself, and had gone away again. Then she heard a creak, and a dark figure rose from a large leather chair that had been drawn into the sun. *Mr. Maitland.*

But he made no move toward her: just stood there regarding her, his hands clasped behind his back, his expression stern.

He cleared his throat. "Now, Mrs. Harrison," he said, "as you know, the inoculation experiment is over, and you are free to go. I, too, am off. I go to Hertford next week."

Without warning, the wail that had been coiled in her stomach all morning sprang long and thin through the parlor, and she burst into tears.

Mr. Maitland watched Lizzy Harrison with alarm. Where had such sorrow come from? The girl was free to go—full king's pardon—surely a joyous occasion. He dug through his experience for some likely explanation, but he was a bachelor. Even his servants—at least, those with whom he came into contact—were men. He was a surgeon, of course, to many ladies, but their tears were different. They cried like crocodiles or falcons—or a chimeric combination of both—when they wanted something. Or they cried in pain. But Lizzy was neither maneuvering nor suffering—not bodily, anyway.

He crossed the room and installed her, still sobbing, into one of the chairs in front of the fireplace. He produced a handkerchief for her, and then paused. What to do next? Best, really, to press on.

"Now, Lizzy," he said again, "I hope you will listen carefully. As I said, I'm off to Hertford. The smallpox is very bad there, and they are in dire need of nurses."

The weeping stopped as suddenly as it had begun. She hiccuped and blew her nose.

"You have shown a commendable diligence and willingness to learn in the past month," he said. "And, I must say, a most admirable talent for nursing."

She was watching his every move, her face wary.

"I serve as surgeon to Christ's Hospital—a charity school for orphans. If you like, I will secure you a place there as a smallpox nurse." His throat tightened as he made the offer. How was he to convince such a girl that it was a good idea? He was not so sure himself that it was a good idea, at least not for her.

The smile that burst across her face took him aback. Like rainbows, or sun suddenly pouring through a break in the clouds. *Really*, he told himself sharply, *you are becoming quite absurdly sentimental.*

"Oh, sir!" she exclaimed. "You would find me a place?"

He nodded.

"In the country?"

"Hertford is not exactly the country," he cautioned, but she was rattling on. Clearly, to her, anything beyond Cripplegate and Bedlam was the country. "And will there be larks? I've always wanted to see larks, sir, though I suppose one 'ears 'em, don't one? And daffodils—in the ground, like."

"Larks I can promise you," he said. "But not daffodils, at least, not until spring." *What was he doing, promising her flowers and birds?* He steered his voice back to gravity. "I must warn you: the engagement is by no means risk free." She tried to press the smile from her mouth, but did not quite succeed. "It is, in fact, an extension of the experiment you have just passed through. We—Sir Hans Sloane, Dr. Steigerthal, and I—believe you are now safe from the smallpox. But we are not sure."

Dr. Sloane and Dr. Steigerthal had not wanted him to be so forthright; they had predicted she would refuse out of hand—and they wanted this experiment badly, as the final seal on their success: the guarantee that inoculation offered reliable protection from acquiring the smallpox in the natural way. So badly, in fact, that they had joined their purses to pay for it.

But Mr. Maitland had been adamant. Lizzy had made a bargain to risk her life in exchange for a full and free pardon. He would not now try to attach an anchor chain. He would offer her an entirely new agreement, to take or leave as she pleased, or he would make no offer at all. Besides, he had been fairly sure that she would only agree under those circumstances. She had more intelligence than the physicians credited, and could smell deceit from four miles off. He was certain, he had said, that without forthright honesty, she would flee.

Sir Hans had sniffed. If Mr. Maitland lost her, he said, the Princess of Wales would be disappointed. As would, no doubt, His Majesty the king.

His Majesty, thought Mr. Maitland grimly, had made a promise.

In front of him, Lizzy sniffled. "You mean you are not sure, or you mean that prig of a Dr. Droop-staff is not sure?" she said with a spark of her old spirit.

"Some say that the distemper was not genuine. That it was merely the

chicken pox, or some other spurious pox. Or that it was not strong enough
to afford you protection. We believe it was. But we are not sure."

"And this will make you sure?"

"Yes."

She bit her lip. "I will have a place? Bed and board?"

He nodded.

"You will teach me more about nursing?"

He nodded again, feeling like a feeding duck. "All those things."

"And it'll be proper? No gentlemen?"

"There will be boys, but not men. Girls too. It is a school."

The smile came back. "Then, sir, I'll go with you to where there's larks."

"You realize you will be risking the smallpox?"

"I'd be risking worse, to stay 'ere." Darkness flickered through her eyes,
and was gone. "I trusted you before; why should I stop now?"

Lizzy had thought the Press Yard fine; within twenty minutes, she decided
the house of Mrs. Priscilla Moss, matron of Christ's Hospital in Hertford,
was paradise. There *were* larks, and though it was not the season for their
angelic singing in the realms of the moon, still, they sang. There were also
sparrows and robins bustling about in their red-feathered waistcoats. Almost as chattery were the children running or walking in their lines, in
their long blue coats flapping up to show yellow skirts beneath. There were
no daffodils, but there was more green than she had dreamed the world
could hold. And wide skies shifting minute by minute and hour by hour
through blue, pink, lavender, silver, sapphire, and velvet black.

"Don't breathe so hard, child," Mrs. Moss had said, catching her at a
window her first day. "You'll faint."

But it was hard not to gulp the strong, sharp sweetness of that air.

Mrs. Moss was kindness and patience itself. Her daughter Sarah was a
little less so—she followed Lizzy nervously with her eyes whenever she
came downstairs, as if she might nick a bit of silver, but she was less sure of
herself than her mother was.

So it was not perfect—but then Lizzy had never imagined paradise to
be perfect either: it had had lying serpents in it, didn't it? She'd take the
work at Christ's, anyday. Which was not to say that it was easy, or always
pleasant. One of Mrs. Moss's serving girls had broken out in confluent pox;
after that first day, Lizzy was set to care for her, and was largely confined to
a room in the attic with her. But it was a big room, with three gabled windows that flickered with the dances of leaves: an elm stood just outside.
She felt quite like a bird herself sometimes, as if she, too, lived in that tree.

The food was filling and hot, and could be counted on—right down to the minute. And she quite liked her patient, though for much of the time the poor girl could not talk. Lizzy cared for her as she might have cared for a mewling infant.

The windows she kept open. Even on the worst stinking days, when the pocks oozed bloody pus over the sheets, the birdsong buoyed Lizzy up, and from time to time little breezes would sweep the room clean.

Mr. Maitland came every other day, at least as interested in Lizzy's health as in the maid's. On the worst of days, when flushes crossed her skin like high, thin clouds on a spring day, and a small crop of pimples sprouted around her incision scars, his concern made her feel that she'd let him down. But the incisions stayed closed, and she felt no pangs of headache or fever, so presently he was pleased again.

Best of all, he spoke to her of other things, which she much preferred to the topic of herself. At the beginning of October, for instance, he began inoculating again, this time among the Hertford quality. His first patient was the two-and-a-half-year-old daughter of a Quaker at Temple, which he said was about three miles from town. The girl, Mary Batt by name, had passed through the inoculated smallpox just as expected, he said: mild first fever, twenty or so pocks, no second fever at all, and the pocks very quickly drying up and falling away.

He was so buoyed up that he tried again, on two brothers, seven and three, on October 12, this time right within Hertford. He inoculated them at the same time, with the same matter: but that was where the sameness ended. Young Benjamin Heath, the three-year-old, was eager to please, clean of habit, and easily governed; he had a very gentle case, quite like Mary Batt's.

But Joseph—well, he said, shaking his head, "he is a fat, foul, and gluttonous boy." Lizzy had nearly dropped the pile of clean sheets she had just folded; she had never heard Mr. Maitland say anything so uncomplimentary. He must have surprised himself, for he exclaimed, "I do not exaggerate! The child has a voracious appetite, and is constantly filling his belly with the coarsest food—cheese, fat country pudding, cold boiled beef. He looks like all three, come to think of it, molded into one lump."

Lizzy began to laugh.

"He will not obey the simplest rule, nor will his parents restrain him—not even to keep him indoors in cold, windy, frosty weather; if he wants to go out, then out he goes, or the house resounds with it. I tell you, he once wet his feet in the water!"

Lizzy had to sit down on the edge of the maid's bed, she was laughing so hard, though she did not know what was funniest: the fat, foul little boy, Mr. Maitland's consternation, or the notion that wet feet was a catastrophe.

"It is not a laughing matter," he said reproachfully. "The boy is very ill. A high fever before the eruption, and now a great load of small, coherent pocks. Had he taken the disease in the natural way, I doubt a worldful of doctors could save his fat, froward life!"

Lizzy glanced sharply at Mr. Maitland's face. So that was the problem. Guilt.

Lizzy's servant-maid patient was no sooner getting well than one of the boys in Mrs. Moss's care came down with ominous symptoms. The servant girl was removed to another room to convalesce, and he was installed in her place. Mr. Maitland expressly directed her to lie in the bed with him every night—but she would've done it anyway, without the asking. Poor little tyke. He clung to her for as long as he could, and then, even when it hurt to move or to be touched, still, he would scrape his arm along the sheets and touch her with one finger: just to know that someone was there.

Sarah Moss began to relax. One day, she offered to teach Lizzy her alphabet and her numbers.

Lizzy practiced as long as there was daylight. Real nurses must be able to read the doctor's instructions, after all.

She did not see Mr. Maitland again for some time. When she did, she was surprised at how haggard he looked.

"What's 'appened at the 'Eaths'?" she asked.

"Heaths'?" he asked absently from the window. "Oh. Both boys at last recovered . . . I did not think it was catching," he said, dropping into a chair. "So much of the arguing, you see, has centered on whether or not inoculation produces a true smallpox or a spurious one—the chicken pox."

He shook his head and dropped it in his hands. "You'd have thought, given my position, I would have foreseen this. But I was as lulled into false understanding by the lightness of inoculated cases as Dr. Wagstaffe. And now six people are ill, and one of them is dying."

Mr. Batt, he said, had six domestic servants—four men and two maids— who had all cared for little Mary while she was down with the inoculated smallpox. He shook his head. Even with the pocks full upon her, they had hugged and petted her daily. Two weeks or thereabouts after the height of the girl's rash, they had all been seized at once with the telltale fever, backache, and nausea.

As if that weren't enough, Mrs. Heath's infant, still suckling at her breast, had also caught the natural smallpox—distinct, thank God. And Mrs. Heath, too, who'd had the distemper many years before, had grown several pimply pustules on her face and hands, though without any sickness attending them. "As often happens to smallpox nurses—and even to the laundresses who must wash their linens," he said. He smiled ruefully. "Just as has happened to you."

It was strange, he said, how different the Batt servants' cases had been, though they had all been infected from the same source—and that a light case of inoculated pox, no less. But the servants had suffered varying degrees of distinct pox, mostly bad, and two had turned confluent, with all its calamities. "But they all did well," he said. "God be thanked."

"All?" she asked gently.

"All except one," he said gruffly. "But she would not be governed."

He turned his back on that death; there was nothing to be gained by stewing over it. The best he could do was to try and understand it.

It was in talking to Lizzy that he began to order his arguments. Lizzy, of course, was proving that smallpox could not reinfect the inoculated, in the natural way. Inversely, these unforeseen accidents had shown that inoculated smallpox *could* infect the unprotected. What better double-underlined proof could there be that the inoculated smallpox was indeed a true smallpox?

By the beginning of November, Mr. Maitland was sure of his success. He waited impatiently, however, until midmonth, when Lizzy's boy was all but recovered and she was still free of fever and spots, before he sat down to write his official report.

> *Having understood, since my retirement into the country, that the late experiment of inoculating the smallpox at Newgate has been pretty much talked of; and finding withal that the reports of that matter are various and oftentimes contradictory: I thought it became me to give the public a plain and honest account of the truth of facts.*

There were so many issues, so many questions, findings, scruples, and doubts. How was he to marshal them all into neat soldierly rows? One at a time, he thought, take them one at a time, beginning with the most important. What was the ultimate reason for making this latter experiment?

Following the success of Newgate, he wrote, *I still had one difficulty left, which I took to be the most considerable; and which, if not fully cleared, would render, in my opinion, the whole of the process but trifling and precarious: and that is, whether everyone who had undergone this operation is really secured against all future danger of catching the smallpox by infection? Were I but well assured of this, I should then, I thought, be at liberty to practice it myself, and likewise with confidence recommend it to others.*

He sighed with satisfaction. He was now in a position to answer his own question, and to answer it strongly.

I myself have lately made open and repeated trials on one of the six inoculated criminals of Newgate, reserved for that purpose, sufficiently to convince anyone that there's no danger of their catching the disease by any future infection. This is one Elizabeth Harrison, of about nineteen years of age. Here I must observe to you that this girl had the fewest eruptions upon her of any of the five that were inoculated at Newgate, but had a more than ordinary discharge at the incisions.

Referring to his notes, he described in detail her trials in the house of Mrs. Moss, nursing the servant maid and the boy. It was all neat and good. More than that, it was incontrovertible.

Even as he thought this, however, he heard in his mind Dr. Wagstaffe scrupling to doubt that so much as a single word was true. The mere memory of the man's voice irritated him.

There's no ground to question these facts, he scribbled, *being attested by a cloud of witnesses.*

He took a breath and put his aggravation away. He was a surgeon from Aberdeen, and though he was proud of his work, he was an honest man. He knew he did not walk among the great geniuses of the age. He had played his part well, he hoped, but he had not sought it out. He had even sought to avoid it. The discovery had tapped him on the shoulder; he had not, like Sir Isaac Newton, dared to run along the shore of some vast ocean of truth, chasing down a particular shell. Nevertheless, it had fallen to him to call forth the trumpets. He must somehow rise like a poet, a prophet, and declare the Truth.

He closed his eyes and thought of a falcon he had once seen, winging over the heather at home; he thought of another he had seen soaring below him, and beyond that, the flower-strewn plain of Turkey, as he descended from the crags of the Bulgarian mountains. Then he leaned forward, biting his lip as he wrote.

Hence, if any regard be due to facts, I am persuaded that all impartial people will allow this method to be not only safe, but useful, and highly worthy to be received with esteem and applause.

He drummed his fingers on the table. That was good, that was accurate and rational, but it did not have a heart-sweeping wheel and swoop.

Is it not a matter of the greatest importance to us, to know how to prevent the mighty contagion of the smallpox, and how to preserve our children and families from the violent attacks, and fatal effects of it? What would not tender parents give to secure to them the lives and features of their beloved offspring, when they behold them disfigured by the loathsome disease and struggling with the pains of death? Do not we oftentimes see great families extinguished by it, as by the plague, and their titles and estates thereby transmitted to strangers? And if they have the good fortune to escape with their lives, what an ugly change from what they were before! What pittings, seams, and scars in their faces! What films and fistulas, and sometimes blindness in their eyes! What ulcers and abscesses in their bodies, contractions of the nerves, and even lameness of for life! Again, to avoid the infection, what uneasiness and disquiet of mind, what fears and apprehension do not even grown people labour under, especially the more delicate and tender? Don't they renounce all commerce with their best friends and dearest relations? And if by chance they meet an object that has but lately recovered, how susceptible then are they of the distemper? And how few thus seized do ever escape?

In short, then, to prevent the havoc made by that mighty disease, which has hitherto seemed to go forth like a destroying angel, subduing all before it and contemning all human means used to stop its career, I may truly venture to affirm that the method here recommended is the safest and, I am sure, far the most infallible.

He tossed down the pen, caught up his coat, hat, and walking stick, and went out for a long winter walk.

❧ 9 ❧

RAW HEAD AND
BLOODY BONES

Boston
September 25, 1721

JERUSHA found Zabdiel sitting in the parlor the next morning, his
head in his hands. He looked up blearily as she came in. "Mary
Dixwell died last night."

She crossed the room and knelt by his side.

"I don't think I killed her, Jerusha. But I cannot stand before my Maker
and swear I did not."

Dr. Douglass rubbed his hands with glee, and sat down to write a letter to
Dr. Alexander Stuart of the Royal Society. *The smallpox rages here epidemi-*
cally: about a thousand persons are decumbent with the disease. Above sixty persons
of all ages, sexes, and conditions have been inoculated, of which several had the
confluent sort, and I am sorry to say, one—and here he paused. Mrs. Dixwell's
death he was sure of. But the number might be considerably worse. Might
double, in fact. From what he heard, Mrs. Nichols was not doing well at
all. She might very well die herself in the next week or two. He did not,
however, wish to hold his letter that long. Lord knew when another ship
might sail for London.

He smiled and dipped his quill in the ink once more. *I am sorry to say,*
one or two have died.

HMS *Seahorse* returned from her northern voyage; this time, nobody con-
gregated to see the plume of her sails. A few anxious wives and parents
slipped down to the Long Wharf, handkerchiefs to noses, averting their

eyes from each other to avoid exchanging greetings that might also exchange contagion.

With the rolling gait of a sailor and the confidence of a man, Charles Paxton strode down the gangplank.

"Where is Hector?" asked Captain Paxton as his son stepped onto the dock.

Charles was taken aback. "Why, with you, Father. Where should he be?"

Captain Paxton's grip on his walking stick tightened. "I am in no mood for banter."

"But he never rejoined the ship."

"Never—?"

"He met Captain Durell himself the morning we left, and showed him a letter from you, requesting him to be discharged—"

Captain Paxton did not hear the rest. His face and neck purple with rage, he pushed past his son and stormed aboard.

If there were one or two hearts about the ship that lifted and one or two minds that thought, *May you be far away, with a fair wind behind*, they kept their eyes down and their smiles shadowed.

As the sun rose over Dock Square, crowds surged through the streets, flinging themselves in ragged bands at Zabdiel's house. *"Raw Head and Bloody Bones!"* they screamed, peppering their cries with pebbles, rotten fruit, and eggs. *Murderer! Devil take you, murdering fiend! Go to hell!*

Zabdiel did not show so much as his shadow at a window, though most of the mob melted into soft shadows of dusk. "Hiding like a snail in his shell," he said bitterly as Jerusha came to bed and blew out the candle.

At midnight, a knocking on the chamber door sent him shooting back out of the bed. Jerusha sat bolt upright, clutching the sheet to her chin.

"Not meanin' to fright you, Doctor," said Jack quietly, his face flickering in the light of a candle at the door, "but Mr. Nichols's man is downstairs."

"What's wrong?"

"Don't know. I expect it's the missus. At least he had enough sense to be quiet-like. Came and scratched at the kitchen window."

Zabdiel threw on a dressing gown and went downstairs. The man rose, tall and black, gripping his hat in front of him.

"I'm to beg you to come quickly, sir. She's flooding."

Zabdiel ran back up the stairs and dressed. Jerusha sat, gripping her knees, her eyes huge in the moonlight. He drew to the bedside and took her hand.

She turned her eyes slowly to his. "Don't go," she whispered. "Zabdiel, please don't."

He smoothed down a few wisps of hair that had escaped her nightcap. "Beth Nichols is losing a child, Jerusha. What would you be saying if she were one of our girls?"

She bit her lip, swallowed hard, and blinked. "Come back to me."

"I promise." He kissed the top of her head and left.

Jack had saddled Prince. He had also saddled his mule. And he had muffled their hooves, in the Indian manner.

"Stay here," said Zabdiel tersely. "Jerusha and the children need a man in this house."

His prodigal son stepped out of the barn. "They have one," said Zabdiel junior. "Though to tell you the truth, I think Mother is easily as good with this thing as I am," he said, hefting the musket in his hand. Then he looked up and dropped his facetiousness. "God go with you, Father. And also with Jack."

Their faces muffled in dark cloaks, they rode quickly up to the Nicholses'. No one stirred in the streets, though the moon hung huge and ominous in the sky. A rat or two scuttled at the edge of the sewer channel, and a stray dog slinked along behind for a while. Once a door banged open, and drunken singing spilled into the street, pressing them farther into the shadows on the opposite side. They rode on.

Mrs. Nichols was worse than Zabdiel had dared to imagine. She was clammy and cold. Blood coursed from between her legs while her mind wandered through the visions of Ezekiel and Isaiah.

"Behold waters issued," she half sang, half sighed. "Waters to ankles, to knees . . . to the loins. A river I could not pass over, waters to swim in." Her voice trailed off in high girlish giggles. "When thou passest through the waters, I will be with thee."

Seizing her husband's collar, and pulling him down to her with startling strength, she rasped, "Wilt thou be with me?"

"I am here, Beth," he said, disentangling her fingers from his throat. "I am here."

Pocks were scattered thickly over her body: small ones, but ominously close together and flat; they were ringed in livid red. Her eyes were swollen nearly shut, her face gray, and her breath rank. Her pulse was so faint that it was hard to tell by feel that her heart still beat.

Zabdiel had Jack mix up a cordial that would knock a horse back on its feet: laudanum sweetened with sugar and heated with a liberal sprinkling of oil of cinnamon.

Twenty minutes later, her heartbeat had sped up to a light flutter. "Come hither," she murmured fretfully, "I will show unto thee the judgment of the Great Whore that sitteth upon many Waters."

"No, Beth," said her husband, "think of the Spirit of God moving on the waters."

"*God,*" she whimpered, curling into a ball as a cramp crossed her belly.

"What can we do?" stammered her terrified husband.

Zabdiel shook his head, and looked at him with pity. "Pray." Though he had been awake the whole night before, Zabdiel remained at the Nicholses', nodding in a chair by the bed until Bethiah's bleeding slowed to a trickle, and then one hour more. Contractions were still rippling across her belly, but nothing other than thin blood had come forth. "There is no more I can do here tonight, Bill," he said. "I will leave you with some cordial: give her one or two drops, if her pulse weakens. Otherwise, leave her alone to sleep: nature must take care of her now."

For the nurse, he left other instructions: "Keep the sheets."

Just before dawn, he returned to his own bed, where Jerusha wrapped herself around him so that he dropped into a leaden sleep in her arms.

Later that morning, he rode out to the Nicholses' again. Frayed lines of children and beggars whipped around him like tentacles of rage. *Raw Head and Bloody Bones! Murderer!*

While Mr. Nichols had prayed through the cold hours of dawn, the nurse had dosed Mrs. Nichols with the cordial two more times; each time, they said, she had regained strength for a while, but then drifted farther into twisted dreams. At ten o'clock she was awake but groggy. At least her pulse was normal.

And the flooding had stopped. Zabdiel sent Bill out of the room for a brief rest, and asked the nurse for the sheets. She gave him only one; inside its folds he found the drying placenta and the tiny half-formed child, two inches long and most of it head and huge eyes, curled over itself in permanent sleep, one tiny thumb, as it seemed, in its mouth. It was covered in pocks.

He had seen women die in childbirth; he had cut still-living children out of just-dead mothers. He had amputated breasts and legs and arms; he had slit into abdomens to pluck out bladder stones. But none of that was as this.

For the first time in many years, he went outside and vomited.

Cotton Mather rose early, slipped away from the still-sleeping Lydia, and went to his study. Two days after losing his newest grandchild, aged one week—during the Sabbath meeting, no less, and only hours before she was to be baptized—the infant's mother, his dear Abigail, his Abby Nabby Nibby as he had babbled to her as a child, was dying too. *G.D.* he wrote. *To strengthen a dear Child in the Agonies of Death is a sad Work, which I am again called unto.*

He had spent so many hours consumed with terror for Sammy and Lizzy, who stood in the way of the smallpox, that he had almost forgotten that the Angel of Death had other weapons. A creeping, malignant fever was slowly fraying Nibby's life. Even in death, the Lord set the Mathers apart.

Dr. Mather spent the day on his knees before his daughter's bed, strengthening her grieving husband with prayer. Not until sometime between ten and eleven that evening did the dear child at last let go.

She was his twelfth child to die; around her, death was mowing down his neighbors, his friends, his family, and his flock by the hundred. Dr. Mather was far beyond tears. At home, he added one sentence to his diary: *A long and hard Death was the Thing appointed for her.*

Dr. Mather threw himself back into his work. His *Account of the Method and Success of Inoculating the Small-Pox, in Boston in New-England* had been finished and dated three weeks before, in gratitude for Sammy's recovery. Nibby's long, scraping death had pushed it aside. At last, he sent it winging away within the wooden walls of a ship named *Friendship*, with a request that the captain deliver Dr. Mather's papers personally to Jeremiah Dummer, Esq., agent in London for the province of Massachusetts.

The Fellows of the Royal Society had not shouldered the burden of testing inoculation: but they should know that one of their number in Boston had dared to roam where they had feared to tread. They should know that it worked.

But that knowledge could no longer remain confined to them. He meant to publish his treatise to the world.

As Dr. Mather's confidence rose, Zabdiel's sank. Across the next two weeks, the trees flamed through their autumn glory; at night, the stars burned ever brighter as the harvest moon waned. Somehow, the world's extravagant beauty only made Zabdiel feel worse. Bethiah Nichols had lost a child, and now she was losing her sight.

The rash oozed into her eyes, swelling them tightly shut. Not until too late did he realize that the swelling was not just around the eyes; pocks had grown up inside them. Then one of them burst, taking the eye with it.

There was no telling whether the other might follow suit; there was nothing to do but wait.

Save for slinking to the Nicholses' at odd hours, Zabdiel stopped trying to go out. A few patients braved the screaming crowds to duck into his shop and beg advice or medicine; he gave it with a grave smile, but his heart held nothing but sawdust. Even Cheever could not rouse him to more than a flicker of a smile. For the most part, he let Jack run the shop, while he retreated to the parlor, where he read everything on the smallpox that Jack could scour up, and he reread everything he had already memorized, as if somewhere an answer, an explanation, an absolution, must be lurking.

He ate when Jerusha required it, but tasted nothing. He slept when she directed, but did not wake refreshed.

"You are fading to a ghost," she said quietly one evening. "The very bogeyman the mobs threaten you with. Raw Head and Bloody Bones."

"*Raw hands and bloody bones,*" he said absently, holding his hands before him. "You don't know what I have done, Jerusha."

"No, but I know what you are doing: you are giving up. You have a gift, Zabdiel, and you are giving up."

He shook his head. "*Thou shalt not kill.*" He looked into her eyes. "I had a gift. It is gone."

On October 2, Captain Paxton advertised a £5 reward for the return of Hector, alive.

"He is not coming back, Father," said Captain Paxton's elder son, Roger, begging to join the ship's company in Hector's place.

Much against his will, Captain Paxton swallowed his pride and agreed. *His boy in the place of a slave.* But with trade stagnant, every halfpenny counted. Roger's enlistment meant one more set of wages trickling in to the office, and one less mouth to feed at home.

He tried to ignore the voice in his head that mocked, *two less.*

Tom Boylston began to cross Dock Square to join his brother's family for dinner every afternoon. "Zabdiel needs you," said Jerusha quietly. "The children need you." To herself, she clucked, "And you need the food." *When was the last time a Boylston had not been able to afford enough to eat?* Tom's nieces and nephews did not seem to notice that he had grown gaunt. Whenever he appeared, they skidded across the room and threw themselves at their favorite uncle; Tommy climbed him like a tree. Top heavy with children and laden with laughter, he would lumber into the garden and wear them out until it was time to say grace. Which was just as well, sighed Jerusha to herself; for Zabdiel had forgotten how to play.

On the sixth of October, the selectmen again sent men scurrying from house to house, counting the sick and the dead. In two weeks, they reported, the death toll had nearly doubled, from 110 to 203. In all, 2,757— a quarter of the city—had fallen ill with the smallpox. At the Old North Church alone, prayers were requested for 202 people sick; in one day, Dr. Mather had prayed with 130 of them. *Surely*, he thought as he dragged himself home near midnight, *the epidemic has reached its height.*

The doctors were no better off, driving from one patient to the next with the horses at a gallop, when they were not inching door to door. And still, untreated multitudes cried out through windows, stretched thin grasping hands from foul doorways, and hobbled breathless and howling after them through the lanes. Other doctors were visiting eighty or a hundred patients each day, but Zabdiel sat in the parlor, reading.

That afternoon, Mrs. Eunice Willard skirted the shop and the house and knocked at the kitchen door. "Wait, Jack," said Jerusha, as she heard him turning her away. "Let me talk to her."

She heard young Mrs. Willard out in the kitchen and then ushered her upstairs to Zabdiel. "I cannot say what he will do," she said quietly on the stairs, "but I wish you luck."

Zabdiel looked up from his page and opened his mouth to refuse the caller, but Jerusha was already shutting the door behind her.

Reluctantly, he rose and bowed. "Mrs. Willard."

She curtsied. "Dr. Boylston."

"To what do I owe the pleasure of this visit?" Her brother Josiah Willard was the secretary of the province. The official mouthpiece, in other words, of the governor and Council. Surely, the government would not stoop to apprehending him through the offices of a woman.

She held both hands, still gloved, clasped in front of her; her dress was noticeably simple, though made well and worn neatly. "I would be inoculated, if you please."

"I am no longer performing that operation," he said.

"Then you must begin again."

Had she said what he thought he heard? He focused on her face. She was plain. Homely, to be honest. But her eyes gleamed with intelligence.

She drew herself as tall as she could. "I am a woman, sir, but I am not cut out for life as a wife and mother. I love my nieces and nephews, but that is enough. Thankfully, I have been well enough provided for by my father's will to make such a decision without fear of poverty. But I would like to do some good in this world, beyond needlework. I am told I have a reputation for learning, but the ministry and medicine are both closed to me. I have no aptitude for children not related to me, and sometimes, not even those: I would make a poor schoolmistress. However, I find I am quite patient with the sick."

She said all this without rancor or bitterness: just a cool assessment of the way the world was, untainted by sorrow or anger over how it ought to be. "I would become a nurse, and there are no nurses in more dire need now, sir, than smallpox nurses. But you see, I have not had the smallpox."

"For which you should be thankful."

"There we disagree."

"What does your brother say?"

"It is not his affair."

"It will be, when you bring the smallpox into the family. In any case, I am no longer inoculating." He turned his back on her abruptly and walked to a side window.

She sighed. "Then I must take matters into my own hands."

He looked at her sharply. "You will do no such thing."

"I am sorry, Dr. Boylston, but I must. You see, I assumed that you were not likely to have a supply of fresh matter." She tugged on a chain around her neck, and pulled a vial out from her bosom. A small bit of dull yellow matter clung to the side of the glass.

He strode over and yanked the vial from the chain around her neck. She did not flinch, even as the chain flew off against the wall.

"What have you done?"

She held his gaze calmly. "Collected my own this morning. From a nephew just at the stage described in Timonius. A boy of clean living, now doing as well as can be expected under the distinct pox. Except that he could do with more nursing. As could all my family. My family, as you know, is rather large. So you see, my plan is not so altruistic as I have represented."

"What have you done?" he said again, as if he might turn in her first answer for another.

"Crossed the Rubicon, sir. Waded right on out into trouble without bothering to take my shoes and stockings off first, as my father used to say. I know the dangers—"

"You most certainly do not."

"I know the dangers as well as one might who has not spent time in smallpox sickrooms. Fanny Webb was one of my girlhood friends," she said quietly. "Against that, I have seen the results of your operation: the Melvilles are my niece and nephew; Sammy Mather is a cousin by marriage."

"No."

"I am of age, sir. It is my risk to take. It is equally your choice to help me, or not. But you will not stop me from taking the gamble."

Zabdiel found he was breathing as if he had been racing. "Sit down," he ordered. "Don't move."

Jerusha, Jack, and Moll were suspiciously busy in the kitchen, a little too carefully not glancing up as he went by into the shop and emerged a few moments later with his lancet and some bandages. He knew, as he climbed the stairs again, that they would be quietly celebrating in the kitchen.

The next morning he returned to a full practice, though he still held off from inoculating. Picking his way through the catcalls and jeers, he could not have said precisely what made him return, except that anger seemed to have scythed through the despair. The despair was not gone: but there was now a narrow path through it.

What a week I must look for! Dr. Mather wrote wearily on the eighth of October. The week before, he had thought the epidemic had reached its screaming peak when he had 130 parishioners sick. But in one week that number had more than doubled, to 315. *Surely*, he groaned, *surely the contagion cannot grow thicker than this.*

One evening a few days later, Zabdiel put his paper down and said, "Daniel Loring wishes me to inoculate his family."

"What did you tell him?" asked Jerusha, without slowing her stitching.

"That I will give him an answer tomorrow."

In and out, up and down, went Jerusha's needle. "Susanna Loring is my cousin," she said.

"My eldest son—Daniel, my namesake—is living in safety in the country," said Mr. Loring in the shop next morning, fiddling with various instruments on the shelves. "He is at Harvard, and doing well. Knows your boy, I hear. I sent him two weeks ago, you know, to stay with my wife and some of her younger children. But the distemper has broken out in Roxbury."

He stood in half shadows, but Zabdiel could feel his eyes. "You know what it is like," Mr. Loring continued. "I cannot bear that they should suffer through it."

Zabdiel sighed. "If the crowds will let me through, I will operate."

As if they could smell the new matter hung around his neck, the crowds congealed and penned him in the house till well past dark, chanting *Raw*

Head and Bloody Bones. The man with the sailor's gait and the noose was back; others swung steaming buckets of tar and old feather pillows.

Next morning, early, Zabdiel slipped through streets splattered with unused tar and feathers. Most of the Lorings were huddled together weeping in the parlor just off the front door.

"Mr. Loring, sir, is upstairs with Dan," said a young woman, curtsying even as she sniffled. "He begs you to come up, so soon as ever you arrive." She plucked at Zabdiel's sleeve. "Sir," she whispered, "Dan came home just yesterday evening to be inoculated, but in the night as we waited for you, he was taken all of a sudden-like with sweating and shivering, vomiting, and backache. We are worried he might already have caught the distemper, in the natural way."

"Let us hope he has not," said Zabdiel.

But quite unmistakably, he had.

Zabdiel inoculated Mr. Loring's twelve-year-old younger son, Nathaniel, at once, as well as the anxious girl, his sixteen-year-old stepdaughter, Hannah Breck. That afternoon, young Daniel broke out in his rash; by nightfall, Zabdiel saw grimly that it would be confluent: even at the rash stage, when they should have been well-spaced small flecks, they were packed so tightly that his rash was more like a flush.

On his way home, he went by to see Eunice Willard; she was sitting up in a chair, reading a book of sermons and tapping one toe against the floor. Her face was a little pale, but her fever had been light, and there had been no nausea. "I am waiting as patiently as I can for my rash," she said.

The following morning, the Honorable Thomas Fitch's carriage rolled up to the door, and a footman descended. "If you please, sir, my master would have a consultation with you, as soon as convenient."

Zabdiel's heart raced. He had inoculated Mr. Fitch's son the day before Mrs. Dixwell died. He had sped through the distemper nicely: had he now had a relapse?

"Now is convenient," he said, his mouth dry. He ducked into the carriage, leaning forward at the edge of his seat, as if it would make the horses pull faster. He did not wait for the footman to open the door, but leapt out himself as the wheels came to a stop and raced up the steps. Mr. Fitch, likewise eager, opened the door himself.

"How is the boy?" gasped Zabdiel

"Fine, fine," said Mr. Fitch heartily, shaking his hand and ushering him inside. "So fine, Doctor, that I must beg of you to inoculate my daughters, Martha and Mary. My wife cannot abide another day without knowing them safe."

"No," said Zabdiel. "It is not safe."

"Because you have had one death and two confluent cases?" The councilor waved off Zabdiel's protest. "Piffle, man. The whole world knows Mrs. Dixwell came by it through her own children. Dix says so himself to any who asks. And Mrs. Webb and Mrs. Nichols are no different—though I must say, bad luck for the Webbs." Mr. Fitch steered Zabdiel upstairs and down a long passageway.

Just outside a door, he stopped and lowered his voice. "I mean no disrespect to your concerns, of course. But you hear the bells every evening same as me, for all Dr. Douglass touts the strength of his cold method of treatment. Any fool with ears can tell you: inoculation's the better risk."

Zabdiel sighed and inoculated the Fitch girls.

He stopped in to see Eunice Willard on his way home; she had erupted into a lovely light scattering of pocks. She felt fine, she said. Laying her book aside, she insisted that he stop long enough to drink a glass of wine with her.

From the North Battery down to the Neck, the death toll kept rising. Funerals were pared to the barest essentials of prayer, so that all of them could be accommodated in the churches. The bells gave death a deep voice every evening; in the morning, said some, you could trace death's tracks by hearkening to bursts of weeping, and in the afternoon you needed no bloodhound to follow the stench. The grass of the burial grounds was pocked with fresh mounds of dirt, and the gravediggers wondered morosely where they would put all the bodies. "Dying keeps on as it is," said one, "sooner or later, we'll be burning 'em in pits, like they's doin' in France."

In daydreams, in prayers, and in nightmares, Cotton Mather was haunted by his vision of the Angel of Death looming high over the city, brandishing God's firebrand, casting the stars from the sky and spilling them across the land, where they burned and bled. Behind the Angel, the Great Adversary, Satan himself, breathed dark fire into the mobs.

On the eighteenth of October, Madam Checkley, the wife of town clerk and Cooke ally Colonel Checkley, died. Up near Salutation Alley, Selectman William Clark's brother-in-law Mr. Bronsdon lost three children in the space of one week; Bill Merchant lost two. The mistress of the charity school, Mrs. Martha Cotes, was buried, along with many of her pupils.

Bethiah Nichols survived.

More noticeable still, the Boylstons, Webbs, Adams, and Langdons, Mr. Cheever and Mr. Helyer, Mrs. Pierce, Mrs. Willard, and young Mrs.

Dodge—all his inoculees who could not be suspected of having taken the disease before the operation—walked through the contagion unharmed.

At the Loring house, Zabdiel watched young Nathaniel and Hannah break into light shivering on the nineteenth, as Daniel's skin bubbled and frothed, and fever ground away at his mind.

Not far away, Eunice Willard shed the last of her scabs. Zabdiel gave her leave to care for her cousins, and she gave him a firm handshake and matter-of-fact thanks.

"It is I who owe you thanks," said Zabdiel.

Very early in the morning on the twentieth, a heavy, wet snow blanketed the ground, following a drenching rain the night before that had sent the last of the leaves shivering from the trees. Without much food and precious little firewood, hunger and cold crept into town in the shadow of death—and it was not just the chronically poor who suffered. With trade at a standstill and heads of families dying, the ranks of the needy were swelling with people who had never thought to find themselves hushing children whose bellies ached with emptiness.

On the twenty-first, Nathaniel Loring and Hannah Breck both erupted. In the following days, they careened through stages their brother was inching through in agony. By the morning of the twenty-third, their blisters were already ripening. Daniel's had spread into what seemed to be one livid pustule that covered most of his body; he had swelled to near twice his size.

Mr. Loring quietly pulled Zabdiel into the parlor. "He is not doing well, is he?"

"I am sorry," said Zabdiel. "He is not."

Mr. Loring had paced for a moment, and Zabdiel had looked away. Presently, Loring blew his nose loudly.

"I should like to read you something."

Zabdiel steeled himself to hear a Biblical passage, a prayer: relatives of the dying, especially parents, often had a desperate need to share some faint shadow of their grief.

Mr. Loring cleared his throat. "It is from this morning's *Gazette*."

London, July 29

On Monday, several physicians and surgeons belonging to the Prince and Princess, attended by Mr. Lilly, their Royal Highnesses' Apothecary, came to Newgate to treat with the felons about undergoing the operation of inoculating into them the smallpox, for an experiment, and agreed with three of them, viz. two men and one woman, who are to be removed into

the most airy part of the prison in order to have their bodies prepared for
the said operation . . .

Mr. Loring looked up. "Did you know of these experiments?"

Zabdiel was startled speechless; all he could do was shake his head. Mr. Loring set the paper in his hand, and he read it twice through, his mouth moving as he read.

"I would say you—perhaps I might be permitted to say we—are running in very high company," said Mr. Loring with a wan smile. "The very highest."

It was true—if the article could be trusted. Zabdiel was not alone: the practice whose merit seemed so clear upstairs, but so muddied out in the streets, had drawn royal attention—not yet approval, perhaps, but enough attention to merit experiment. *At Newgate*, said an arch little voice in his head. *Among felons.*

"And the lowest," said Zabdiel.

He hurried to the post office, to purchase his own copy. At the door, Mr. Musgrave, postmaster and proprietor of the *Boston Gazette*, hailed him with the heartiness he reserved for people from whom he wished to wheedle something.

It was as Zabdiel expected; the postmaster had a whole pile of *Mercury*s, and knew perfectly well what came next. He winked at Zabdiel. "Sometimes, you have to dole out excitement in mere drams, like opium, eh? Keep 'em coming back for more."

It was all Zabdiel could do to keep from leaping over the counter and seizing him by the collar. *"What came of the experiment?"*

"Not so hasty, not so hasty," said Mr. Musgrave, pulling out a bottle of Madeira and two glasses. "I must ask a favor in return. Fair's fair, you know, and I owe both Mr. Campbell and especially Mr. Franklin a drubbing in the matter of sales."

Forty-five minutes later, Zabdiel departed only a little unsteadily, leaving behind a promise and carrying with him a copy of the day's paper and, even better, knowledge that made him so giddy he thought he might float.

"Look," said Zabdiel, setting the paper down on the parlor table as the family gathered for prayers just before dinner.

Tommy scanned through the ship notices and the advertisements, and looked up with shining eyes. "Papa! A camel!" He ran his finger along the page word by word, reading carefully, *"Just arrived from Africa, being above seven foot in height and twelve foot long."*

"I am not talking about the camel, child," said Zabdiel.

Young Jerusha and John snatched the paper to their end of the table. Tommy shrugged and ducked under the table, which made a good treasure cave.

"*Operation of inoculating,*" read John carefully, and then his eyebrows rose. "*Newgate!*" he blurted. A sharp rap came from under the table; Tommy reappeared, rubbing his head. "*Felons . . . experiment . . .*" continued John.

"*The Prince and Princess of Wales,*" breathed his sister, looking up at her father in awe.

Peering over their shoulders, Zabdiel junior read the article aloud from beginning to end.

There was such a commotion of shouting and laughter that no one heard Tom ride up; his face just suddenly appeared, floating pale and staring in the doorway. Jerusha took one look at him and sent the children downstairs to Moll. They obeyed in stricken silence.

"Sarah?" asked Zabdiel, steering Tom to a chair.

"She has given birth to a boy. Both healthy."

"But what?" asked Zabdiel.

Tom rubbed his eyes. "But one of the maids went visiting a beau on the sly, and came back with the smallpox. . . . It was several days before anyone knew it, though. She helped at the birth." He sat forward, his hands on his knees. "Sarah's near hysterical to be inoculated, Zabdiel. I don't know what to tell her. Will you come?"

He left at dawn on October 26, Governor Shute's Day of Thanksgiving, glad for the excuse to be absent.

The consultation was brief. Zabdiel explained the procedure and the risks to them both, and then he laid down his sole condition: that the infant should be sent elsewhere with a nurse while Sarah recovered. Perhaps to their brother Peter's out on the family farm in Brookline, he suggested. Sarah nodded, but tears poured silently down her face.

Zabdiel withdrew from the bedchamber to let the two speak in private, only to find himself besieged by his sisters. The house was full of Boylston women, some having taken refuge there with Sarah from the first, some having arrived lately to help with her labor and lying-in. Now, though, with the disease lurking in the house, they were preparing to scatter.

It was no more than a minute before Tom emerged and begged his brother, for both of them, to inoculate Sarah.

It took no time at all. After it was done, as Tom arranged for the nursing of his newborn son, Zabdiel inoculated the daughters of two of his sisters: eleven-year-old Rebecca Abbot and twenty-year-old Mary Lane.

Just as he was finishing, Mrs. Blague, Dr. Mather's younger sister, came to call. "The dowager duchess of Matherdom," groaned Mary, glancing out the window. "She will expect tea just so, and tipsy cake. And us in the middle of packing, with cabbage plastered over our arms."

But Mrs. Blague surprised them all.

"Poor thing," she clucked from the doorway of Sarah's chamber, watching the tearful farewell between mother and newborn. "She belongs in her own bed, cared for by her husband, she does."

"She must have a coach for that," said Zabdiel.

"And how do you think I arrived here, Doctor?" snapped the lady. "On a broomstick? She shall have mine, of course."

Mrs. Blague's coach returned not two hours later, fitted with a bed for Sarah's comfort. In thanks, and more than a little shamefaced, Zabdiel rode over to the widow's place on his way home, and inoculated her new little black girl, just five years old.

In town, Dr. Mather dared to hope the epidemic might be receding: *The Sick of the Small-Pox in the Notes to be prayed for sunk to 180*. But not even he had the heart for a full day of Thanksgiving. All across town, the usual services were scaled back from two sermons to one.

In the Brattle Square Church, Jerusha tried not to think dark thoughts while the prayers rumbled on: *Amidst the various awful rebukes of Heaven with which we are righteously afflicted in the contagious and mortal sickness among us, still, Lord, we owe gratitude for Your Divine Goodness vouchsafed to us in the course of the year.*

"What goodness?" she wondered. *For the king*, proclaimed the prayers, and she sighed. *For the Prince and Princess of Wales*, they continued, and suddenly Jerusha found herself absorbed in fervent supplication to heaven, for the Prince and Princess, for their experiment of inoculation, and for the lives of six felons in Newgate.

In the small hours of the morning, young Daniel Loring died, even as Nathaniel and Hannah shed the last of their scabs in their sleep. Zabdiel attended the funeral, but regretted it. All his grief had been drained from him; he could only mask his face with solemnity, behind which washed regret and an unseemly relief. *But for the grace of a howling mob*, he thought, *I would have notched another death on my soul tonight.*

On October 30, the *Boston Gazette* reported the story Zabdiel had been hugging close to his heart for a week, waiting for the rest of the town to learn:

The smallpox have plainly appeared upon some of the persons in New-gate who underwent the experiment of inoculation on Tuesday last Sev'night; and 'tis concluded from appearing symptoms that the rest will have them, except one man who was known to have had them before, on whom the engraftment of them hath made no alteration.

The royal experiment with inoculation had been a success. Or just as good as a success, he told himself.

Below that came the piece Mr. Musgrave had coaxed from him, in exchange for an early peek at the news. It did not have his name on it; Mr. Musgrave wanted to maintain decorum and the semblance of neutrality. But it was filled with Zabdiel's knowledge, his arguments, and his conclusions:

A Faithful Account of what has occurred under the late Experiments of the Small Pox managed and governed in the way of Inoculation. Published, partly to put a stop unto that unaccountable way of Lying which fills the Town and Country on this occasion, and partly for the Information and Satisfaction of our Friends in other places.

I. The Operation within these four months past has been undergone by more than threescore persons. Among which there have been Old & Young, Strong and Weak; Male and Female; White and Black; Many serious and virtuous people, some the children of excellent persons among us.

II. Concerning five or six of these, we had all possible demonstration that they first received the infection of the Small Pox in the Common way; and these (as none would imagine otherwise) underwent the distemper in the Common way: However, there is cause to think that the discharge at their Incisions was of use unto them. Only one gentlewoman so circumstanced died, but her nearest friends and all that knew her case do firmly believe the transplantation was not the least occasion of it.

III. Of all the rest that have passed under the operation, there has Not so much as One miscarried. It has done well in all, and even beyond expectation in the most of them.

It went on, detailing their symptoms and answering the objections of the doubters, point by careful point. With particular satisfaction, Zabdiel read through his conclusion once again:

But for a further confutation of all the opposition, and that all the Raw Head and Bloody Bones with which our good people have been practiced upon may vanish, let this One Passage be considered. We are not only credibly informed that this New Practice *is now begun in* England *with success and that persons of quality are coming into it, but also that a person of too much honor to have his veracity questioned asserts that the* English Ambassador at Constantinople *brought his two sons under the* Inoculation *of the* Small Pox. *And that same gentleman also adds that if God Almighty had not mercifully taught the poor people there this way of encountering the* Small Pox *the mortality was thought so great as to have threatened an extreme dissolution to those countries.*

It was too late for Boston, he thought, but God willing, other towns might take warning in time to preserve themselves.

But let us beseech those that have called this method the Working of the devil, *or a going to the* devil, *no more to allow the cursed thought or utter the horrid word, lest they be found* Blasphemers *of a most merciful and wonderful work of GOD.*

It was better, he thought, than his earlier efforts. He was learning. But then, he ought to be, seeing as he had had Dr. Mather's help in going over it. If only Zabby would apply himself at college, as he was doing under Dr. Mather's tutoring. The boy might make something of himself yet.

Zabdiel turned the page and found yet another snippet from Newgate. A second experiment had been tried: the doctors had dipped a bit of cotton in smallpox matter and thrust it up some poor woman's nose. The opposition screamed that it was done nefariously, while she was asleep, and that she was deathly ill—as good as murdered, they implied: but the latest news denounced these shouts as lies intended to discredit—and he read this part twice—*the safe and universally useful experiment of inoculating the smallpox.*

The papers flew out of the post office; people could be seen huddling at corners under gray skies, stepping in puddles or bumping into posts, reading while they walked. They read it over tea tables, and spread the sheets across shop counters. They gathered around tables and heard it told aloud in the taverns.

That afternoon, Judge Addington Davenport's carriage swept through the gabbling crowd to Zabdiel's door. The judge and his son descended, and right there in the street, for all to hear, he said, "I beg of you, sir, the favor of inoculating my son John." Captain John Osborne and his wife Sarah rolled up next. Elder Caleb Lyman, founder of the New North Church, and his adopted daughter Susannah, were not far behind. "Elder Dixwell," he said, "has recommended me to your service."

The following day, Dr. Mather's nephew the Reverend Thomas Walter and two friends arrived from Roxbury to be inoculated. Mr. Loring's brother Nathaniel, who had lost all his children but one to the epidemic, brought his last son and namesake, Nathaniel, to submit to the operation. The next day Councilor Edward Bromfield brought his young daughters to be inoculated. "It was my Fanny's last request," he said. "I should have done it before now."

Day by day, the number of his patients swelled: not to a flood tide, to be sure, but to a steady stream. More remarkable was the rise in their stature and power, and the coincident rise in stature and power they granted to him. They did not come in the dark; they did not ask for discretion or secrecy. They did not send for him to attend them at home, as any of them could have demanded. They drove up in broad daylight and requested the operation in full view of the street.

Even as the crowds grew more stately and decorous during the day, they grew more vicious at night.

"But the distemper is diminishing, Jer," said Zabdiel. "I don't understand it."

"They need someone to blame," she answered. "In the last month alone nearly twenty-five hundred people have fallen ill, Zabdiel. Over four hundred are dead. Still more are staring starvation in the face. As for your considered opponents, they are more dangerous now than ever: before, they were fueled with the hope of victory; now they are burning with the hatred of the vanquished."

"They are not vanquished yet, you just said so."

"They will be," she said.

On the fourth there was a contentious town meeting, in which the anti-inoculators drove through a vote making it illegal to enter Boston with the intention of being inoculated. As if that weren't a direct enough attack on Dr. Boylston and Dr. Mather, they picked up the plague bludgeon again. Anyone caught disobeying, the law announced, would be dispatched immediately to Spectacle Island, *lest the Town be made a Hospital for that which may prove worse than the Small Pox, which has already put so many into mourning*.

Never mind, Cheever observed angrily to Zabdiel afterward, that the multitudes fleeing Boston had driven up the price of food and housing in all towns round about. Never mind that Bostonians had trailed the disease into Roxbury, Cambridge, and Charlestown. No stranger was to find either prevention or cure in the suspicious bosom of Boston.

Zabdiel, as usual, ignored the huffing and puffing as much as he could.

He focused on Sarah Boylston, who erupted that morning, and looked to do well. All his new inoculees looked to do well.

On the seventh, the General Court crowded into the pews of the First Church of Cambridge, just across the street from Harvard, to hear the governor open the session, displaced and late as it was, with the shortest speech anyone could recall falling out of his mouth, formally or informally.

> *Gentlemen,*
> *Since it hath pleased God in His wise Providence to suffer the smallpox to spread very much in this province; and being also informed that many members of the Council and the House of Representatives have never had the distemper; I shall therefore only recommend to you at this sessions, the quick dispatch of those affairs which will be absolutely necessary for the present welfare of the government.*

Hear, hear! called the House, stamping the floor in agreement—especially the men who had not had the smallpox. It was quickly resolved that all minor affairs should be postponed to the next session.

But Mr. Cooke, Dr. Clark, and the governor nonetheless found plenty to bicker about, including how much to pay the governor and where to stow the Indian hostages from the war up in Maine, since the smallpox was rampant at the Castle, but the jail in Cambridge was not judged to be secure against the wiles of the Abenaki.

A week later, they were still squabbling, when the smallpox broke out in the heart of Cambridge. On the thirteenth of November, fear dissolved even House solidarity against the governor. A delegation was sent up to beg the governor to call an end to the session.

The governor refused.

That same day, Daniel Loring's second wife Susanna and her twelve-year-old daughter Mary Breck returned to Boston from the no-longer-safe country, and Zabdiel inoculated them.

That afternoon, James Franklin made a face as Dr. Mather passed him on the other side of King Street; the knot of young men he was walking with sputtered into laughter. The sound of it chipped and hammered at the minister's self-control; suddenly, the wrath that he had caged for so long leapt free and roared through him like a whirlwind. "You there!" he cried, striding across the street. "Young Man! Mr. Franklin!"

Mr. Franklin turned, startled at the outburst. His companions disappeared, while all along the street, heads craned from windows and doors.

Dr. Mather pitched his voice at the crowd. "You claim to edify the public with your *Courant*, but it is plain to all that your chief design is to abuse the ministers of God. You would do well, sir, to remember that God's blessing on the priestly tribe of Levi contains these words: *Smite through the Loins of them that rise against him, and of them that hate him.*"

A sudden awful stillness settled up and down the length of King Street.

Dr. Mather raised his voice in triumph. "I would have you know that the Faithful Ministers of Christ in this place are as honest and useful men as the ancient Levites were, and are as dear to their Glorious Lord. If, sir, you resolve to go on in serving their Great Adversary as you do, you must expect the consequences. Good day." With that, Dr. Mather strode quickly away.

Zabdiel smiled ruefully as he told Jerusha the story in the parlor that evening, as she sewed, and he toyed with a book; Zabby was reading a Bible story to the younger children, drawn around the table. "He has a good heart, Jer. And he means to do well. Only he gets himself so balled up with rage that he does himself and his cause more harm than good. Little boys chased him home taunting, *Loin-smiter.*"

"It's not funny, Zabdiel, not in the least," she said, her forehead crinkling.

A rumble in the street below made everyone look up.

"Papa," said Jerusha, walking to the window, "there's—"

Shards of glass and a scream cut her words short. Several rocks hit the floor, and then, in slow motion, something heavier and harder arced through the window, spitting fire. It hit the chair where Zabdiel had been sitting moments before and fell against the floor with a heavy thud. The brightness slithered across the floor to the wall, filling the room with acrid smoke.

In a single motion Zabdiel threw his coat on the line of fire, scooped up his screaming daughter, and herded everyone else back into the hall. Tommy rushed over and stamped another bit of fire out, before being hauled out by Zabby. Even as he was dragged out, he bent and picked something up.

Jerusha was scratched and hysterical, but not badly cut. They heard more glass, and more rocks.

"Papa," said Tommy in an odd little voice, "it's an iron ball. Are they shooting cannon?"

"*Tommy,*" croaked Zabdiel, "gently, now. *Give me that.*" His hands shook as his son set the metal, still warm, into his hands.

Jack and Moll ran up the stairs, carrying Jackey. Downstairs, more glass shattered, and then a regular thudding began slamming against the door to the shop. *Raw Head and Bloody Bones!* screeched a tangle of voices.

Zabdiel and Jerusha looked at each other; they had discussed this, had rehearsed it once, but he had never believed it would come to this.

Her skirts suddenly seemed made of clinging children.

"Go," she said. "They will not dare to touch me or the children." But she handed the musket to Zabby to load, in any case.

"Go."

❧ 10 ❧

JUST RETRIBUTION

Dock Square, Boston
November 13, 1721

TO turn from his family, slink down the stairs, and into the shadows was the hardest thing Zabdiel had ever done. But he and Jerusha had gone over this possibility again and again. They were looking for him, not her or the children.

If he got away in time, they would never find him; if he stayed, he was one man against a mob: and that kind of heroism was not heroism, she said. It was foolishness, to put your children into the position of watching you torn from their arms and strung up in the street.

Jack opened the back door and walked out before him; it was clear. Odd, Zabdiel thought with clarity, how single minded and stupid a mob could be, even when consisting of intelligent men.

He crunched across the icy ground to the stables. Talking softly, he stepped into Prince's stall, and squeezed around the stallion. There in the back corner he found the latch to the door obscured behind Prince's feeding bag. It opened on a cupboard that had not been meant for a person, but would hold one, just. Zabdiel was not sure what it had been meant for: it was an odd nook in the barn's space, and someone long ago had made use of it. Probably to store valuables. Where safer, than behind the iron hooves of a stallion?

Lately, he and Jack had been keeping fresh water in there, along with blankets and some food; Jack had been changing it every day, when he fed Prince. Zabdiel had added a Bible, too, though it would be too dark to read. He slipped in and shut the door.

Only then did he realize that he was still holding the missile. He could not see it, but he knew what it was; he had seen it with terrible accuracy as it arced through the window. It was no cannon ball, as Tommy had thought. It was a grenade. The fuse had been knocked loose in its fall, or it would have exploded in his son's hands.

Zabdiel began to shiver, and then to shake. He set the grenade down in haste before he could drop it, and curled himself into a ball. It took every ounce of his strength to keep rage from exploding through him with all the force that had failed the grenade.

From down the street, on the other side of the mob, Dr. Douglass rapped on the carriage for his man to stop. He sat at the window watching the mob engulf the inoculator's house. It was not how he would have chosen to win; but really, the man had brought it on himself.

What could one do, one man against a mob?

He heard a thundering of hooves, and a company of men rode up on horses, tossed themselves off, and waded into the fray with their whips. The crowd began streaming in the other direction.

Up ahead, the shattering and wrenching, the yelling and screaming, gradually stopped.

Dr. Douglass stepped down from his carriage and into the house. Possibly, he could be of some help.

In the house, Jerusha, too, heard the pounding of horses, followed by the thud and crack of bullwhips. Harsh men's voices, and a sudden scuffling and quiet.

Then she heard a clomping on the stairs. There was a knock on her chamber door. The children all ducked behind the bed, and she lowered her musket. "Who is it?"

"Elisha Cooke, madam," said a deep voice. The door slowly opened, pushed in from the outside. She saw him glimpse the musket, and then look up at her face. "At your service," he said, with a deep bow.

He was not alone; by his side stood Captain Durell, and behind them crowded several constables. She grimaced as she saw Dr. Douglass, who inclined his head. But she let the musket tip up toward the ceiling.

Mr. Cook took a step into the room; behind her, the children edged their noses over the bed. "We should like a word with your husband."

"He is not here."

"He is not safe in this house, madam. We are offering him safe escort."

"Where?" Her voice, she thought, sounded harsh as a crow's.

"To the Town House. It is the strongest building in town."

So you can accidentally let the mob have him on the way there—or give them the key? She did not say it aloud. "Unfortunately for you, he is not here."

"Where is he?"

"I don't know." *It was, carefully, quite true. Of course, she had a mighty fine guess. But she did not know.*

"You will pardon us, madam, if we ascertain his absence for ourselves."

"You will no doubt ascertain it, whether I pardon you or not, so perhaps you will pardon me if I don't waste my breath."

Mr. Cooke smiled at her. "We will also be looking for illegal inoculees."

"By all means search," she said. "You will not find any."

She led the way to the guest chamber, where they kept sick patients who needed round-the-clock care. From there, they checked every room, every closet, even the attic and cellar. They searched the stable and the hay loft. Prince snorted in warning as they drew near, and gave one good kick to the outside wall of his stall. They steered a wide course around him.

"As I said," she said icily. "He is not here."

"Let us hope, madam, that he may come home safely."

"No doubt he will, if you control the rioting in the streets. Good night, gentlemen."

She closed the outer door, banging it back into place where it was loose. Then she picked her way through the shop, icy air knifing through the windows, and shut the door that separated it from the house. Sliding the bolt across, she turned and leaned back against it, and then she slid down on her haunches and sobbed.

After a few minutes, she dried her eyes and went upstairs. The girls were sitting wide eyed in the bed; Jack and Moll had made pallets for the boys and for Moll and Jackey on the floor.

"Where will you sleep?" she asked Jack.

"Don't you mind me, missus," he said. He took the musket and went downstairs. Zabby went with him.

Jerusha dropped into the bed, led the children in brief prayers, and lay staring at the ceiling with her three girls pressing themselves around her.

Come back to me, she thought.

The screaming pierced his dreams first, followed by showers of glass. Thomas Walter awoke to the smell of burning, and a billowing of smoke. He and his companions leapt out of bed.

Pox on your house! Someone cried in the night. Dogs, horses, and roosters awoke as footsteps scattered through neighboring yards.

Dr. Mather was pounding at the chamber door. Somewhere outside, a bell was tolling 3:00 A.M.

They stamped the fire out, and examined the missile. It was not a rock, it was a bomb. A grenade. But the fuse had hit the casement on its way in and fallen loose.

Wrapped around the metal was a strip of paper with rough writing on it: *COTTON MATHER, you Dog, Dam you: I'l inoculate you with this, with a Pox to you.*

Very nearly, the night had cost him his life, thought Dr. Mather, wrapped in a blanket and a dressing gown, his fingers like needles of ice despite the gloves.

He rubbed his hands until his fingers warmed up enough to write. *G. D. This night there stood by me the Angel of the GOD, whose I am and whom I serve.*

He did not return to bed. He wrote till daylight, welcoming the glorious martyrdom for which the Lord was preparing him. Then he rang for his chocolate early and took himself off to the ferry for Cambridge, to harangue the governor into revenge.

At dawn, Zabdiel opened the door to the cupboard. Prince snorted and shifted his weight, twitching his tail in greeting. Zabdiel gave him a rub down the neck, and slipped out.

The entire world seemed silent and deserted in the gray light. As he drew nearer the house, he saw that Moll had already laid the fire and begun breakfast; she handed him a hot cup of chocolate as he walked through the door.

"Jack's sweeping up in the shop," she said. "Missus still sleeping."

Zabdiel put his finger to his lips and crept up the stairs. In their bed, Jerusha was coiled around the girls. He stood for a long time, watching them. Felt eyes on him, and turned to see Jackey, bright eyed, sucking his thumb and watching.

The family woke and prayed together in the bedroom, and then Zabdiel went downstairs to take stock of the damage. Jack had finished sweeping up the big pieces and was setting overturned things to rights. Moses Pierce was already there, replacing the broken windows.

Mrs. Bath, the poor widow of a needlemaker, appeared in the doorway, open mouthed, with her fifteen-year-old Mary firmly in tow.

"We had a bit of excitement in the night, Mrs. Bath," said Zabdiel. "But everything is fine now. May I help you?"

"I want you to inoculate my Mary," she said. "I have sold my wedding ring," she added hurriedly, as if he might send her packing on the assumption she could not pay. "I have the five pounds." She picked her way across the crunchy floor and laid the coins proudly on the counter. "I would like it as soon as is ever convenient, if you please."

"Now is convenient, madam," said Zabdiel.

As soon as the women had left, he tried to give the money straight across to Mr. Pierce, but he would not take it.

"My Liza that you inoculated, she's alive, and my two other children nursed through their sickness by her," he said without stopping. "My sweet youngest, our baby Lizzy, died where she ought, in her mother's arms. If anything, I ought to be paying you the privilege of replacing these windows."

Later, a delegation from the governor stopped in to speak with Zabdiel about the disturbance. They looked around at the new sparkling windows and the neat shop, and were confused. "Was there not a riot in your street last night?"

"Boys," said Zabdiel with a shrug. "A drunken sailor or two. That is all."

"If you will not help us, sir, we cannot press charges."

He was tempted; he was sorely tempted. But had already taken his measure of revenge; he had resumed inoculating. "Charges for what?" asked Zabdiel.

In Cambridge, the General Court voted £1,000 to be paid out of the public treasury for the relief of families nearly reduced to gnawing leather.

The following afternoon, the governor and council coaxed the House into issuing a reward of £50 for discovering "the Author and Actor" of the wicked attack upon Dr. Mather's person and property. They did not mention Dr. Boylston.

Crane Court, off Fleet Street, London
November 16, 1721

Just east of Fetter Lane, on the north side of Fleet Street, coaches lined up near the entrance to the narrow courtyard of Crane Court. Like an immense ornate egg, each coach in its turn rolled to the entrance, shed lines of footmen in silver lace, and then popped open with a click, hatching gentlemen with luxuriant plumes of hair into the glow of lamplight. One by one, they unfolded themselves to proud stands, retrieved walking sticks and gloves from impassive servants, stowed hats under their arms, and stalked across the courtyard, disappearing up the fanned stairway and into the pale stone house. Emptied of its treasure, each coach pulled away to the crowded coach-house and full stables, and the next coach drew up.

In the foyer, gruff laughter and the long, leaning snorts of snuff-taking mingled briefly with the clink of glasses full of fine old Madeira, but the men soon drifted into the grand meeting hall. Irascible old Sir Isaac Newton limped his way to the president's chair, rapped upon the table, and the meeting of the Royal Society came to order.

Dr. Alexander Stuart waited impatiently through run-of-the-mill reports and ho-hum everyday business. At last, he judged the restlessness to indicate a certain willingness for fireworks, and he rose. "I have here a letter dated September twenty-fifth, from Dr. William Douglass, who writes from Boston, in New England, upon the subject of the smallpox." He cleared his throat. "On inoculation for the smallpox, to be precise."

The fidgeting stopped and heads turned. One or two men who had been dozing snorted awake.

"We trained together in Leiden. I can vouchsafe for the man's education and intellectual capacity." He read the letter through, reveling in the dropped jaws and raised brows certain sentences elicited. "A thousand people ill in the month of September," for instance. He knew what they were thinking: *Why, London goes years at a time without so many ill of a single distemper in one month—and London must be fifty, maybe sixty times the size of Boston!*

He continued: "Above sixty persons of all ages, sexes, and conditions have there been inoculated—"

A collective gasp swept the room. *Sixty!* Under the leadership of Sir Hans, the Royal College of Physicians had lobbied hard for permission to inoculate six prisoners at a go—and the doctors had thought themselves daring.

Dr. Stuart, a Scottish Tory who disliked Sir Hans and the Whig ministry, purred his way through the end of his sentence: ". . . of which several had the confluent sort, and one or two have died."

There was a drumming of feet on the floor, an outburst of hollering, as the Tories faced the Whigs with conquest in their eyes.

Sir Hans sniffed and stood to face Dr. Stuart. "Perhaps now might be an opportune moment to give a report of our own trials of inoculation, at Newgate." Dr. Stuart sat down, and Sir Hans turned to smile at Dr. Freind and Dr. Wagstaffe, who were looking smugly at nothing.

"They have been an unmitigated success," Sir Hans continued smoothly. "All those who were inoculated had the distemper communicated thereby in a very gentle degree."

Dr. Wagstaffe's attention snapped back into focus. "So gentle," he cried, "that it must be doubted whether what you communicated was indeed the true smallpox!"

"Do stop speaking of 'the true smallpox' as if it were the true cross, Wagstaffe," grumbled someone in the back, and a dangerous silence enveloped the room.

"Facetiousness aside," sniffed Dr. Freind, "you cannot deny that the operation presents grave risks whose nature and consequences you do not understand. What assurance do you have that it works?"

Angry voices and local quarrels erupted across the space. Sir Hans raised his voice above it all. "The question, gentleman, the question has been put whether the inoculated smallpox indeed secures a person from any future return of the infection." The very walls of the room seemed to hunch in tighter around him.

"I am happy to report that one of the women who suffered the experiment in Newgate has since undertaken to nurse other persons down of the distemper. Mr. Maitland assures me that she has been put to bed with two different patients for six weeks now, without any ill consequence whatsoever."

More gasps crossed the room, along with some significant *oh-ho's* and a little satisfied chortling as well: the tussle over inoculation appeared to be heating into a royal battle with room for all.

"As for Boston," said Sir Hans as he sat down, "I am expecting further news imminently."

He had been well prepared for such boisterous nonsense. Only a few days earlier, he had drafted his report for the princess and translated it into French. *One can assuredly communicate the infection to suitable subjects, without danger of any relapse or recurrence. The entire operation is not only absolutely without danger, but also very easy and practicable.*

He had also caught wind of the Boston controversy from Mr. Jeremiah Dummer, who had a letter—no, a treatise—from Dr. Mather.

He sighed. Dr. Mather wrote incessantly and voluminously about American oddities to various Fellows of the Royal Society. That he had chosen this particular moment to approach the Society sideways, through the roundabout door of the provincial agent—and demand anonymity, no less—was vexing indeed. Sir Hans had done his best to persuade Mr. Dummer to ignore that demand, in light of necessity. Surely royal urgency counted for something. The lawyer had promised to consider it.

Cambridge, Massachusetts
November 16, 1721

William Hutchinson, selectman and representative for Boston, woke in the night with a splitting headache and spinning nausea. Dr. Thomas Robie, physician and tutor of mathematics, astronomy, and natural philosophy at Harvard, was sent for, but he had no alternative diagnosis to offer. Mr. Hutchinson had come down with the smallpox.

Dr. Clark, his fellows howled. *Despite all the speaker's care to cleanse himself from the contagion after visiting his patients, he has carried the disease in among us, and passed it to Mr. Hutchinson. Who might be next?* By morning, so many members of the House were packing in panic that the governor found it necessary to put a dignified face on the chaos by proroguing the General Court until March.

The following day, November 18, five people rushed to Dock Square in Boston to put themselves in Dr. Boylston's care.

Russell Square, Bloomsbury, London
November 18, 1721

Mr. Dummer regretted it, said his disappointing little note, but he could not countenance the breach of confidence that Sir Hans had requested. He would send back to Boston directly, begging for permission to use Dr. Mather's name on his pamphlet.

Sir Hans took his spectacles off and sighed. Mr. Dummer had intimated that he could make what private use he might of Dr. Mather's glowing report from Boston, but public proclamation would have to wait the length of two ocean crossings. In winter, no less, when the North Atlantic would scream with icy anger that quelled even the bravest hearts from setting sail for long stretches of weeks. It might well be February before he had an answer.

He drummed the table with impatient fingers. Why must proclamations that would do good lie silent, while those aimed at nothing but panic could be plastered through the gossip-mongering papers? Spread before him on his breakfast table were two of the vile rags, both proclaiming a further experiment to be made on every last orphan of St. James's.

He did not know where such leaks came from. Almost certainly not from anyone within the princess's counsel, for they were considering inoculating a few children. The princess had suggested an en masse inoculation, but he and Lord Townshend had reasoned her out of it: until the operation should be known to be safe, they could not make it a requirement. It must at least appear to be voluntary. Besides, they needed a success rate of one hundred percent, and some of those children were already on the downhill slope toward death.

Some! Sir Hans snorted. His inspection of the charity children of St. James's had presented such a bleak picture of misery that he had postponed the entire affair until a few of the ragamuffins could be given enough food, warmth, and sleep to stand a chance of fighting off even the attenuated infection of inoculation.

Cambridge, Massachusetts
November 20, 1721

The appearance of the rash dissolved Mr. Hutchinson's last refuge of hope. Watching the red speckles thicken, he called for paper and ink and made out his will.

The following morning, Dr. Robie inspected him in the gray November light and his face grew grim. Already, the rash had sown itself nearly solid.

"It is not of the best sort, is it?" asked the selectman.

"I am sorry," said Dr. Robie. "It will be confluent."

Mr. Hutchinson blinked and looked away out the window. "Have you had news of my wife?" he asked. "And the children?"

"She is distraught for your sake, but still safe. Far in the country, where the air is still clean."

Dr. Robie heard a sharp intake of breath. *"Vengeance is mine, saith the Lord,"* said Mr. Hutchinson with a bitter laugh. "What do you think of Dr. Boylston's operation of inoculation?"

"I do not know what to think. I cannot conceive how it works."

"But does it work?"

"It would appear that it does."

Mr. Hutchinson sighed and turned back to the doctor. "It is just retribution—" Dr. Robie moved to protest, but Mr. Hutchinson waved him off. "You do not know what hell we have put him through, in our pride and vainglory." He leaned across the table. "It is too late for me. But not for others." He gripped Dr. Robie by the arm; his own was red and thick. "You must learn to inoculate."

The doctor stepped back, but Mr. Hutchinson's grip strengthened. *"Without delay."*

The dissolution of the General Court dispersed panic throughout the province. Even as deaths tapered off in Boston, people began flocking to

Dr. Boylston, begging to be inoculated. On the twenty-second of November, Zabdiel inoculated ten people. The next day, Dr. Robie appeared from Cambridge, ushering in three students from Harvard and a plea that Zabdiel had thought he would never hear from a fellow doctor: *Show me how it is done.* "With pleasure, sir," he said, and two heads bent over the glint of his lancet. The next day Dr. Robie returned with eight more students, a fellow, and Mr. Edward Wigglesworth, the Hollis Professor. The day after that, three more students arrived. In three days, Zabdiel inoculated almost the entire student body and faculty of Harvard—most of those, at any rate, who were still untouched by the speckled beast. In addition to the Bromfields and Fitches, Lorings and Lyndes, he had already inoculated, Sewalls, Foxcrofts, and Danforths now came to call: the most exalted names in the province begged for his time, bowing and scraping about convenience.

They were not alone. Day by day, the number of inoculees rose: 10, then 12, 13, 14—as many as 15 in a day. In the three weeks following the attack on his family, Zabdiel inoculated 119 people in Boston and Roxbury: more than doubling the number in the previous five months. Since the people of Roxbury could no longer come to him, he went to them. When he could, he went to Charlestown and Cambridge as well. Waiting—anything to do with stillness—ceased to be part of his days, which were devoured by inoculating, by checking up on his inoculated patients, by riding back and forth across the Neck, or sailing hither and yon on the Charlestown ferry.

In Cambridge, Mr. Hutchinson's skin swelled and frothed, flushing from red to yellow and then fading to an ominous ashen gray.

The ministers, meanwhile, threw their heads back and roared. Increase Mather published *Several REASONS Proving that Inoculating or Transplanting the Small Pox is a Lawful Practice, and that it has been Blessed by GOD for the Saving of many a Life.* To it was attached another essay: *Sentiments on the Small-Pox Inoculated.* The second, as everyone knew, was by Dr. Cotton Mather, though still he refused to put his name on it. His father's was what was needed, he told himself.

Mr. Colman provided *Some Observations on the New Method of Receiving the Small Pox by Engrafting or Inoculating,* and Mr. Cooper—under the guise of "A Minister of Boston"—offered *A Letter to a Friend in the Country, Attempting a Solution of the Scruples and Objections of a Conscientious or Religious Nature, Commonly Made against the New Way of Receiving the Small-Pox.*

As Boylston gained the rich, the powerful, and the poor, Dr. Douglass's practice drained away. His cold method, a strict interpretation of Dr. Sydenham's theories, was not doing as well as he would like; nor was his liberal use of opiates and the spirit of vitriol. Not that he was doing poorly.

There were still so many sick that only the most powerful could be choosy; most people were properly grateful to have a physician (or to have a doctor at all, thought his slave Pompey). "I shall seclude myself from all other company but that of my patients," sniffed Dr. Douglass to himself as his carriage passed by lines patiently waiting outside Boylston's door, "and commit to writing—for my own reminiscence and private use—the remarkable cases in what is, after all, still a very extensive practice."

On the thirtieth of November, Selectman William Hutchinson died of the smallpox in Cambridge, contracted in the service of the House of Representatives. He was thirty-eight years old. At his side, Dr. Robie bowed his head and then rose, walking across Harvard Yard to inoculate his first patient: his fellow tutor, Nicholas Sever.

Two days later, the funeral for Mr. Hutchinson in Boston was a great one, deep, dark, and sonorous with mourning pomp. Dr. Boylston did not attend; he saddled up Prince and rode straight up to the beacon on Beacon Hill. Up there in the cold wind, he listened to the tolling of the bells below and sent his own prayer heavenward—for the deceased and for his widow and young children, but mostly, truth be told, for the anguish of Dr. Clark.

He watched the sun set, and thought of a burning angel folding his wings and slinking away. The petty nastiness would not slip away so quietly, he knew that. There were still skirmishes to be fought, and no doubt sputtering ugliness to endure. But the dark fury was subsiding, chased out of town by the steady stream of footsteps, wheels, horse hooves flowing to his door.

Later, he withdrew to the Salutation Inn, where Cheever, Helyer, some Webbs, and several Langdons were gathered around the big fire.

"Where've you been?" cried Cheever, calling for a fresh round of rum punch.

"Giving thanks," said Zabdiel, stamping snow from his coat and boots, and crossing the room to stretch before the fire.

"Alone?" protested Cheever. "Without us? Without trumpets or harps?"

"I had my horse," said Zabdiel, gratefully accepting a steaming tankard of hot rum punch from Mr. Dodge, and cupping cold hands around it. "What would I do with a harp?"

"And there you have him," said Cheever to the crowd. "Dr. Boylston, at the height of celebrating his part in revealing inoculation to be the greatest blessing Providence has ever afforded mankind . . . Be as modest and monosyllabic as you like, my friend, but tell us this: Would you do it again?"

Zabdiel set down his tankard, pulled his pipe from his coat, filled it, and lit it. "Let us hope," he said, "that I never have to answer that question."

"Hah!" said Cheever. "Dizzy with optimism at last." He waved his own pipe in the direction of the front door. "There will be an 'again,' you know. Because that wide darkness out there would be the sea, just in case you forgot. Sends the golden talents of Ophir streaming our way, for the most part. But every now and again, it spits up the Beast." He leaned forward to Zabdiel. "When that happens, will you start this whole fury anew? Will you inoculate again?"

Around them, the whole circle of men leaned in.

Zabdiel pulled the pipe from his mouth. *When it shall please Providence to send the distemper among us again*, he had prayed as he sat atop Prince, up on the hill, *may inoculation revive, be better received, and continue a blessing*. He had even liked the words so much that he pulled out his case notebook and scribbled the sentence in the margins. But he did not repeat it aloud.

Instead, he released a slow ring of smoke. "Of course," he said quietly.

❧ 11 ❧

IN ROYAL FASHION

London
February 1722

AT last, the seas smiled again, sending a ship from Boston scudding up the Thames.

Mr. Dummer slit open the long-awaited letter from Dr. Mather and groaned. With a most unfortunate and emphasized certainty, Dr. Mather did not wish his name to be bandied about in print concerning this matter. But he did wish his little treatise to be published.

Applebee's was rather more pleased at the bad news its editors received from Boston. *Four hundred dead every week!* The epidemic was still raging in Boston, the Tory paper screamed, and the Americans had had precious little but bad luck with their project of inoculation: perhaps, the article insinuated, the preposterous death toll might be laid at the feet of this new-fangled practice.

Mr. Dummer was outraged. How could anyone accidentally confuse four hundred dead in a month with four hundred in a week: a number he doubted that London had ever known, except in time of the plague?

Mr. Maitland shrugged it off and put the final touches on his account of inoculation (and his name into the title) and sent it off to the printers.

"Poetry is dead, and Physick had replaced it," grumbled Pope, hard at work on his translation of the Odyssey.

"You are jealous," teased Lady Mary.

"Only of you, my lady," he said.

There had been a lull in the inoculation controversy since early December, when the *St. James Evening Post* whispered that "a Noble Duke in

Hanover Square" had undergone the operation; two days later, the *Weekly Journal or British Gazetteer* added Charlotte Tichborne, woman of the princess's bedchamber, to the list. Somehow, notice of Mr. Maitland's inoculation of the children of Mr. Colt, colleague of Mr. Dummer at the Middle Temple, escaped the newspapers' notice. Then the Christmas holidays arrived, and smallpox receded from view as halls were decked, and gentlemen made merry.

On February 23, 1722, the wrangling came back with a roar. Under royal sponsorship, Mr. Maitland inoculated six more people. "The curious," announced the papers, "may be further satisfied by a sight of those persons at Mr. Forster's house in Marlborough Court, at the Upper End of Poland Street and Berwick Street in Soho, where attendance is given every day from ten till twelve before noon, and from two till four in the afternoon."

Though nominally open to view, the Newgate experiment had essentially been closed to all but the most intrepid: many who were safe from smallpox had refused to attend for fear of jail fever or distaste for the rude antics of the prisoners. The six new subjects, however, were genteel enough to offer safe viewing to anyone not vulnerable to the smallpox. The curious, the suspicious, and the horrified began to drift in, clutching copies of *Mr. Maitland's Account* still damp from the press.

That very day, Jeremiah Dummer at last signed and dated his introduction to Cotton Mather's unacknowledged *Account*, and sent it forth, dedicated to Sir Hans Sloane, President, and the rest of the Royal College of Physicians. "Gentlemen," he began with a sigh, "I receiv'd the following Account of the Method and Success of inoculating the *Small-Pox* in *New-England* from a Person there of great Learning and Probity, who desir'd his Name might be conceal'd." The gentleman in question, he assured them, had "no other View than a charitable Inclination of doing Good to the World." To New Englanders, thought Mr. Dummer, that sentence was as good as a name: there was only one Dr. Dogood. But Londoners, no doubt, would likely miss the reference.

To Dr. Mather's arguments he added three observations of his own: first, in Boston, there had been virtually no preparation of patients' bodies, but they seemed to do well in any case. Secondly, the discharge of matter at the incisions was surely a boon to bodies needing to vent poison. And third, for his part, he suspected some of the ease of inoculated smallpox stemmed from knowledge: the dread of a monster that might lurk unseen in every breath could now be dissolved with a welcome—and watched—stroke of a lancet.

Mr. Dummer was not alone in his willingness to press the success of inoculation in New England. The Reverend Mr. Daniel Neal followed suit by reprinting the work of his friend and fellow dissenting minister, Benjamin Colman, along with the still anonymous work of Mr. Colman's associate, Mr. William Cooper.

The Princess of Wales spoke to both of them. In one respect, Mr. Dummer had been easier: he was no court intimate, but he was, nonetheless, a gentleman who appeared now and again in the Drawing Room. He proved irritatingly resistant, however, to being opened by her intellectual knife. Though born in the colonies, he had long been a London lawyer and the agent for the province of Massachusetts. He was, in other words, a polished diplomat, trained in the fine art of saying nothing.

Mr. Neal, on the other hand, was not regularly present at court, and required to be summoned. As a proudly dissenting Puritan, though, Mr. Neal prided himself on being outspoken—in a gentlemanly way—in the service of Truth. He told the princess what he knew, and he gave her names. He also reiterated, in his rough way, a recommendation she had found in his work: "The chief scene of action, Your Highness, has hitherto been New England: within these last six months, there having been more persons inoculated in Boston than in all of Europe. It seems reasonable—I might even say *necessary*—that we should become acquainted with their method and success of this practice among ourselves. Surely their inoculator should be called upon to provide an accurate account?"

Such forthrightness, the princess remarked that evening, when Mrs. Tichborne carried in a late supper, was no doubt furthered by the fact that the fellow was not a physician; no London doctor would have made such a claim, no matter its truth, to the detriment of the Royal College of Physicians.

The princess sighed, toying with a bit of bread. She prided herself on her ability to ferret out truth—but in her position, it did so often require such a lot of ferreting through flattery, half-masquerades, and tangles of desires, plans, schemes, and frankly Machiavellian maneuvers. Sometimes she grew tired just thinking of it. And then came along a minister who would probably tell the truth if it killed him. Shout it all the louder, for that matter. Oh, for a golden mean.

She held out her glass for a splash more wine. "Mr. Neal's suggestion, now, that the Boston physician—what was his name, Tich?"

"Dr. Boylston, madam."

"—His suggestion that Dr. Boylston be induced to publish *his* account to the world: surely that would be as valuable as Mr. Maitland's fine account. More valuable—for all their well-meaning—than the twaddling ministers'." She pushed the tray away. "Remind me to mention it to Sir Hans."

Sir Hans found his next conversation with the princess ruthlessly steered toward Boston, though to be frank, the subject annoyed him as much as it fascinated him. *Sixty!*

"I should be glad of a chance, one day, to speak to this Dr. Boylston," observed the princess. "In this business, the colonies seem to be outstripping the capital entirely."

"Their goals are different," said Sir Hans sourly. "They are colonists, Your Highness, fighting for the survival of their children in an epidemic such as London has not seen since the last great visitation of the plague. They are not trying to induce a crowned head to risk his heirs."

"Their goals are exactly the same," said the princess. "And their children will survive to adulthood."

Several days later, Sir Hans arrived home in Russell Square to find a hurriedly scrawled note from Claude Amyand, the king's principal sergeant-surgeon in ordinary, awaiting him.

> *To Sir Hans Sloane*
> *March 14, 1722*
>
> *Honored Sir,*
> *The parish of St. James has tendered five children to be inoculated. These children are very miserable, and their Royal Highnesses apprehend that the ill state of their bodies does not make them the fittest for an experiment. However, I submit that to your better judgment.*
> *What I thought proper to urge was that these fresh instances might reconcile those that were yet diffident about the success of the inoculation, and I hoped might be brought over to the experiment by the beginning of April. The princess will be glad to know whether you think these wanting, and therefore I came to wait on you on this account.*
> *I am with all respect,*
> *Your most humble and obedient servant,*
> *Claude Amyand*

Damnation, thought Sir Hans. Sergeant Amyand, it was clear, wanted to go through with the experiment, to convince the still undecided king and council—"those that were yet diffident," hah!—as soon as possible. But the princess had misgivings.

As well she might, he concluded, when he saw the children. One was downright scrophulous, and another a mere two months old. And the stakes were so very high: they needed more successes, preferably among children, but they could not afford a single loss. How they were to get through without a single loss, starting with this sorry set, he did not know.

He gave the nod to proceed, and proceeded himself to pray.

Despite his misgivings, all the children went through the smallpox with pleasingly favorable symptoms—save one girl who had no symptoms at all. Upon further inquiry, which he suspected included a well-deserved hiding, she admitted that she had had the smallpox before, but had pretended otherwise so as to get the reward.

The Royal Society heard from Boston again. From Dr. Mather again, to be precise, thought Sir Hans, though the minister still chose to maintain his mockery of anonymity. This latest paper, like his treatise, had come through Mr. Dummer, this time via his colleague at the Middle Temple, Henry Newman. Very odd, Sir Hans grumbled to himself, given that Dr. Mather allied himself so closely with their inoculator as to make it sound as if they held the lancet together. For all that, Dr. Mather had written an admirably concise and clear paper, giving a detailed account of inoculation as it was practiced by Dr. Boylston. *Why the devil wouldn't the fellow put his name on it?*

The only part that bothered him was Dr. Mather's unqualified praise for the operation. The man went so far as to claim that patients actually had their overall health improve as a result. Sir Hans shook his head. He approved of the operation; he counted himself one of its staunchest supporters. But he was not at all sure such extravagant buoyancy was the best way to win suspicious converts.

At the beginning of April, Sir Hans received his own summons to Leicester House. As he was announced, the princess dismissed all her women except Mrs. Tichborne and Prince William's nurse, and these two withdrew to a window seat to play with the baby.

The princess paced about for a while, and then came to the point directly. "I should be grateful, Sir Hans, for your frank opinion in the matter of inoculating the young princesses."

He liked her. Not just as a princess, but as a woman. Fair of hair and fair of temperament, she had gray-blue eyes that were sharp with intelligence, without being hard. She loved her children, but without going loose in the brain over them, as most women did. At thirty-nine, her skin was still remarkably taut and so pale it was nearly translucent; at the moment, a rosy glow of excitement or anxiety or both was beating in her cheeks.

He bowed. "By what has appeared in the trials, Your Highness, it seems to be exactly what is claimed for it: a method to secure people from the great dangers attending the smallpox taken in the natural way."

She was tapping an exquisitely shod toe in front of him. "I know what inoculation is, Sir Hans. I am asking for your opinion of its dangers. Of its worth."

He continued. "For private persons, madam, I cannot think the practice anything other than very desirable, given the proper preparations of diet and body. Not being absolutely certain of the consequences, however, I cannot persuade or advise you to make trials upon patients of such importance to the public as the princesses."

She turned away from him, hands on hips as she regarded her son in the distance; the boy was laughing as he held himself to a wobbly stand by the edge of a low table. "To me they are also children, Sir Hans. My children."

He watched her with pity, but said nothing. On his side of the balance hung no less than his career, his livelihood, and possibly his life. It was all he could dare, to connive with her in the matter of luring the king into a favorable decision; the decision itself would have to be royal.

Other women might have raged or cried. Caroline of Ansbach, Princess of Wales, came to a standstill and stared at him, cocking her head. "Let me ask my question another way: Would you dissuade me?"

"No, madam, I would not. Most certainly not, in a matter so likely to be of such advantage."

A smile of such sweet blue and gold flashed across him, that he had a sudden impression of a bluebird in spring. "I am resolved, then," she said. "It should be done. It *must* be done." She came forward and linked her arm in his, leading him to the door. "You will go to the king, and you will find some way to convince him."

He bowed. "I have already received a summons."

"What a charming coincidence," she said, with a much more discreet sort of smile.

At St. James's, Sir Hans went on a brisk late-afternoon walk in the silver-green park with the king and the earl of Sunderland, first lord of the treasury, the three of them huffing and puffing through crisp, still-wintry air. *At least,* thought Sir Hans, *Sunderland is huffing and puffing as much as I am.*

The king seemed impervious to either the cold or the length of the walk; he seemed rather to grow larger with goodwill and pleasure, the farther they went.

"So you are here to recommend this practice, Sir Hans?" he said, stooping for a stick to throw for his dogs.

"I am here to advise on any questions you may have, Your Majesty." *Damned awkward, trying to bow and trot through damp grass at the same time,* he thought.

"You are a wise man," said the king. "Irritating, perhaps, but wise. Let me think how to put my questions." He fondled the dog who had outraced the rest of the pack to return with the stick; its tail wagged so hard there appeared to be ten of them. "It is a risk?"

"It is, sir."

"And why do you think it works?"

"There are many theories," he began, but a sharp look from the king made him change his answer. "We do not know why, sir."

"But you have reason to believe it will work, though you cannot tell me why?"

"We have made a number of trials, all of them submitted to you in report. Every trial has indicated that inoculation for the smallpox produces a very favorable case, which bestows the usual survivor's protection against reinfection."

"And how far can we be sure that it will not harm?"

"It is impossible to be certain. Raising such a commotion in the blood might produce unforeseen accidents—"

"Accidents are always unforeseen, Sir Hans." He threw the stick into the distance once again.

"And some, sir, are dangerous. Even fatal."

The king walked on, motioning to both of them to stay back. He went forward to a small copse, and watched with pleasure as his dogs roused several startled pheasants into the air. He came back. "Physic is always dangerous, is it not? People might well—no—people most certainly have lost their lives by a bleeding or a purge, let never so much care be taken, no?"

Sir Hans nodded.

"So you see, I am not asking if it is infallible. I am asking whether, as a gamble, it is a good one."

They walked on in silence for another ten minutes, and then rounding a bend in a hedge, Sir Hans saw that they had come full circle; secretaries galore were rushing out from the palace to meet the king; Mehemet was stalking behind with a warm coat.

The king headed for his servant.

"Majesty?" Sir Hans dared to say.

"Eh?" said the King, stopping. "What?"

"Might I inquire whether you have come to a decision?"

"What? About inoculation? Wasn't I clear? Must be done. Without delay." He allowed Mehemet to put on his coat. "What do you think, Sunderland?"

The earl, who had purposely said nothing the whole length of the walk, and had had high hopes of getting out of it without a word, now sighed. He had lost his first wife to smallpox; his own face was a map of its cruelty. He was no fan of letting the disease anywhere near his children: he did not believe it could be tamed. His third wife, Judith, though, had been pestering him to have her son inoculated for months now. Judith's sister-in-law, Charlotte Tichborne, had tried it herself, and was an intimate of the princess, and they both knew Lady Mary—though *liking* was not precisely the right term, he supposed. Charlotte liked the duke of Kingston's eccentric daughter; Judith, thank the Lord, was content to respect her head. It made for a mighty bustle of women.

Women he could withstand. However, if the king was going to begin hinting that inoculation was a good plan, he would have to surrender. "I will arrange for Mr. Maitland to inoculate my son William immediately," he said.

"Excellent," said the king. "You see, Sir Hans? Decisions are to be made quickly."

On April 2, Mr. Maitland inoculated the Honorable William Spencer, two-and-a-half-year-old son of the Earl of Sunderland.

Almost two weeks later, on April 17, 1722, as young Master Will's pustules were scabbing over, Princess Emily and Princess Caroline dressed for an occasion of state, save that the sleeves were removed from their satin bodices. In the private sitting room in the nursery suite in St. James's, the royal family, the princesses' governess, the countess of Portland, and a medical council of war gathered, goaded on by the sounds of Princess Anne at the harpsichord, tripping furiously through a series of Mr. Handel's sonatas.

The wide doors remained open to the larger receiving room where Lady Mary and her miraculous daughter, Charlotte Tichborne, the duchess of Dorset, and other ladies of the Princess of Wales's household milled about with sundry men of the King's Council and the prince's household. The earl of Sunderland was not feeling well, so he had begged off for the sake of the princesses, as he put it; his wife was attending their son, and it was thought best not to toss any chance of infection about.

After an early-morning visit with his granddaughters, the king made himself busy elsewhere, though Mustafa, the junior of his two Turkish servants, made himself unobtrusively useful in the outer room, serving wine.

In the inner room, Dr. Sloane and Dr. Steigerthal were supervising, while trying to allow the prince the appearance that he was in charge—which he mostly maintained by marching about rapping on things with his riding crop, finding fault with everyone and everything, especially his wife. Mr. Maitland was there, of course, to advise, to point, to hold the lancet and the crystal vial of matter ready, and even to pinch the royal skin together, ever so gently. But it was Claude Amyand, principal sergeant surgeon in ordinary to His Majesty the king, who cut the royal skin.

Her Royal Highness, Princess Amelia, age eleven, demanded to be first, by right of seniority. She stepped forward, as if to a dance, and solemnly gave Sergeant Amyand her hand to kiss. But she did not offer to minuet; she turned sideways, just so, so as to offer the best view of her right arm, instead.

Sergeant Amyand winked at her, told her she was a brave princess, and proceeded through the operation step by step, while Mr. Maitland stood there instructing—for Sergeant Amyand of course had never done this operation before. Mr. Maitland pressed the little girl's muscle together just a bit, so as to loosen the skin, and Sergeant Amyand opened the upper layer of skin—the length of barleycorn, no more. In popped a bit of lint, and around the whole popped a bandage.

The princess presented her other arm; it went just as fast.

"It's easy, Caro," she whispered, as she stepped back. "And it doesn't hurt. Or it hurts just a little. Not like we thought."

"It does not hurt at all," said her father, giving a table a good whack with his crop. "You will admit of no such thing."

"It does not hurt at all," said Emily, as Amelia was known to the family. With the precision of long practice, her obedience was precisely modulated between abjection and exaggeration. But the ghost of a smile played around her mouth—such that Caro could see it, but their father could not.

Princess Caroline, just nine, stepped forward clutching her favorite doll.

"Deeper," said Mr. Maitland had said quietly, during the brief moment the family's attention was distracted. Mr. Amyand nodded, and this time he cut a bit deeper and longer, so that the princess gasped a bit, and a tear came to the corner of her eyes.

"May Anne-Caroline have a bandage too?" whispered the princess, as Sergeant Amyand finished.

It was all the surgeon could do to keep from wrapping her up in his arms, against the strutting rooster of her father. "Who?"

"Anne-Caroline," she said, thrusting out her doll. "She has the names of my first sister and my lady-princess mamma."

"*Bien sûr!*" cried Sergeant Amyand. "What was I thinking? La Princesse Anne-Caroline must be inoculated as well."

"What about Pierre?" asked Emily.

"No," said her mother. "Most certainly not."

Sergeant Amyand looked up in a silent plea, but the Princess of Wales was fighting off a smile. "Pierre is a spaniel," she said. "Though most certainly he is a prince among dogs."

"*Ah, non, ma petite princesse.* What is good for you, Highness, is not good for the dog, and vice versa."

"Is that is all?" exclaimed the Prince of Wales from the far window. "Is that what all this fuss has been about? Perhaps I shall ride after all."

In the outer room, Lady Mary noted that Mustafa had silently disappeared.

Sergeant Amyand sped home and inoculated the only two of his children who had not yet had the smallpox; if anything happened to the princesses, he must be seen as having taken the same risk.

To his horror, his youngest son, George, only seventeen months old, was struck with a bout of vomiting and a pretty sharp fever for four or five hours in the morning. He did not even wait for their own physician to arrive; he gave his wife a quick kiss and scuttled to the palace.

Finding everything calm, he dropped into a chair until the sweats evaporated. By then, though, the city had somehow got hold of his family's news, and were praying for his son and even harder for the princesses.

So later that day, when Lady Mary's friend Allen, Lord Bathurst, asked Sergeant Amyand to inoculate his six children, Sergeant Amyand came quite close to kissing him in the French manner of delight. He obliged that very afternoon—four daughters and two sons—at the Bathurst home in St. James's Square.

Perhaps the city's prayers did some good. At any rate, when the surgeon arrived home, he found his son's fever and nausea gone off, though the incisions had already begun to fester. His two-and-a-half-year-old daughter was as yet entirely unfazed, and was amusing her bedridden brother by spinning like a top and shrieking at the top of her lungs.

On the nineteenth, the world was shocked from the topic of smallpox by the sudden and quite unexpected death of the first lord of the treasury, the earl of Sunderland. Two days later, as little Princess Caroline began to grow tetchy under a light fever, the earl's young son, the honorable William, went into convulsions and died. A messenger went galloping to the palace.

"Was it the inoculation?" asked the king, after being pulled from a most delightful meeting with his architect. "Did he die of the smallpox?"

"We do not know, Your Majesty," said one of the council.

"No," said Sir Hans, "he did not. He was already shedding his scabs. How could that be?"

"No one knows how it works, Sir Hans," said the king. "You told me so yourself. So how can anyone possibly answer your how-can-it-be question? I hope, however, that you will discover an answer for me directly."

By morning, half of London seemed to be weeping and moaning outside the palace gates. Inside the nursery, though, the little girls were kept oblivious and as cheerful as possible under the circumstances. Little Princess Caroline was slightly feverish, and wan enough with nausea that even the doll Anne-Caroline was pushed away. But though she was miserable enough to make a mother's heart ache, she was not in any real danger, said Sir Hans.

Emily grew impatient. "When will I be sick?"

"Do you wish to be sick?" snapped her mother.

"Only to get it over with."

"I am sorry, *ma petite*," said her repentant mother, bending down and stroking her hair. "I am as impatient as you are, you see, but less kind this morning. You are a fine brave little heart of Hanover. And Britain," she added as her eyes met Sir Hans's.

In another room of the palace, the surgeons opened young Spencer's body in hopes of finding some reason for his death. There was some water on the brain, they reported. But they found nothing to quash the screaming of bloody murder in the press.

"You would think they were glad of the boy's death," grumbled Sergeant Amyand.

"They are," said Sir Hans.

The next morning, on the twenty-third, Princess Emily had her wish to be ill. Having been first snapped at by both father and mother, and then praised for being brave, she was absurd, heartbreaking stoicism itself, in a pale shade of green. Little Ann Amyand—just the age poor Sunderland's child had been—fell ill the same day, Sergeant Amyand was unutterably happy to report. Lord Bathurst reported his four girls ill the next day.

"Your sons, then, do not groan?" asked the Prince of Wales.

"Not yet," said Bathurst.

"My son will be even so," said the prince. "You will see."

No one bothered to remind him that he had two sons; he and the princess did their best not to think of their eldest son, Frederick, made a stranger by long absence in Germany.

On the twenty-fifth, Caro's rash appeared; by afternoon, her flecks were rising into blisters.

"When will I have some pocks?" fretted Emily.

"You don't want them," said Anne with a shudder. "Loathsome, squashy, smelly things."

"I do," protested Emily.

"You want a few small ones," specified her mother, as Emily curled tight against her.

The Princess of Wales had insisted upon spending a rare evening with her daughters. Even more rarely, the king and Prince of Wales took some very deep breaths (as well as a break from Sunderland's funereal solemnities) and shoved their deep dislike and distrust of each other as far as possible beneath the fragile family truce. For the sake of a mother who wished to be alone with her sick daughters, and for the sake of a front of family solidarity, they went to the Haymarket Theater the same night, and listened to Mr. Handel's marvelous new opera, *Floridante*.

Just before Emily went to bed, the rash began to flow across her; by the afternoon, she, too, was sporting blisters. All day long, the sisters watched each other, counting. By sunset, Caro had hit three hundred; Em was still far behind with sixty.

"I assuredly hope the princess Caroline's rash stops where it is," said the Princess of Wales, walking with Sir Hans to the outermost room, as he departed. "Where does your daughter stand?" she asked Sergeant Amyand.

"At eighty or ninety, Your Highness."

"What about your other little one?"

"George presents an interesting case," said Sergeant Amyand, his distress increasing both visibly and audibly. "His mother had the smallpox when young, madam; when another of our children broke out in the distemper, she nursed him through it, though she was then pregnant with George. As she recalls, the boy soon became more restless and unquiet in the womb than I understand is quite usual—and though she did not miscarry, she tells me now that she believes George had the distemper in utero. At any rate, he has never had the hint of a rash, and his incisions healed on the fourteenth."

"Don't tell that story as if it's an apology, sergeant," she said kindly. "You make me feel quite the fiend."

The next morning, Lord Bathurst triumphantly announced that his youngest son, Master Harry, had fallen ill at last. The girls were sprouting spots. His elder son, however, still had no sickness whatsoever, though his incisions festered. The family's apothecary—he frowned—had chosen this moment to divulge his suspicions that a rash he had treated the young master for a year earlier had actually been the smallpox—and had rendered him immune. "I must say I doubt it," said Lord Bathurst, "but I cannot make out any other reason why the boy should not be ill."

He neglected to report that the same day a nineteen-year-old servant— the children's favorite groom, Bert—had been laid low by flashing pains in the head, aches in his bones, and a high fever. Bert had come up to town from their estate near Cirencester in order to be inoculated with his young summer charges, but he had arrived too late, and the venom used for the children had curdled. So he had been drumming his fingers in the servants' quarters, waiting for fresh matter to arrive.

Dr. Mead ordered him blooded and vomited, and postponed the inoculation till after his recovery: "If it is still necessary," remarked the doctor gravely. For his symptoms had all the signs of the smallpox.

"How?" barked Lord Bathurst. To the fury of small stomping feet, he had forbidden Bert's visits to the nursery until fresh matter could be procured.

"The smallpox, my lord, is insidious," replied Dr. Mead. "It does not follow orders."

Bert was removed to the house of the smallpox nurse in Swallow Street.

In the palace, Emily stopped complaining about being first. She began to think that *first* might really mean best, and that in the matter of pocks, perhaps that meant fewest. The girls drew pictures of each other spotted— some of the pocks very large, others small—but Lady Portland insisted they burn their drawings.

A few days later, Emily at last was first: she lost the first scab. She decided first was fine, after all.

"Not fair," exclaimed Caro. "You have fewer."

"I'm first, I'm first," crowed Emily. "First, first, first."

* * *

Watching all this from afar, through the eyes and ears of Mr. Maitland, Sir Hans, and occasionally her old friend Dr. Arbuthnot, who attended the Bathurst family, Lady Mary wrote to her despondent sister in Paris: *I shall say little of the death of our Great Minister because the newspapers say so much. I suppose the same faithful historians give you regular accounts of the growth and spreading of the inoculation of the smallpox, which is become almost a general practice, attended with much success.*

To the doctors and surgeons, she kept asking, "Why must you cut so deep?"

And she kept being greeted with hemming and hawing that amounted to no answer at all.

In their house in St. James's Square, the Bathurst children developed mild cases. To much rejoicing in the nursery, after two days of care under Dr. Mead's supervision, Bert's smallpox was declared a false alarm and he was brought home to the Bathurst servants' quarters. Lord Bathurst, Dr. Mead, and Sergeant Amyand were almost as exhilarated as the children.

Even as their tension eased, however, a particularly rabid *Applebee's* began shouting about unchristian murder, claiming that the poor honorable toddler William Spencer had died "of *inoculations,* a new kind of distemper not known in former days, and an unhappy experiment to this young nobleman, who might in all probability have lived many years, if this operation had not been practiced upon him."

In a nose-thumbing answer, Mr. Amyand inoculated Lord Bathurst's Bert two days later.

On the second of May, the Bathurst children's smallpox ripened quite nicely. "You reduce me to uselessness," declared Dr. Mead with satisfaction.

By the third, both princesses were out of perceptible danger. Two days later, the last of Emily's pocks had disappeared, though Caro did not begin to shed hers till the following day. "Perhaps they will cling forever," said Em, in a temper, after Caro pulled Pierre's ears.

In St. James's Square, Lord Bathurst's children began to scab on the seventh, only twelve days after their inoculations. On the eighth, Bert's smallpox appeared—so favorable and distinct, and so firmly shooing away his nausea and fever, that congratulations were had all around.

The next morning, however, the singing and laughing stopped as Bert took a sharp turn for the worse. He began vomiting bile and his bowels went loose. His fever returned, carrying his mind into ravings, and then all of a sudden the infection boiled over and pocks fluxed all over his body, until there was no space for another pock to crawl out.

Despite near round-the-clock care by Dr. Mead and Dr. Arbuthnot, and the weeping prayers of children, Bert died on the twelfth of May.

For one day, all of aristocratic and royal London hunched in stunned silence. "It was a death," sighed the Princess of Wales at last, "and no death should go unmourned. But it was not an inoculation death, surely."

On the fourteenth, the earl of Berkeley took her point, and had Sergeant Amyand inoculate his two children; their mother, a legendary beauty, had died of smallpox a year after Lady Mary had battled it. His wife, remarked the earl grimly, had been one of the Princess of Wales's ladies while she lived; she would surely be urging him to proceed.

On the seventeenth, Mary sat at the Townshends' holding Dolly's hand as four of her pretty chickens were infected. On the twenty-second, she sat with Charlotte Tichborne and Lady De La Warr as they submitted their babies to this trial by fire. Suddenly, Lady Mary was run ragged.

In the palace, the girls' maids slathered heavy cream on their most stubborn sores, but to no avail: on both girls, two or three festered. Those, unfortunately, left their marks: but not badly, and in no material place—on the arm, the leg, the back. Their incisions kept running for about five weeks. In the end, Caro had the last laugh; her incisions stopped running on the twenty-third. Anne Amyand's had dried up two weeks earlier, a fact Sergeant Amyand did his best not to mention. Princess Emily's dripped for two more days, until the twenty-fifth. That day, Dr. Sloane, Dr. Steigerthal, and Sergeant Amyand examined them carefully, and pronounced both little girls free and clear.

Their mother held them close for what seemed like hours. "We will not see her so often anymore," said Em to Caro as they watched her depart.

"Could we be sick again?" asked Caroline.

"Not with the smallpox," sighed Emily.

The next day, they were seen in the park, taking the air with their sister, Princess Anne.

The incisions on Lord Bathurst's children healed much sooner than their grief. The earl of Berkeley's son did marvelously well: only seventy or eighty small pustules that clung to him a mere nine or ten days and then scurfed off, leaving no trace of their passage. His sister, Lady Betty, did not fare quite so lightly. Her pocks were numberless and larger, and she had a swelling on her right shoulder: a large abscess lodged under her deltoid muscle, which eventually had to be lanced.

"*You must stop all this cutting,*" Lady Mary said in cold fury to Sir Hans, drawing him out of the girl's bedchamber. "You must! That poor girl's incisions resemble suicide gashes more than cuts."

"The poison must vent, my lady, and the longer incisions are widely thought to help."

"They do *not* help. Lady Betty may have received the smallpox by inoculation, but her case is no different from a severe case of the distinct smallpox, received in the natural way. The Turks do not cut at all—only scratch, and they do not have such complications."

"You must allow us to improve somewhat upon the Turks."

"*But you are not improving it!*" she cried. "You are turning it into a physician's bloody goldmine."

Sir Hans had known Lady Mary most of her life. She saw him try his best to forgive her, as he drew himself tall, his nose pinching into a thin disapproving line.

"I am afraid you are thinking with your heart rather than your head, Lady Mary. The college—and I daresay the nation—owe you thanks for your part in promoting the practice. But in matters of medical knowledge, my lady, you must allow the college to make the decisions it sees fit."

She fled, shaking with rage. In Covent Garden, she hurtled up the steps and into her Turkish sitting room, where she paced furiously around the room, picking up this trinket and that, on the edge of hurling them all in a grand shattering rain of china, crystal, and silver. As she began to calm down, she stood panting at the window, fighting back tears of fury. This would never do. What was the good in weeping or breaking things?

In the window, she caught a faint reflection of a Turkish robe draped over a chair on the other side of the room. She stalked over to it, swirled it around her shoulders, and sat down cross-legged at her low writing desk. Then she rang for paper, ink, and pen.

How could they dismiss forty years of practice that worked, for the sake of theories that eminently did not? *How?*

She had been a Turkish merchant before, when she wished to tread where no woman was allowed; by Mahomet and his crescent, she would do it again.

I am determin'd to give a true account of the manner of inoculating the smallpox, she wrote, *as it is practised at Constantinople with constant success, and without any ill consequence whatever. I shall sell no drugs, nor take no fees . . . that is, I shall get nothing by it, but the private satisfaction of having done good to mankind, and I know nobody that reckons that satisfaction any part of their Interest.*

Two people had been *murdered*, she raged. Not by the operation, but by the physicians: by their "preparations" that weakened bodies just when they needed all their strength to fight off infection, by the miserable gashes they slashed through their patients' arms, and by the vast quantities of purulent matter they pasted into the wounds by the tankardful. She scratched through her conclusion without pause, sanded it, and rang for a glass of wine. All that was left was figuring exactly how to circulate it so that everyone should know it was hers, but no one would be able to prove it.

The physicians and surgeons among her friends were not amused; Dr. Arbuthnot, Dr. Mead, Sir Hans, and Mr. Maitland called upon her in a grand unsmiling delegation. She received them in an impeccably English drawing room.

"Surely, my lady, you can see that physicians per se are not your enemies?" Sir Hans began gruffly.

"Whose enemies?" she asked.

"Drop the masquerade, if you please, my lady," said Mr. Maitland. "Such subterfuge does not become you."

"And stubbornness does not become you, gentlemen."

"Will you not see that the inoculators are not your enemies?" pleaded Dr. Arbuthnot. "I must tell you, Lady Mary: you have flung down the word *murder*, but the two who died most certainly did not die from inoculation, no matter what you want to argue about incision length. Young Spencer was well through the distemper, and Lord Bathurst's servant had caught it in the natural way, before being inoculated—though to be sure, he may well have caught it from the inoculated children, or from being sent to the smallpox house. A niggling point, you may say, as you might still like to lay those deaths at medicine's door: but they did not come about through inoculation."

"I do not know why you feel the need to lecture me on this point, gentlemen, but seeing that you are, perhaps you will allow me to engage you. I hear what you have said about the deaths, Dr. Arbuthnot, and I must say your reasoning is convincing. But I tell you, I agree with this Turkey merchant: by your changes, you are making the operation far more severe and dangerous than necessary." She turned to Mr. Maitland. "Surely *you* can see that?"

"What I see most clearly, my lady, is that those of us who support inoculation would do well to stick together just now. The opposition screams with the fury of a storm from the sea."

She looked at them all, one by one, and then she rose. They hurried to stand in her wake. "If it comes to a battle for inoculation's survival, gentlemen, you can count on my support."

* * *

It did come to that, and soon. All summer long, jeering mobs followed the inoculators through the streets, and slurs began winging through the press. "Mr. Maitland is grubbing for money and patronage," sneered some.

"A new way to murder with impunity!" screeched others. "Guardians will poison their wards in order to come to rich estates."

"An artificial way of depopulating a whole country," shouted still others.

The most resounding thunder among the physicians came from Dr. William Wagstaffe, who had been reading certain pamphlets from the colonies quite carefully. Inoculation does not and cannot communicate smallpox, he argued. Inoculation produces something much closer to chicken pox: so how can it be expected to give protection from smallpox? Infusing the blood with such malignant matter, he argued in the next breath, may lay the foundation for many more terrible diseases.

But what really riled Dr. Wagstaffe was the absurdity of learned men listening to women and foreigners: *Physicians at least, who of all men ought to be guided in their judgments chiefly by experience, should not be over hasty in encouraging a practice, which does not seem as yet sufficiently supported either by reason, or by fact,* he roared on paper. *Posterity will scarcely be brought to believe that an experiment practiced only by a few ignorant women amongst an illiterate and unthinking people should on a sudden—and upon a slender Experience—so far obtain in one of the politest nations in the world as to be received into the Royal Palace.*

The Reverend Edmund Massey made pulpits ring with almost as much condemnation as the presses, working himself and his congregation into a froth of righteous hatred. *So went Satan forth from the Presence of the Lord, and smote Job with sore boils, from the sole of his Foot unto his Crown,* he thundered, proving that the devil himself was the first Inoculator.

Against the paranoia and the prejudice, the Royal Society—or most of it—called for patient reasoning. Dr. Arbuthnot and Dr. James Jurin, the society's secretary, listened to the arguments of a country doctor from York, and set a move underfoot to apply the cool precision of mathematics to the question of whether or not inoculation worked. Dr. Jurin began to peruse London's official bills of mortality, and to beg surgeons for their inoculation records.

Someone—Lady Mary never discovered who—leaked her Turkey merchant's letter to the press. In September, the *Flying-Post: or, Post-Master* printed a heavily edited version. Two weeks later: Isaac Massey, apothecary of Christ's and Reverend Massey's nephew, railed at it as "a sham Turkey

Merchant's letter"—but though he sensed a mask, he could not see behind the disguise.

Throughout the year, the squabbling whirled on in the press, crossing the Atlantic, and the Channel as well.

But the issue was decided slowly and steadily, below the chatter. It was decided by numbers.

In a quick assessment of London's official bills of mortality, Dr. Arbuthnot figured that living in London gave one a 1 in 9 chance of succumbing to smallpox. Dr. Jurin's more careful long-term study of both natural and inoculated smallpox—presented to the Royal Society in January 1723—concluded that 2 of every 17 Londoners died from smallpox. During epidemics, 1 in every 5 or 6 of those who fell ill died. In comparison, by the end of 1722, 15 inoculators throughout England had operated on 182 people, mostly children, and only 2 had died. Against the 1 in 6 chances offered by natural smallpox, inoculation's 1 in 91 risk of death looked inviting.

Numbers decided the case, but it was the sound of feet that reinforced it: the echoing footsteps of ranks of footmen running before carriages to send for inoculators, the light kid whisper of Lady Mary's slippers rising gracefully up grand staircases, the step of surgeons in the halls, and the patter of children in nurseries. People voted with their feet, and staked their children's lives upon their decisions.

The high and mighty were particular: they wanted Sergeant Amyand or Mr. Maitland to make the incisions, but they wanted Lady Mary in the room. Many of these were Lady Mary's friends, or currying favor with the Princess of Wales.

Others lived for nothing more than to make the inoculators' lives a sojourn of groaning, jeering, and gnashing of teeth.

And so the controversy went, tumbling into the next year, tattered with screaming and with pleas.

On the morning of thirteenth of May, 1723, a brilliant company gathered at Leicester House. The great names in the Prince and Princess of Wales's household, of course: dukes and duchesses, earls and countesses, lords and ladies aplenty. Mrs. Howard (the prince's mistress) and Mrs. Clayton (power-monger). Lord Townshend and many of the council, deputed from the king. Sir Robert Walpole and several others deputed from Parliament.

They could open Parliament, quipped someone among the prince's ushers, if Parliament only had papist leanings enough to worship a Madonna and child, rather than priding itself in bickering with kings.

For the center of attention, seated on a chair little less ornate than a throne, were the Princess of Wales, with Prince William Augustus on her knee. "They do look rather Raphael," remarked someone else.

"What is so amusing in that corner?" demanded the princess.

The chortling disappeared beneath deep bobbing bows.

"Leave 'em alone, woman," said the prince. "Look at old Amyand there, preparing to do battle with his lancet. St. George jousting with the speckled monster." He puffed with such obvious pleasure at his own jest that courtiers hurried to feed him with laughter.

The princess held her son close, drawing in the scent of his hair. All boy, he loved nothing so much as his hobby horse and was impatient to be off her lap, until he caught the gleam of the small knife.

"Be my brave, little general," whispered the princess, but Prince William did not appear to hear. Fascinated by the lancet, he watched the whole operation in silence.

"That all?" said someone in the back when it was over. "Why ain't every last body in the kingdom clamoring for it?"

A short distance away, in the Piazza of Covent Garden, a crowd surged forward, hooting and jeering as the doors to the Wortley Montagu house opened to reveal a phalanx of footmen surrounding Lady Mary and her small daughter. The shouting mounted, and a few turnips and a rotten egg or two arced over the carriage, splattering Lady's Mary's skirts as she disappeared into the waiting coach.

The mob trailed her coach all the way to Lincoln's Inn Fields, though blessedly, at the duchess of Ancaster's gate, she left everything but their noise behind.

"Oh, Mary, there you are," cried the duchess from the top of the grand staircase. "What is that horrid din?"

"My admirers," said Lady Mary. "Do you suppose I could borrow your maid?"

"Oh, my dear, what have they done?" said the duchess, arriving breathless at Lady Mary's side. "There is quite half an eggshell perched atop your wig, as if it has just hatched."

"Is there?" Taking her small daughter's hand, Lady Mary allowed herself to be steered toward the duchess's dressing room. "I only noticed the turnips." They sped up the hall, the servants impassive, but looking askance as they passed. *Unnatural,* hissed one or two, but Lady Mary affected not to notice.

The maid straightened her hair, removing a few foreign objects, and brushed out her skirts, while the duchess glared out the window. "Is it always like this?"

"Not always, no. They always seem to know, though, when I am headed toward an inoculation."

"Don't they recognize an angel when they see one? I was telling Ancaster only this morning that you are nothing if not an angel."

"They believe they see a devil, my dear. Or perhaps the Scarlet Whore of Babylon." She looked ruefully at her skirts. "They do have a penchant for tossing cherries in season, which unfortunately necessitates the wearing of red." Suddenly, she was very tired. *If I had foreseen the tenth part of the vexation, the persecution, and the obloquy heaped upon me day to day*, she told herself, *I would never have attempted to bring this operation into fashion.*

"If they had only known my poor Meg," said the duchess, stamping her foot. She turned and plopped down on the window seat. "Do you remember those days, when we used to peep over the garden wall at each other, Brownlows and Pierreponts?" She sighed. "It's a strange world, Mary, isn't it? I am so happy with Ancaster, you know—it is not all bad, to be a duchess. But it could not have happened but for poor Margaret's terrible death. I say a prayer for her every day, I do. Such a monstrous distemper, the smallpox. Took your Will, didn't it? And it nearly took you, too, poor dear. Sometimes in the night I cannot sleep, wondering when it will pounce upon my Louisa. She looks so much like Meg—even talks like her. It is quite eerie, at times." Tear welled in her eyes. "I could not bear it. I could not."

"Nor shall you," said Lady Mary. "I expect Sergeant Amyand will be here any moment, with his load of precious poison. Just think: Lady Louisa will have no less than a royal dose of the smallpox—same as Prince William."

The duchess sniffled and smiled, and Lady Mary took her arm.

"Let us go and find your pretty child."

"Lady Albina, my niece—her cousin—only, that goes without saying, doesn't it? Ancaster is always telling me I say things four times, when I need only say them once. Where was I? Oh, yes. Lady Albina is to be inoculated today as well. And Miss Selwyn—her mother, you know, is one of the princess's women of the bedchamber, and her father is something to the prince, I can't recall what."

Lady Louisa's inoculation went by in a twinkling. In a chattering, thought Lady Mary: Jane did love to talk.

As soon as was polite, Lady Mary and her daughter headed for the door. The duchess accompanied them, clasping Lady Mary's arm. "Are you quite sure you will be safe, my dear?"

"I do not think anyone has yet been killed by a rain of elderly vegetables, Jane."

"Is there nothing I can do for you?" insisted the duchess.

Lady Mary nodded and the footmen opened the door. "Admire the heroism in the heart of your friend," she said, and stepped into the screaming.

Aftermath

❦ 1 ❦

MEETINGS AND PARTINGS

The Boston Neck
July 26, 1723

ZABDIEL took Tommy and rode south across the Neck to race through wheeling clouds of birds far out into the salt marshes at low tide. It was a form of worship, he thought, this exhilaration in God's glories of wind, wings, and horses, though he knew neither Jerusha nor the Reverend Mr. Colman would agree. But it was how he liked to give thanks to the Lord for His delivery of Tommy two years ago.

When they returned home bright eyed and glowing, Jerusha smiled and said, "There is a letter for you in the parlor. From London."

He retrieved it and went out to the garden, to sit on a bench where he could watch his favorite mare nuzzling her new foal.

The letter sat lightly in his hand, as if it were a bird that would presently fly off. But it went nowhere, not even floating on a breeze, though dandelion gossamer skimmed about in the late afternoon light. Eventually he slit the seal and opened it.

> *Pleased to have the honour . . . Royal Society . . . a grateful world . . .*
> *Superior person . . . Your devoted servant, Sir Hans Sloane.*

He looked across the garden. The gooseberry and currant bushes were bending under their loads; roses and lavender were sighing their scent into the soft air. Most people would brandish such a letter aloft in triumph. Why, then, did he want nothing more than to curl up beneath this tree and sink into sleep?

After Mrs. Dixwell's death—*could that already be nearly two years ago?*—

he had reluctantly taken up his lancet again, only to find a grateful world suddenly clamoring for his services. It had by no means spelled the end of all difficulty, though. *Difficulty!* He scoffed at himself. A fine, mincing euphemism for death. For there had been more deaths: five more, to be exact. He had grieved sorely for every one of them, though he knew that most were probably due to the infection taken naturally before he had inoculated. The few that he reckoned were the result of poor doctoring, he bore as scars on his soul: but unlike Mrs. Dixwell's death, they had not paralyzed him.

Nor had they stilled the tumult in the streets; after the General Court had scattered in panic, the mob's frenzy for stopping him had transformed—overnight, it seemed—into an equally tireless enthusiasm to hound him into operating. His learned opposition, on the other hand, had relished each new death. In the press, the shouting dived gleefully into libel and even doggerel. Through it all, Zabdiel had done his best to keep his head down and his tongue silent; very little of the shouting deserved the dignity of a reply.

In any case, the demon disease had soon folded up its scaly wings and slunk out of Boston to terrorize neighboring Roxbury, Cambridge, and Charlestown. From December on, most of his inoculations had taken place in those towns. In Roxbury, people flocked to him after ten of the first thirteen head-of-household men to contract it had died; the place had thereafter been largely passed over by the angel of death. Cambridge, too, had clamored for his services, but in Dr. Robie, that town soon had an experienced inoculator of its own. In Charlestown, though, where people were more suspicious, they died in shoals. The Charlestown Boylstons and Webbs, along with their relations and trusting friends, had been conspicuous exceptions.

Meanwhile, in Boston, the urgency to inoculate had faded in the wake of the disease's disappearance. Dr. Douglass had ignored this connection, preferring to compare the waning interest in inoculation with the sudden dissolution of the witchcraft furor thirty years earlier. Massachusetts, he sneered, had at last shaken itself awake from yet another Mather-induced nightmare. Under Mr. Cooke's direction, the House of Representatives had tried to outlaw the operation, but the bill had died a swift, silent death upon being sent up to the Council.

In April and May, there had been one last stutter of excitement, as those who had fled drifted back into town, and a few more cases of smallpox flared up. Just as trade was returning to normal, it had shuddered and paused once again, as country towns heard rumors that the smallpox was back in Boston. Zabdiel took up the lancet once again, and inoculated six more people.

The selectmen promptly banished all six to Spectacle Island, while Dr. Douglass railed that the operation was once again crawling abroad, like serpents waking in summer. As the inoculees were Sewalls and Alfords, Zabdiel knew the blow had been struck as much in retaliation against the Council as against him. But it riled him, even in memory, when he thought of poor Joanna Alford dragged from her own house, her husband pinned helpless against the wall by five men.

Mr. Cooke and the rest of his selectmen had hauled Zabdiel before a meeting—again. This time, however, it was a full town meeting. They had demanded his word that he would stop. The danger was virtually past; wishing for nothing more than a cessation of the infernal, uncivil squabbling, he agreed.

In public, Dr. Douglass kept right on spitting rage. But in private, he had been heard, once or twice, to admit grudgingly that the smallpox "seems to be somewhat more favorably received by inoculation than received in the natural way."

The numbers were grim enough: in May 1721, 2 men had walked down the gangplank of a single ship, sick, into a bustling town of about 11,000 people. So far as could be figured in the ensuing chaos, 6,689 of those who did not flee had not had the smallpox before. By the end of January 1722, 5,989 of them had caught it. Only 700 people known to be vulnerable—just over one in ten—had escaped unscathed. Among their less fortunate fellows, no fewer than 844 had died—nearly half of those in the single dark month of October. There was no accurate count of the other casualties: the blindness in one or both eyes, the scarred faces, the miscarriages, the long-lasting boils, ulcers, and arthritic aches—but Zabdiel put those in the hundreds as well.

Against those numbers, he could set his own: he had inoculated 247 people, and had lost 6. All but one or two of those—along with most of his serious complications—he strongly suspected had taken the infection before he operated. At their best, then, his numbers suggested that inoculation offered better than a 1-in-100 chance of dying. Even taking his numbers at their worst, the risk of death looked to be only 1 in 41. Natural smallpox, on the other hand, threatened 1 in 7. "Somewhat more favorable," indeed.

By June 1722, his last patients were trickling back from Spectacle Island, having all recovered nicely under the care of Dr. Robie. Zabdiel had not been allowed to visit them with so much as a note—for fear, he supposed, that he might scrape out a pock and store up some matter with which to continue.

Finally, the press had let go and moved on to juicier topics: not necessarily to the press's benefit. For printing a satire suggesting that the government was collaborating with pirates, James Franklin got himself tossed into jail by order of the Council. His father, Josiah, had come hat in hand to Zabdiel. His son's imprisonment, he thought, might be—in some measure—belated punishment for his publishing of so many anti-inoculation columns. Josiah had tried to reason with the boy, he said, his voice cracking. He had once or twice succeeded in getting him to quash a really rank piece—but, for the most part, James had been imperviously coated with the stubbornness of the young. Money was not the problem; Josiah's younger son Ben could run the press. But the stone dungeon in which James had been shackled was a pit of darkness. He was like to lose his life of jail fever or the bloody flux before he ever saw the light of day again.

That afternoon, Zabdiel delivered to the Council a terse letter pronouncing it paramount that James Franklin be allowed freedom of the Press Yard, for the sake of his health.

Mr. Franklin was duly transferred, and eventually released the first week in July.

By that time, Zabdiel was consumed elsewhere, for his mother was dying. She passed on July 8, firm in the belief that her middle child could do anything. Later that month, full-scale war broke out with the Abenaki Indians up in Maine; closer to home, the petty war between Governor Shute on one hand and Mr. Cook and Dr. Clark on the other rattled on.

In September, Zabdiel had kinder news. At noon on Sunday the sixteenth, one year to the day after he had inoculated Mrs. Adams, she gave birth to a son named Samuel. "He looks to thrive," said the infant's startled father, who had not yet seen a son born healthy enough to survive. "He has a lusty yell, I can tell you that. Mary and I have great hopes for him."

In the Town House, the mood had not been so glad. All that long autumn, the governor exasperated even those who were disposed to support him for the sake of the office, if for nothing else. In the face of increasingly open hatred, Governor Shute secretly boarded HMS *Seahorse* one night in December and absconded for London.

"Zabdiel?"

He started. Jerusha was standing before him, hands on her hips, smiling at him as if he were a wayward child. He handed her the letter, watching her tip it toward the fading light, squinting to see.

"*London,*" she said with hushed wonder, as if it were an earthly Eden and Canaan, Sodom and Gomorrah, flowing with milk, honey, and abomination all at once.

He made room for her on the bench.

"It is a great honor, Zabdiel."

"Curious, Jer. I have wanted to see London for many years. But now that this place is slipping back into civility, I find I don't want to leave."

"I am not sure you have a choice," she said quietly. "I suppose you had better ask Mr. Colman or Dr. Mather, but surely Sir Hans Sloane's reference to 'a superior person' means royalty."

"I was afraid of that." He stood up and held out his hand to her, drawing her up beside him. "If I must go, my dear, may I hope that will you come with me?"

She looked slowly about the garden. Its color was draining, but its scents were ripening into sensuous riot. "My place is here, Zabdiel. So is yours. If you must go, I will stay here with the children." She smiled up at him. "That way, you will be sure to come back."

In the morning, Mr. Colman confirmed his fears. "No doubt about it," he said cheerfully, clapping him on the back. "Sir Hans has issued the invitation, but the force behind it is royal. While you may delay, I am afraid you may not refuse."

"It seems like a dream," said Zabdiel shaking his head in wonder as he took his leave. "If you don't mind, I would rather not spread the word of this invitation until I know for certain what it produces."

"All manner of honors, I expect," said Mr. Colman. "But I shall be as secret as the grave."

At the beginning of August, Zabdiel advertised in the papers for people to settle their debts with him, as he was designing a voyage to London in a very short time. Meanwhile, he replied to Sir Hans, both to accept the invitation and to apologize for the unavoidable delay in doing so; it would take time—as much as a year, perhaps—to make suitable arrangements for his practice, his shop, and his family.

A few weeks later, Jerusha found her husband pacing back and forth in front of his bookshelf in the parlor one evening.

"I have had a word with Captain Barlow," he said. "I do not know, Jerusha, how we will pay for my passage. . . . I must sell either my books or my horses."

"The books," she said without a second thought. "Did you think I would say anything else?" she cried, as relief flooded his face. "Books are replaceable. A fine bloodline such as you have spent years refining is not." She crossed the room to put her arms around him. "But I do think you ought to consider parting with a few of your horses. Three or four." Ignoring his dismay, she pattered on. "You must take some with you, Zabdiel. I don't know how it's done, though it must be possible, since horses are shipped this direction."

"*Take some*—? Have you taken leave of your senses entirely?"

"You must go bearing some American gift worthy of royalty. I am not saying you will need it," she said, laughing at the consternation on his face. "But surely you must go prepared. I have seen the stock that comes to us from England; we are no provincial backwater in the matter of horse breeding. And I cannot think of anything else we have that might be suitable."

By October, Zabdiel had caused a small stir among the province's literati, by selling his fine collection of books to a recent graduate from Harvard.

Sir Hans replied to Zabdiel's note with a suggestion. Perhaps, during the delay, Dr. Boylston might consider submitting to the Royal Society some paper likely to be of interest to the Fellows?

Zabdiel considered consulting Dr. Mather. Instead, he rode up to the Salutation Inn.

"What the devil can they want?" he grumbled to Cheever. "What could I possibly know that they might find of interest?"

"What do they talk about?"

"Wonders of the natural world, I think. Curiosities like inoculation for the smallpox."

"How about ambergris? There's a curiosity for you."

There were always whalers from Nantucket in the Salutation; he began his research that very night, over tankards of the Webbs' best brew.

In February 1724, he began advertising for someone to rent two and a quarter acres of his garden, containing gooseberry, currant bushes, fruit trees, and an asparagus bed, among other useful plants. Also on offer was the right to sell its produce—as well as imported drugs—from his shop.

That spring, the king dispatched Mr. Maitland to Hanover to inoculate His eighteen-year-old Royal Highness, Prince Frederick, second in line for the throne after his father, the Prince of Wales. As a consequence, Prince Frederick received one light fever, five hundred pustules, and indemnity from the natural smallpox. Mr. Maitland received the lavish sum of £1,000. Inoculation had received the highest commendation the kingdom could offer.

Sir Hans retreated to the Repository, the Royal Society's triangular nook of a library—strange but lovely design of Sir Christopher Wren—to open the letter from Boston. That it was not addressed in Dr. Mather's crabbed handwriting had given him particular excitement; perhaps he would at last discover what he yearned to know, after being put off so long.

Dr. Jurin found him there a quarter of an hour later, laughing so hard that tears were streaming down his face. "I wrote to ask Dr. Boylston of Boston whether he might grace us with a paper sure to be of interest to the Fellows, as his voyage has been postponed so long," he gasped. "He has earnestly obliged." He slid the paper across to Dr. Jurin.

The good doctor had written about the oceanic mystery of ambergris.

"Not bad, mind you," said Sir Hans, wiping his eyes. "Indeed, I think it quite publishable. But how can he possibly have missed my reference to inoculation?"

The long-avoided day of doom was fast approaching. In November 1724, Zabdiel realized that perhaps a gift for the Royal Society would be in order, so he advertised for a large quantity of ambergris. Only he spelled it as New Englanders pronounced it—"ambergrease"—in an admittedly hurried scrawl—and the *Courant*'s typesetter got it confused with bear's grease. "A most malodorous mistake," sighed Jerusha, wrinkling her nose as she surveyed the pails full of hairy bear's fat that kept appearing, as if by magic, every morning on the kitchen steps. But she couldn't blame the donors, who carefully noted their names and the weight of their offerings. Ambergris was worth ten times what bear's grease went for.

It was the least he could do, thought Dr. Mather, putting pen to paper in the middle of December, to help open doors into learned society for his beloved physician. No doubt Dr. Boylston would have tales of inoculation that the Royal Society would wish to hear from his lips. But Dr. Mather was hoping he might also prime the doctor with a few more personally useful tales as well. For he needed help—preferably help bodily present in Crane Court—to conquer once and for all a particularly vexing tribulation the Lord had lately poured upon him.

Suspicious of the fact that Dr. Mather claimed fellowship in the Royal Society but did not receive their journal, Dr. Douglass had induced some of his minions to pry into the Society's official membership records. They had come up empty.

Dr. Mather, that odious Scot had begun crowing, was no member at all. His "F.R.S.," was a miserable sham.

Dr. Mather was deeply hurt. He would never have adopted such august initials of honor had they not been offered to him by the bona fide secretary of the Society. He had written to the present secretary, Dr. Jurin, to say so, and to apologize for having trespassed—if indeed he had trespassed. He had also steadily offered the suggestion (so deeply wrapped in black velvet that he himself could barely discern it) that the Royal Society owed him an apology in return, not to mention a clarification of their error, trumpeted to the world.

He had at last received the clarification—his failure to appear on the membership rolls was a mere oversight of procedure. Not to worry, he was indeed entitled to his F.R.S. He had not, so far, had the apology, however.

Yes, providing Dr. Boylston with a letter of introduction was a fine thing to do.

To Dr. James Jurin
December 15, 1724

Sir,
Having lately addressed you with some number of letters, I have just now nothing to add but that I have an agreeable occasion of introducing to your knowledge and kindness a friend that has been to me as the golden wedge of Ophir. 'Tis Mr. Zabdiel Boylston, the sight of whom will doubtless be the more welcome to you because his name has already reached you.

He is a gentleman whose performances as a chirurgeon (and very particularly in lithotomy) have hitherto been equaled by no person in these parts of the world. And as a physician he has been to an uncommon degree successful, and so beloved and esteemed that his absence for a few months from us, on his present voyage, is a matter of uneasy apprehension to a multitude.

But that which will more particularly recommend him to your notice is that this *is the gentleman who first brought the way of saving lives by the inoculation of the smallpox into the American world.*

When the rest of our doctors did rather the part of butchers or tools for the destroyer to our perishing people, and with envious and horrid insinua-

tions infuriated the world against him, this worthy man had the courage and conscience to enter upon the practice; and (generously beginning with his own family) he alone, with the blessing of Heaven, saved the lives of I think several hundreds; yea, at one time he saved a whole town from a fearful desolation, after the smallpox had begun to do the execution of a great plague upon it. With an admirable patience he slighted the allatrations of a self-destroying people, and the satisfaction of having done good unto mankind made him a noble compensation for all the trouble he met withal.

You having done so much to oblige the public in your candid essays to procure a just reputation for a practice, which if mankind were not obstinately bent upon self-destruction would soon save the lives of millions, it cannot be unacceptable to you to have an opportunity for inquiring of this gentleman what has occurred in his own experiments, and particularly, how far he can justify the account I have given you of those few who died after the inoculation.

Yes, Dr. Boylston was just the person to attest to his accuracy. This was very satisfactory, indeed. So satisfactory that he thought he might venture quite a daring recommendation.

Yea, perhaps the Prince and Princess themselves, if informed of such a one coming to London, may not be unwilling to take some cognizance of a person so distinguished by an operation of so much consequence.
Your most hearty servant,
Cotton Mather, D.D., F.R.S.

The letter was such a good idea that he directly began another, to Sir Hans Sloane.

"He thinks the Royal Society is all his idea," said Zabdiel to the Reverend Mr. Colman. "I don't have the heart to tell him otherwise."

"You do him a kindness," said Mr. Colman, adding letters of introduction to the merchant Thomas Hollis and the minister Daniel Neal to his stack. "And in any case, it is most certainly his idea that you should defend his honor before the Society . . . I must confess, I also have a request to make of you." He closed the door to his study. "Someone, you see, must talk sense to the governor. I am sorry to say that Elisha Cooke has announced his plans to sail to London; no doubt he will seek to sever all Governor Shute's ties to this country. I am only afraid that he will sever other things as well. Possibly including most of whatever may be left of the goodwill the court bears us. May those of us in favor of peace between Council and town count on your discretion as an emissary?"

Zabdiel groaned and nodded in agreement.

So, early one morning at the end of December, Zabdiel, Jack, and Jackey—now six and, to Tommy's everlasting envy, going along as page to Zabdiel—drove four of Zabdiel's horses up the gangway and into a specially built pen on the deck of Captain Barlow's ship. In his tiny cabin, Zabdiel stowed a stack of letters, the diary that held all his case notes for inoculation, a light waxy gray ball of ambergris, and a heavy burden of responsibility. Not long afterward, he kissed Jerusha and the children goodbye, while Jack and Jackey bade farewell to Moll. An hour later, they were under sail for London.

"I am sorry that the man's practice has fallen off so drastically here at home that he feels he must seek his fortune abroad," sniffed Dr. Douglass at a meeting of the Scots Charitable Society. "I am sorrier still that he has had the overweening gall to think he will make a splash in London's medical milieu." He took a sip of rum punch and leaned back with satisfaction. "He'll be back soon enough, tail between his legs, I tell you. London has plenty of highly trained inoculators. What need have they of one more quack?"

In the intolerable quiet of Leicester House just after the New Year, the Princess of Wales was obeying tradition and good hygiene by keeping to her bed during the six-week period of lying-in after delivering the newest princess, Louisa, to the nation on December 18. In reality, she was fretting and fidgeting—and, as soon as her ladies turned their backs, up and pacing about the chamber.

Sir Hans was sent for, to see if he could calm her down.

For him, she was induced to sit in a chair and take a glass of wine.

He did his best to bring her news of the subjects she liked. "My grandson Stanley was inoculated on the twentieth," he said. "Seems to be doing quite well."

"Inoculation," snapped the princess, fidgeting with the coverlet that Tich had insisted upon tucking around her. "Why does that man Boylston not come?"

Sir Hans sighed. "Boston is a long ways away, Highness. And not without peril. They say he once lost a brother bound for London by sea. Perhaps he is reluctant."

"A man like that? Afraid of the sea? I do not believe it. Besides, we are going back and forth on the sea to Hanover all the time. I see that look, Sir Hans, you will tell me that crossing the Atlantic is different from crossing the Channel. But I am sure that wretched man Shute has done it four times."

"Only once, madam. Though I will agree that it seems like four times."

In Covent Garden and Twickenham, Lady Mary was enjoying a respite that very nearly amounted to retirement. The smallpox had waned across 1724, and the pluckings at her skirts and her sleeves, the notes that chased her down and said *Please come* or *Please stay away* had disappeared with the disease.

The physicians had wrested the practice away from her—they even came in for most of the praise for the discovery, at least in the serious matter of the saving of lives. Lady Mary found her name relegated to decorating poetry as a rescuer of beauty and wit.

She affected a relentlessly arch cheer and wrote flowing letters to her sister Frances, Lady Mar, sinking ever farther into despondency in her Parisian exile: *I see everybody but converse with nobody but des amis choisies.* Though, to be honest, a terrible number of her friends were slipping into long, silent conversations with death.

But Frances would not wish to dwell on Lady Mary's creeping sadness for the passing of friends. She forced herself back into brightness: *We have assemblies for every day in the week, besides court, operas, and masquerades.* She thought of the absurdities of the rising generation, and shook her head. *For my part, it is my established opinion that this globe of ours is no better than a Holland cheese, and the walkers about in it mites. I should be tolerably easy though a great rat came and ate half it up.*

Lord, she sounded little less gloomy than her sister. How was such a letter to cheer up poor Frances?

Near the end of January, Zabdiel, his servants, and his horses at long last arrived in the metropolis. On the eleventh of February, 1725, he dressed carefully in the new suit that Jerusha insisted he have made for him, freshly powdered his best wig, and went off to Crane Court, to be introduced to the Royal Society.

There were many men milling about outside the meeting room, some hurrying to clap old friends on the back and draw them off to quiet corners, others standing about in proud poses and eyeing one another surreptitiously. He had the feeling that he was going to be miserable, when two men walked up together.

The younger and less imposing smiled and said, "Dr. Boylston, I presume?" At his nod, he introduced his elder companion—none other than Sir Hans Sloane—and was in turn introduced as Dr. James Jurin.

"Delighted, delighted to meet you I am sure," they said all around, and Zabdiel thought that perhaps they might even mean it.

Soon afterward, they all filed in to the hall. Sir Hans—as vice president—took the chair in Sir Isaac Newton's absence, and the meeting began. It was both dull and brilliant, as they read old minutes and moved to new ideas. They spoke first of a new French study of suppuration, and then of a home-grown treatise on vegetables; at last, they gave the floor to Dr. Jurin, who introduced him to the gathered company as "Dr. Boylston from New England."

With some trepidation, Zabdiel rose and gazed over the gathered crowd. Briefly, he recalled the hostile faces leaning toward him at the select-men's meeting in Boston, but these faces—some a great deal more grand, others a great deal more dissolute, and some equally serious and sober—were for the most part politely interested. No doubt he himself formed part of their interest, he thought dryly. They were probably regarding him as just another exotic specimen.

Carefully, he unwrapped the immense lump of ambergris he had hauled all the way from New England, and presented it to Sir Hans and the Society, regaling them with a tale of Nantucketers discovering the stuff in a bag near the formidable genitals of a male sperm whale. It was moist and most offensive smelling when first found, he assured them, though after proper curing, its scent was legendary for its sweetness.

At Sir Hans's request, the lump was broken open, so that they might see what was inside. It proved solid throughout, but the breaking proved valuable. A bit was designated for the Repository, but the rest was shared out among members with their own collections to feed.

Dr. Boylston was formally thanked, and the meeting broke up. Men crowded forward, all eager to speak with him—quite a few about ambergris, but many more, he found, about inoculation. Zabdiel was astounded to find that Dr. Richard Mead wished to speak to him. So did Dr. John Arbuthnot and Mr. William Cheselden, the developer of a promising new technique for extracting bladder stones, and the man Zabdiel regarded as the greatest living surgeon. Amid a cluster of fellows, he was swept across the Strand to their unofficial home at the Grecian coffeehouse, to indulge in conversation both more leisurely and more intense.

One morning later that month, Lady Mary sat at her dressing table in a long Turkish robe and idly pinned up her hair while her daughter galloped in noisy circles about the room. *She will be a hoyden just like you*, Mr. W had said upon hearing that Lady Mary had given their daughter a hobby horse, but Lady Mary thought the more the girl took after her and the less after Mr. W, the better.

Behind her, the doors to her chamber suddenly flew open and two footmen stepped inside. Footmen in new and entirely extravagant gold lace. A man's heels clicked on the floor. Her daughter had fallen silent.

"Mr. W—" cried Lady Mary in annoyance, half rising as she turned.

But it was not Mr. Wortley.

Her sleeve swept a jar from the table, splattering glass and white cosmetic paste across the floor in a long dash of surprise. An odd little squeak came from her throat, and she sank to her knees, filled with the old terror.

"Forgive me, Father. I did not expect you."

"Of course you did not," said the duke of Kingston irritably, stalking up to her to proffer his hand to be kissed. "How would you? I never find myself accidentally in this quaint corner of town, and you never invite me."

It was true she did not ask him often. But she most certainly did ask him. He always regretted, however, without any apparent regret.

His hand withdrew, but he remained in front of her, talking to the top of her head. "Servants in a deplorable state of disarray. One insolent fellow actually tried to stop me from entering. Ought to dismiss him. . . . But I am not here to discuss the state of your household."

He walked to the windows, skirting the mess on the floor, and Lady Mary realized that her daughter had disappeared. While her father's back was turned, she raised her head and looked surreptitiously about. There she was—eyes big as saucers, gleaming beneath the dark scrolls of a japanned card table. Mary gave her a quick smile and put her finger to her lips. But then her father stirred, and she dropped her hand and looked back down.

He did not turn, however, just stood at a window watching the world scurry by, squawking and singing in the market square below. "I daresay," he mused, "I would never have allowed you to traipse over to Turkey. So I suppose old Wortley must come in for at least that much thanks."

He cleared his throat and turned. "In the matter of inoculation, I mean. I could have wished you had brought home your discovery in time for poor Will. However, it is at least in time for his children." He crossed back to stand before her.

Still staring at the floor, Lady Mary held her breath. Her father did not hold conversations with his children; he delivered proclamations. This, though, looked to become the longest speech he had ever deigned to grace her with. And the closest thing to a compliment too.

He went on. "Sir Hans says he fears that the smallpox may be as strong as ever this year. So I have engaged Mr. Maitland to inoculate Lord

Dorchester." In spite of herself, Lady Mary glanced up. Her father's namesake—Will's son—young Evelyn, Lord Dorchester, was all that stood between her father and the extinction of the dukedom his family had schemed for a century to acquire.

For the first time in her life, he allowed her to hold his gaze. "And the duchess," he continued, "insists that Lady Caroline must join him. . . . Their younger sisters we shall see about later. Might I ask the favor of your presence?"

"I should be honored, Father."

He reached out and laid his hand on her head in blessing. "You have done well, my Mary. Rather more notoriety than necessary, perhaps, but I like your spirit. I may even say I am proud to claim it as mine. God knows neither of your sisters got it." He whirled on one heel and strode quickly out the door, his two footmen—for they were his, of course, she ought to have recognized them—falling into step behind him.

"Mamma," whispered little Mary, creeping out from under the table and looking carefully about the room. Seeing they were alone, she skidded across the floor and flung herself into Lady Mary's arms. "Mamma, was that really the duke of Kingston?"

Tears sliding down her cheeks, Lady Mary stroked her daughter's hair; it still amazed her that Mary was now seven. "Yes, darling. That was my father. Your grandfather." She watched her daughter consider this information. Like a little wren, really.

"He is very grand for such a tiny old man," she said at last.

Lady Mary began to laugh. *A tiny old man! She had not seen that at all.* She kissed the top of her daughter's head. "Yes, my little Moll. He is very grand."

Just after the end of his first month in London, Zabdiel sat down to write his first report home to the Reverend Mr. Benjamin Colman. He had dined several times with the governor, as well as with Mr. Dummer and Mr. Cooke, but alas, what he had to report was not pretty. *I am at a loss what to say about our governor,* he began.

Governor Shute was peacocking about, full of pride and resentment, as if his government would be reconfirmed on whatever terms he chose; Mr. Cooke, quite possibly equally well informed, hinted exactly the reverse. At times, thought Zabdiel, all of London seemed to run on innuendo.

> *The Governor tells me that no one is putting in for the government, or can subvert him if he pleases to return, so we are here just as you are there:*

perfectly ignorant of the great affairs of the court, until they act. . . . I am
under such concern for my country that I would freely give all my horses
for a sudden and perfect healing of all our divisions, together with a good
Governor. Though you know, sir, that my horses are very dear to me.

I pray sir, your continued favours to me and my family.

And am,

Dear and reverend Sir,

Your most Affectionate

and most

Obliged servant,

Zabdiel Boylston

On February 27, Lady Mary attended the inoculations of her thirteen-year-old nephew and nine-year-old half-sister at her father's house in Arlington Street, while the two silly mothers shrieked and shook as if they were already in mourning. The younger girls, of course, caught the hysteria, which brought her father roaring out of his library, at which point the entire household dissolved into chaos.

After promising to return every morning, she went home with a headache.

And so it began again, even as the smallpox reared its speckled head once more. Her friends, her acquaintances, people who had seen her once across the room at court, desperately pleaded for her presence while their children were being inoculated; they wanted young Mary as well, as if she might be some kind of good-luck charm.

Just as desperately, the same people shunned her when she had been attending the inoculations of other children.

On April 2, Zabdiel arrived at Leicester House half expecting to be turned ignominiously from the door. Instead, he found himself ushered into the hushed fastnesses of the unofficial but princely palace, on the occasion of the inoculation of Her Royal Highness Princess Mary, age three.

At a grand set of double doors, his name was announced as he was thrust into a surprisingly crowded reception room, its formal walls and ceiling larded with gilt, carved plaster swags, and cherubs who looked to be diving down on one's head with no good intent. Sir Hans appeared at his elbow, steering him into a slightly smaller inner room, warmly paneled and painted, where he presented Dr. Boylston of New England to the Prince and Princess of Wales.

"Your Royal Highness," said Zabdiel to the prince with a bow.

"Capital," said the prince, turning away to roam the room in impatient circles.

"Your Royal Highness," said Zabdiel to the princess, bowing again and kissing her hand.

"*Enchantée*," she replied. "Your presence is most valuable, Doctor. You must tell me of your battle against this beast presently, but just at the moment, I have a question for Sir Hans."

The princess led Sir Hans away for a tête-à-tête. Why the princess imagined she needed to summon him all the way from America, Zabdiel could not fathom; the room was thick with several more surgeons and at least a half-dozen bona fide physicians of the Royal College. On the other hand, he need not fear calling attention to himself by breaking some arcane rule of etiquette; in this press, he could hardly be noticed. He recognized Sergeant Amyand and Mr. Maitland, inspecting the instruments. Mr. Lilly, the apothecary. Sir Hans, of course, along with Dr. Steigerthal, Dr. Mead, Dr. Arbuthnot, and several others with the patronizing air of London physicians, though he did not know them by name.

By a window, a small boy—four or five, Zabdiel guessed—knelt on the floor, absorbed in lining up small carved infantry and cavalry troops just so according to a battle plan in a large book spread out beside him. He wore a sumptuous military uniform in scarlet and gold, but his unsoldierly tongue was set firmly in the corner of his mouth as he moved from book to floor, placing his figures.

Prince William, thought Zabdiel.

"What battle are you fighting?" he asked, sinking to his knees beside the boy.

"Marlborough at Blenheim." The boy's voice was high and clear.

"Very likely to win . . . that is, if you fight on the British side."

"I always take the British side," the boy bristled. "At least, always when there is a British side. I would like to do Alexander the Great at Gaugamela, but no one has found me a battle plan. But if they do—*when* they do, then I won't be British."

"Because you will be William the Great?"

The boy looked up, suspicious of being laughed at. "Not yet," he said haughtily. "You can be born a prince, says my grandpapa, but you must earn a 'great.' But I will be a general, and then I will conquer France. Already I have a cavalry regiment. Do you like to ride?"

"Always," said Zabdiel gravely. "I would much rather be riding than sitting here just now."

"Ha!" said the Prince of Wales over his shoulder. "The last honest man in London. . . . So you like the riding, my American doctor?"

Groaning inwardly, Zabdiel turned and stood. "Yes, Your Highness. So much so that I have brought my own horses with me from America."

"American horses, eh?" said Prince George, thwacking his crop against his riding boot. He narrowed his eyes. "Do they make good hunters?"

"Yes, sir," said Zabdiel. "Though the hunting they know is surely different from the customs here. I learned to hunt alone in the woods, you see, from my father and an old Indian servant."

"A Red Indian?" squeaked Prince William, his jaw dropping.

"Your stature, Doctor, soars with the eagles," said Prince George dryly. "I do not care one way or the other about Indians, but I would like to see these American horses of yours. Horses, you know, seem to be running in from the most unexpected places these days." His eyes scanned the room. "See that one?" he cried, brandishing his crop in the direction of a woman across the way. "In green and gold, by the door?" Zabdiel winced at this boorishness, but the prince prattled on, oblivious. "Must have you speak to her. Knows Turkish horses. Quite small, you know, but with the stamina of elephants. The horses, I mean, not the lady."

She had dark, glossy hair smoothed into a roll at the nape of her neck. As if their eyes burned her, she turned and lifted one dark slash of a brow with displeasure.

Zabdiel colored and looked away.

"Pity, ain't it?" said the prince. "Lady Mary Wortley Montagu."

Zabdiel glanced back. She had returned to her conversation, with Doctors Mead and Arbuthnot; it seemed to be lively. He saw nothing to pity. To his eyes, she was startlingly beautiful.

"Used to be quite lovely," rumbled the prince. "Fancied her myself, you know. Before the smallpox roughed her up. Come to think of it, horses weren't all she brought back from Turkey were they? The two of you will have more to speak about than bloodlines. . . . Lines of blood, so to speak." He stomped the floor with delight at his cleverness, and a toy soldier disappeared beneath his boot with a brittle crunch.

A wail of dismay rose from Prince William.

"You, sir," barked the Prince of Wales. "Cease that caterwauling. Remove this clutter from my floor and go make yourself useful to your mother directly." Glaring at his son, he kicked the whole battle aside and walked on.

Prince William looked after his father with hatred in his eyes, but his lower lip trembled.

"If it would suit Your Highness to command me," said Zabdiel, "I will shift your battle to that table over there by the next window, while you do as your father wishes."

The boy flashed him a smile, and then withdrew it in pride. "You shall be a field marshal," he said. "I command to you to reorder my field." He strutted away, already a small parody of his father.

"As the prince has so clearly pointed me out to you, I will take the liberty of assuming that we have been royally introduced," said a light, acid voice behind Zabdiel, just as he was finishing.

"My lady," he said, rising and bowing.

"We are supposed to hurl ourselves at each other in animated conversation about horses, I believe," said Lady Mary.

"We could talk about Marlborough at Blenheim, if you'd rather," said Zabdiel. "Just at present, I am up on it."

A smile glimmered at the edge of her expression. "I hear you possess a marvelous stallion named Prince," she said.

He bowed again. "To my eyes, my lady, he is without fault."

"Then he is surely far superior to princes of the two-legged variety," observed Lady Mary.

They took a turn about the room, but it was not about either horses or battles that they spoke. By the time they closed their first circle, they were both laughing.

Not long afterward, Princess Mary arrived, and the operation was performed quickly and well, so far as Zabdiel could see through the gathered crowd.

As word of royal interest in Zabdiel buzzed through London's drawing rooms, requests for him to attend inoculations kept Jack and Jackey busy traipsing from the front door to his study and back with notes piled on a silver tray. He would be happy to attend, he always replied, though he refused all suggestions that he perform the operation. In the ensuing weeks, Zabdiel's path began to cross Lady Mary's at these inoculations. Frequenting the Grecian with Mr. Cheselden and Dr. Arbuthnot, he also met the celebrated portraitist and art theorist Jonathan Richardson, sixty-ish and fond of moralizing, and once or twice their even more celebrated friend, Mr. Alexander Pope. Gradually, Zabdiel found himself invited to convivial gatherings at private homes as well.

Somehow, the prince's interest in Zabdiel's horses trickled out. Offers to buy them, sight unseen, began to arrive—with such outlandish prices attached that Zabdiel assumed they were sent in mockery.

I fear he overvalues his horses, Mr. Hollis wrote home to Boston, *and will never again get the prices offered that he is said to have refused.*

Meanwhile, the small princess fared superbly: growing only about forty pustules, though her incisions ran a great deal and were not healed till the twenty-eighth. Two days later, Leicester House went into pandemonium when a tussle between Prince William and Princess Mary burst open the incision on her left arm. Fanned by much hand-wringing, it healed again by the third of May. On May 8, however, a small boil began swelling in her left armpit. This necessitated another medical council of war. After a great deal of discussion, it was decided to allow nature to proceed without any more help than watching.

"Ah, my American doctor," said the prince as the meeting broke up. "I should like to see these horses of yours. I hunt at Richmond this summer. Perhaps that would serve?"

"I should be honored, Your Highness," said Zabdiel.

"Capital," said the prince, striding off.

"You should indeed be a great deal more honored than you look," said Lady Mary, appearing at Zabdiel's elbow. "Many men would kill for an invitation to hunt with the prince."

"His invitation, I fear, will kill my horses," replied Zabdiel. "Horses must eat, my lady, and sleep warm and dry, if they are to run well. How I am to house them in that neighborhood, I cannot conceive. My connections do not reach to such grandeur."

"I have a summer house in Twickenham," she said, "with room to spare in the stables."

After a little oozing, the swelling under Princess Mary's arm subsided on its own. On the eighth of June, the Prince and Princess of Wales gathered their younger children and trundled westward to the clean air of Richmond.

In Twickenham, four tall bay horses and two black grooms moved into the Wortleys' stable. On the first day the prince was to hunt, three horses were led back out, groomed to a high gloss, their tails and manes intricately braided.

"Where is Prince?" asked Lady Mary.

"In his stall," replied Zabdiel. "Where he belongs."

"Surely you will not leave him behind," she chided. "He is peerless."

"He is also yours, my lady. I am not in the habit of giving the possessions of others away, my lady. Even to princes."

I ride a good deal, she wrote to Frances, *and have got a new horse superior to any two-legged animal, he being without fault.*

*   *   *

At the royal stables, the prince inspected Dr. Boylston's American horses, grudgingly pronouncing them capital, until he was presented with all three of them, when his interest transformed to evangelistic pride.

Trotting behind his father, trying to appear distinct from his gaggle of sisters, Prince William thought them tall. "In America," said Zabdiel, "we make a special saddle for mounting small people atop tall horses. If it would please you, I shall send you one, when I return."

The young prince crowed with delight; then he collected his dignity. "It is the duty of a field marshal, after all—"

"If you are finished," Prince George cut in, "we might ride."

"May I ask a favor of my own first, Your Highness?" asked Zabdiel.

"What?" barked the prince.

"The use of a horse."

The prince snorted in amusement; around him, the roiling pack of courtiers tittered and broke into laughter.

"You are not dressed for riding," said Zabdiel one morning.

"The quarry has shifted from foxes to deer," sighed Lady Mary. "The riding has gone beyond my ladylike skill."

"Then your skill must improve, my lady," said Zabdiel. "I might be of some help, if you would allow it."

All that summer, they chased deer through the green-gold glimmer of sunlight dancing through trees, pausing to let their horses drink at laughing streams while whip-thin dogs flowed on through the grass like white-and-dun water determined to roll to the sea. Sometimes, the princess called Zabdiel to take refreshment with her in some open glade, to tell his tale until her eyes glittered with tears, and her ladies wept openly. At other times the horns and the baying of hounds pulled the company into an ecstasy of flight, skimming together and apart like swallows whittering low over the earth.

When they were not hunting, Twickenham offered them other delights. Not far from the Wortley Montagu's house stood Mr. Pope's palladian villa, where the laughter of Lord Bathurst, Dr. Arbuthnot, Mr. Richardson, and Mr. Cheselden was joined at times that summer by that of Dr. Boylston and Lady Mary.

August 1725

Dear Sister,

I pass many hours on horseback, and I'll assure you, I ride stag hunting, which I know you'll stare to hear of! I have arriv'd to vast courage and skill that way, and am as well pleased with it as with the acquisition of a new sense. His Royal Highness hunts in Richmond Park, and I make one of the beau monde in his train.

I desire you after this account not to name the word old woman to me anymore; I approach fifteen nearer than I did ten years ago, and am in hopes to improve every year in health and vivacity.

"We have had riding enough," said the Princess of Wales as the weather snapped cold, and the beau monde trooped back toward London. "I should like to see some writing, if you please."

"Writing, Your Highness?" replied Zabdiel.

"Your experiment with inoculation, Doctor, is not just a tale to make ladies weep happily in the sun. Dr. Jurin, I am sure, will want the numbers. The details, sir, are what matter. They must find their way into print."

"She wants a book," he groaned later to a small gathering in Mr. Pope's grotto, artfully arranged on a bank sloping down to the Thames. "What am I to do?"

"Write," said Dr. Mead.

"Writing is a skill I have never pretended to."

"Then your skill, Doctor, must improve," said Lady Mary with a small smile. "I might be of some help, if you would allow it."

"By all means, the conquest of smallpox must be immortalized," pronounced Mr. Richardson, as Mr. Pope caught his eye.

"It is not a conquest," Zabdiel protested. "Not yet."

"False modesty, Doctor, will get you nowhere," teased Lady Mary.

Zabdiel turned on her. "If I must tell my story, my lady, then surely you must tell yours."

In this, the whole party warmly agreed.

Lady Mary had long been at work arranging and editing her *Embassy Letters* with their salacious gossip and their sublime descriptions of distant towns, lands, and people. That fall, as Zabdiel labored to transform his notes into a book, she turned her hand to polishing the deeply embedded jewel of her smallpox letter.

Back in London that winter, Zabdiel sloshed through heavy wet snow up to Lincoln's Inn's Fields, to the house Mr. Cheselden had specified; at his nod, Jackey rapped on the door, which was answered by an Irish girl, her green eyes widening to see a small black boy on the step.

They were ushered upstairs into a room filled with the scents of new-sawn wood and paint. Its edges were a dark riot of color and shadow, strewn with bare canvas and frames and unfinished paintings of figures stepping from gray nothingness. But the center of the room was clear, lit by a single slanted shaft of light dancing with bright motes.

In its midst stood Lady Mary, glowing as if from within, in a golden robe with a cloak of blue brocade and ermine draped like a soft stretch of sky around her shoulders.

"Ah, Dr. Boylston," said Mr. Richardson, stepping from the shadows palette, in hand. "May I present my son-in-law and principal assistant, Mr. Thomas Hudson? You know Cheselden and Arbuthnot."

Zabdiel bowed to them all in turn.

"Richardson," explained Mr. Cheselden, "has been charged with a commission to commemorate the battle against smallpox. We could not proceed, of course, without you."

"I am honoured," said Zabdiel with a nod to Lady Mary, "to watch such splendor transferred to canvas."

Mr. Cheselden glanced to the other men and back. "Your *double* battle, sir."

Zabdiel felt heat flush his face. "You surely cannot be suggesting that you wish to put me in your picture," he said, turning to the painter.

Mr. Richardson bowed. "Posterity will wish to look on the faces of its saviors. I only hope I may do you some justice."

"*Justice!*" exclaimed Zabdiel, shaking his head. "I must disappoint you, sir. I will not disgrace any canvas with this face. Especially not one that is to hold Lady Mary."

"False modesty, Doctor," she chided from the middle of the room.

"No, my lady," he said firmly.

For a moment, no one moved, and the afternoon hovered on the edge of disappointment.

Mr. Richardson stepped forward, addressing everyone in turn. "Might I suggest, gentlemen, a symbolic alternative? The origin of your discovery, my lady, is to be represented by your Turkish costume. I understand that the doctor learned from Africans. Perhaps, sir, we could borrow the boy."

"Borrow the boy?"

"Paint him, sir, in your place," said Mr. Richardson, pointing to Jackey, who was peering at the canvases as if they were doors to other worlds.

Zabdiel began to laugh. "You have no idea, sir, how fitting your suggestion is. He is the first fruit of the operation, being one of the first three people I inoculated, along with his father and my youngest son. I would be happy to agree, if it would please Lady Mary."

"The lady will make the best of it," she said, shifting the gleaming blue fall of her cloak.

So Jackey was pulled to a costume rack and put into a fur-lined red coat—far too large, but Mr. Richardson thought it looked properly exotic—and red boots, ditto, and given a parasol to hold. As a final touch, Mr. Hudson clattered through a chest and came up with a silver collar.

"No," said Zabdiel. "That is preposterous."

"It is preposterous that you claim to own him," shot Lady Mary.

Zabdiel opened his mouth to protest, and closed it again. Jackey stood stone-faced as Mr. Hudson snapped on the collar.

All that morning and into the afternoon, Zabdiel stood with his friends and watched the image of Lady Mary bloom upon Mr. Richardson's canvas, as the painter captured the uptilt of her shoes, the light that skated like gold wine from the falls of her caftan, the jewels winking at her waist and cascading over one ear. Most amazingly, Mr. Richardson caught the glitter of her eyes fixed on them all with challenge and with pride. Behind her, in the shadow of his parasol, Jackey peered up at her with much the same intensity, his almond eyes fusing awe and fury.

Lady Mary saw little of Dr. Boylston that spring. He had other projects as well as the book to keep him busy. With Mr. Cheselden, he studied the new method of cutting for the stone. He spent long, happy hours with Doctors Jurin and Arbuthnot, discussing the implications of applying the mathematics to the analysis of disease and its treatment. He visited every relative he could find in the vicinity of the capital, and then traveled north to see more in Birmingham. And still, he inched his way through his book.

Of Mr. Pope, on the other hand, Lady Mary saw more than she wished, for on the afternoon that Mr. Richardson's painting was delivered, he went down on one knee—he was already only knee-high—and declared his grand passion for her. It was so gloriously absurd that Lady Mary laughed aloud, and saw, too late, that he had not spoken in jest.

Having finished her *Embassy Letters*, she began writing a long, winding tale of hopeless love. If her friends noticed her quarrelsome and sad, they said nothing. She had many reasons for low spirits, after all. Her son was already proving himself a young rake; he ran away from school again. Her sister was slipping into madness, and in March, the duke of Kingston quite suddenly died. That, her family could neither have predicted nor stopped—though the ensuing squabble over the young heirs and their money was predictable enough. But Lady Mary railed against the unnecessary deaths of Lady Townshend and her old Sister in Affliction, Philippa Mundy, from smallpox. Lady Townshend—Dolly—had inoculated most of her family, but had ignored herself; poor dear timid Phil had never summoned the courage to put herself through the operation.

* * *

Early in April, just after Easter, Jack laid a letter from home on Zabdiel's breakfast table. The paper was marked with the wind, weather, and rough handling of an Atlantic crossing, but for all that, it was nearly blank. Only four words crossed the page: *Come home to me.*

"I must go soon, my lady," said Zabdiel when he met Lady Mary again.

"Go?" she teased. "You have only just arrived."

"I am not talking about this instant," he said. "I must go home, my lady."

"To America?" she protested. "But you have interest at court, you have friends, you are building a reputation. Why will you not make your home here? In Boston, what will you be?"

There was a silence broken only by a tumble of coals in the grate. "A surgeon, my lady," he said gently. "I belong there. My family is there, and my duty."

"Your duty is to finish your book."

"That is what I came to tell you," he said. "I have finished."

"You must forgive me," she said ruefully. "I do not have friendships to spare just now. I would not lose yours without a fight."

"I finished a book," he said. "I did not say I finished a friendship."

At the beginning of May, Zabdiel's book came back, warm and damp from the printer. In the middle of the month, he was given leave to make a formal presentation of his book to the Princess of Wales, and received the triple gift of a royal blessing, a royal reward, and a royal dismissal.

On the nineteenth, he was invited once more to the Royal Society, where he presented the Fellows with another fine copy. They asked him, as was usual, to give them a short account of what was in it. He had not prepared for this, and momentarily froze. But he forced himself to his feet, recalling their kind reception of his ambergris paper, and took a deep breath. Calmly, concisely, he told them the story, from its beginning in Dr. Mather's letters, to his investigations among the town's Africans, to his terrifying experiment on his youngest son and two slaves. Pitilessly, he laid out before them the shortcomings of both the treatment and his usage of it: Esther Webb's infection from her inoculated parents, Bethiah Nichols's loss of both an eye and an unborn child, Mrs. Dixwell's suffering and death.

But he also gave them—as he had learned from Dr. Jurin, Dr. Arbuthnot, and the other mathematically inclined fellows—the numbers. Numbers that marched in line with Dr. Jurin's calculations for London: inoculation offered somewhere between a one-in-fifty and a one-in-a-hundred chance of dying, depending on how sanguine or skeptical you were about the deaths surrounding the practice. Natural smallpox forced a one-in-six or -seven chance upon its victims.

His audience, he noticed with surprise, was straining forward to catch every word. He cautioned them. It was not a victory: he could not in honesty tell them that. Smallpox still lived and breathed, scattering its terrible spotted death on large numbers of people. And yet—and yet—for the first time in history, it had become possible to say following. He opened his book to a passage he had marked and read: *It is and shall be acknowledged to the praise and glory of God! By this happy discovery of transplantation, also called inoculation, a most wild, cruel, and violent distemper which has destroyed millions of lives is now become tractable, safe, and gentle.*

He looked back up. "So you see, gentlemen, we have tamed the smallpox."

For a moment, no one said anything. Then Dr. Jurin rose to his feet, followed by Sir Hans, Dr. Steigerthal, Dr. Mead, Dr. Arbuthnot, and Mr. Cheselden. On and on around the room, his new friends and acquaintances rose, until Sir Isaac Newton himself rose tottering from the president's chair to join in the stamping and cheering of the standing ovation, while Dr. Boylston watched in utter amazement.

A week later, Dr. Steigerthal nominated him as a Fellow, and he was duly elected. On July 7, 1726, to general approbation, beaming, and applause, a still astonished Dr. Zabdiel Boylston was installed as the newest Fellow of the Royal Society. In the ensuing weeks, he lectured there and at the Royal College of Physicians, the new F.R.S. flapping proud and tall at the end of his name.

He sent a third fine presentation copy to a certain house in the Piazza, Covent Garden.

"I have found but one fault in your book, Doctor," said Lady Mary with a wry smile, as Zabdiel called to take his leave. "False modesty."

A few weeks later, Dr. Zabdiel Boylston, *F.R.S.*, and his two black slaves took ship for Boston and home.

Alone in her sitting room, Lady Mary penned the last sentence of her tale of torn love: *Abandoning the views he had of making his fortune, his interest at court, his friends, and reputation,* she wrote of her hero, *he left the kingdom as soon as possible and went to finish his life in the solitudes of America, where some of his relations were established, secure of less barbarity amongst the savages than (he thought) he had met with in the fairest princess of France.*

* * *

To Sir Hans Sloane
Boston, December 14, 1726

Much Honored and Worthy
    Sir,
    A sense of gratitude for the many obligations you have laid me under will not suffer me any longer to rest in silence. After a long and expensive voyage, I am safe arrived to my family, friends, and country, from whom I have received a hearty welcome. I shall always acknowledge the honours done me by Sir Hans, and as often as I have opportunity to collect anything worthy of your notice, who are so nice a judge of Nature, I shall think myself in duty and honour bound to present you with it.

For starters, he was enclosing a five-and-a-half pound stone taken from a gelding's belly. Had killed the horse, of course. But was hopefully a fine prize for a man so fascinated by bezoars. Perhaps this summer he would conduct some proper experiments on another of their shared interests: rattlesnakes.

    I am
    Dear and honored Sir,
    Your most obliged
    and devoted servant,
    Zabdiel Boylston

    P.S. I have not heard that any one of our anti-inoculators have said any thing against the truth of my account given of the practice, and some of my friends say there is but one fault in it, and that is that I was too modest in debunking the opposers.

❧ 2 ❧

THE PRACTICE

BOSTON remained free of smallpox until September of 1729, when the speckled monster once again invaded from the sea, as a ship from Ireland disembarked infected passengers. The contagion smoldered until early in 1730, when it exploded once again into an epidemic.

Boylston immediately republished his *Historical Account* for the benefit of Bostonians; far more surprisingly, Douglass conceded—however cautiously and ungraciously—that the operation had its merits. Far from apologizing for his slurs against Boylston, however, he remained as churlish as ever toward his old rival, whom he still refused to grant the title of "doctor." *I can but seldom have recourse to Mr. Boylstone's Accounts, because of their being so jejune, lame, suspected, and only in the nature of Quack bills.*

The town government was not yet ready to encourage inoculation, but resigned itself to the operation's inevitable popularity; there were no more attempts made to outlaw it. This time, about 4,000 people fell ill and 500 died. About 400 were inoculated, of whom 12 died—about 1 in 33: as Douglass remarked, these numbers were "not so favourable as in 1721." They were still considerably better than the 1 in 8 odds of dying after catching smallpox in the natural way, however. Possibly the problems came from inexperience: in addition to Dr. Boylston and Dr. Douglass, many of the town's other doctors appear to have taken up the practice. Very probably, some of that dip in its success rate was due to European physicians' tendency to cut deeper and longer, and use more "matter" than was common in the folk practice.

The 1730 epidemic, however, passed off lightly in comparison to the catastrophe of 1721, and seems to have confirmed in many people's minds that inoculation was a lifesaver, though the opposers were by no means silenced. Again, the disease passed, and Boston was safe—from both the smallpox and inoculation—for another twenty years.

Then, on Christmas Eve, 1751, a ship wrecked in Nahant Bay, and the people of the town of Chelsea poured out to the beach to rescue the survivors. In the chaos, the captain did not tell anyone that the smallpox was aboard; within a month many of the rescuers and their families died for their kindness. In Chelsea, somewhere between a fifth and a quarter of the population died.

Across 1752, the infection whipped through Massachusetts. Of Boston's 15,684 residents, 1,843 fled. Among those who remained, 5,545 caught smallpox in the natural way, and 539 (about 1 in 10) died; 5,589 were immune, having survived it before. It's the inoculation numbers that are really notable, though: 2,124 people were inoculated, and only 30 (1 in 70) died. As Dr. Douglass himself admitted, "The Novel Practice of procuring the Small-Pox by Inoculation is a very considerable and most beneficial Improvement in that Article of Medical Practice."

The epidemic was not confined to Massachusetts; it spread up and down the coast through all the major port cities of Britain's American colonies. In Philadelphia, Ben Franklin became an ardent supporter of inoculation, using his editorial control of the press to trumpet the procedure's merits. Six years later, though, his four-year-old son Francis died from smallpox before he could be inoculated; Franklin blamed himself for that death for the rest of his life. After he became a wealthy man, he paid for large numbers of Philadelphia's poor to undergo the expensive operation.

Both directly and indirectly, inoculation had a major impact on the American Revolution. It certainly protected a number of the fledgling country's great statesmen. Boylston's great-nephew John Adams (the grandson of Zabdiel's older brother Peter) had himself inoculated in Boston in 1764. Meanwhile, his fiancée, Abigail Smith, was banished from his side, reduced to disinfecting his letters with smoke before she read them; she was so lonely she threatened to come to the hospital to wave at him through a window. Down in Virginia, Thomas Jefferson had himself inoculated after losing a beloved sister to the disease. When the Continental Congresses convened in Philadelphia in 1774 and 1776, members who had not yet had smallpox had to wrestle with the decision whether to inoculate themselves or stay away; most decided to inoculate themselves. The Declaration of Independence was written and signed in safety as smallpox stalked the streets outside.

After receiving good evidence that the British were using smallpox-infected blankets and refugees as an insidious weapon—and knowing the terrible vulnerability of most of his men—George Washington had the entire Continental Army inoculated in 1777. Washington's own face was already famously scarred from an earlier bout with the disease, contracted on a visit to Barbados in 1751. But Martha had herself inoculated, so that she might visit her husband in the soldiers' camps with impunity; smallpox parties became popular among Revolutionary women—including Abigail Adams and Mrs. John Hancock.

In London, inoculation's popularity waxed and waned through the 1730s, with the force of the disease: in bad years, people flocked to be inoculated; in light years, the practice shrank. Inoculation was a security—the *only* security—to cling to within the terror of an epidemic; in times of good health, however, it looked like a foolish flirtation with danger. (This is not unlike the *vaccination* for smallpox at present: in case of an outbreak of the disease, the vaccination is all that may stand between humanity and a massive, speedy die-off the likes of which this planet has not seen since the Black Death. In the absence of a real and compelling threat of smallpox, the vaccination itself—which kills one to two in a million and can seriously harm many more—is a danger not to be messed with.)

In 1743, inoculation became mandatory for the orphans of London's Foundling Hospital; after the disease ran amok in 1746, a dedicated Smallpox and Inoculation Hospital was established, originally for the "deserving" poor and for servants of its wealthy contributors (such establishments as the smallpox house in Swallow Street proving too small and unregulated). On the Continent, despite early support by such thinkers as Voltaire, it took decades for the practice to break through barriers of conservatism. Holland was the first country to experiment with it and adopt it widely.

In later years, a series of self-proclaimed innovators (particularly James Kirkpatrick and Robert Sutton) announced at different intervals that the practice had died out, but that they had invented a brand new "light" process that would make inoculation safe and easy. In effect, they were reinventing the Turkish, Greek, and African wheels: reverting to scratches or very shallow cuts, and using tiny droplets of matter.

On the other hand, the physicians kept "improving" the process according to the best medical theories of the time. They preferred ever longer "preparations," often involving bleeding, vomiting, and purging, as well as cordials containing antimony and mercury. Many of the scholars who have studied this history most carefully come away shaking their heads, with the conclusion that doctors unwittingly "took a (relatively) safe procedure and made it dangerous."

Its danger and discomforts kept many people from risking it. In 1754, the uninoculated Prince of Wales fell ill with the smallpox, but survived to become King George III; the following year, the Royal College of Physicians formally endorsed the operation. In a terrible twist of fate, in 1783, this king's four-year-old son Octavius died as a result of being inoculated; the young prince was, however, the last royal Briton to suffer the disease.

For all its shortcomings, as Genevieve Miller has written, "Inoculation was the chief *medical* contribution of the Enlightenment, at least in the opinion of the age itself."

In one of the many quirks of medical history, it was the very discomfort and danger of this first "improved" shield against the smallpox that produced a better one: and the birth of modern immunology to boot. In 1757, in the town of Berkeley, in the western English county of Gloucestershire, an eight-year-old orphan named Edward Jenner endured the three months' misery that inoculation had become. From his older sister's perspective, she was saving his life. From his boy's perspective, he was starved, purged, and bled, and then locked up in a stable with other boys undergoing the treatment until the disease had run its course through them all.

While apprenticed to a surgeon in Chipping Sodbury in the rich dairy country of the Cotswolds in the 1760s, Jenner heard dairymaids fearlessly dismiss their chances of contracting smallpox—then rife in the neighborhood—on the grounds that they had suffered the sores of cowpox on their hands. He put the legendarily creamy skin of these women together with their old wives' tales, and something began spinning in his brain concerning the connections between smallpox and the poxes that infected barnyard animals—cows, horses, and pigs—with a far lighter disease.

In 1788, Jenner first came to the attention of the Royal Society for his work on cuckoos, describing the exact process of how the birds lay their eggs in other birds' nests, and the voracious young chicks then eject their foster siblings to monopolize the attention of the unwitting parents. That year, he was already showing a drawing of cowpox-infected hands to medical men in London. In 1790, he inoculated his own son and the boy's nurse with swine pox; later that year he started collecting stories of dairymaids who'd had cowpox and then had resisted smallpox inoculations—though they had never had smallpox. He was an inoculator; he was in a position to see such curiosities in the flesh.

In 1796, a woman named Sarah Nelmes came to him terrified about a rash on her hands; he calmed her down and discerned that her cow Blossom had the cowpox, and had communicated it to her. On May 14, he inoculated James Phipps, the eight-year-old son of his gardener, with matter from one of Sarah's pocks. Young Phipps duly developed a mild case of cowpox. At the beginning of July, Jenner then inoculated the boy with smallpox matter—with no reaction. The boy appeared to be immune. *I shall now pursue my Experiments with redoubled ardor,* dashed Jenner.

In 1797, he submitted his conclusions to the Royal Society, which soon returned his paper with a note recommending that if he valued the solid reputation he had established by his work on the cuckoo, he had best not promulgate such harebrained ideas as using cowpox to prevent smallpox. The following year saw an outbreak of cowpox; not to be so easily discouraged, Jenner gathered matter from the infected cows, and tried again. In June 1798, he published the results himself.

It was, wrote one of his supporters, "as if an angel's trumpet had sounded over the earth." By 1801, over a hundred thousand people had been vaccinated in Britain; in 1802, Parliament voted Jenner a £10,000 reward, and in 1806 another £20,000. President Thomas Jefferson supported the new practice in the United States; at the height of the Napoleonic Wars between Britain and France, Napoleon returned prisoners of war to Britain at Jenner's request—remarking, it is said, "Ah, Jenner. Him I can refuse nothing."

In the press, however, vaccination went through the same baptism of fiery controversy that inoculation had earlier endured. By this time, though, the scientific method of study had become well developed, and the application of mathematics to epidemiology was a standard practice. It did not take long for vaccination to overcome inoculation (more properly "variolation") as the preferred prevention of the smallpox: vaccination was safe enough to practice even outside the immediate threat of an epidemic.

So successful was Jenner's practice that researchers began to fiddle with it in fighting other diseases. The once disease-specific name of "vaccination"—from *vaccinia,* the Latin term for the cowpox virus—has long since become a generic term for inoculation against any disease, in the same way that Kleenex, Xerox, and Levi's have given their brand names to whole technologies and products.

Where smallpox was concerned, vaccinators began aiming at something higher than the protection of individuals, something never before imagined: they began to dream not just of taming smallpox, but of conquering it. First, they concerned themselves with towns and counties, and then with whole nations. In the mid–twentieth century, under the field marshalship of D.A. Henderson, the World Health Organization launched a serious long-term war to eradicate smallpox from the earth.

In one of the last ironies of this struggle, the disappearance of the disease from India—one of its last three hiding places (along with Bangladesh and Somalia)—was hindered by an echo of the same religious objections that high-church Anglicans and conservative Puritans wrestled with in 1721. In 1974, the spiritual leader of a single Indian village in the southern state of Bihar refused to have his family or his flock of followers vaccinated on the grounds that smallpox was the rightful scourge of God. Smallpox kept flaring up in this corner of the world; in the end, he and his family were inoculated by force.

Jenner himself predicted that "the annihilation of smallpox—the most dreadful scourge of the human race—will be the final result of this practice." In 1977, he at long last proved right.

Until and unless human beings prove fool enough to reopen Pandora's box.

Jenner was not the first to experiment with cowpox as a shield against smallpox, but he was the first man with the dogged curiosity to study it systematically, and to have the equally dogged courage to force Europe's scientific world to take notice. He has been justly celebrated ever since as the founding father of immunology, but this father had his own mother and father in Lady Mary Wortley Montagu and Zabdiel Boylston—whether or not he knew them any better than he knew his own parents. In turn, Lady Mary and Boylston had parents from the Ottoman Empire and Africa.

From beginning to end, the conquest of smallpox proved a global endeavor.

❧ 3 ❧

THE PEOPLE

LADY Mary soon broke with Alexander Pope in a long, loud, and nasty quarrel that distressed those like Lord Bathurst and Dr. Arbuthnot who strove to remain friends with them both. If their rupture was rooted, as she claimed, in her laughing refusal of Pope's love, Cupid had his revenge. Not long after, she fell in love again, disastrously, with the wealthy young Italian Francesco Algarotti—who also charmed Voltaire, Pope, and Lady Mary's friend Lord Hervey (though only Hervey appears to have been her rival for Algarotti's attention).

Understandably tired of Wortley, in 1739 Lady Mary followed her brilliant and probably bisexual Venetian beloved to the Continent. Disappointed in him, she fell in love with an even more disastrous Italian, Count Ugolino Palazzi, who was younger than Lady Mary's son and a ruthless extortioner, thief, kidnapper, and possibly poisoner to boot. None of this deterred Lady Mary from reveling in life as an expat; she remained in France and Italy until just before her death, becoming a fixture on the British Grand Tour. Young men with any claim to polish strove to come home with an anecdote of meeting Lady Mary. One scurrilous but not unlikely story has her showing off her commode, painted inside to look like the backs of books by Pope, Swift, and Bolingbroke. She knew them well, she told one astounded young man: "They were the greatest rascals, but she had the pleasure of shitting on them every day." She seems to have either charmed her visitors—as she did Joseph Spence—or utterly repulsed them—as she did Horace Walpole. Either way, they gossiped about her and her love affairs (long past and present) incessantly. Early in 1761, she was shocked to learn—apparently in casual conversation—of her husband's death. Not until she was probably already quite ill with breast cancer did she return to London, where she died at age seventy-three on August 21, 1762.

Edward Wortley junior proved an adventurer like his mother—but lacked her moral courage and fiber: he was an inveterate liar, a rake, and a scoundrel. As a youth, he ran away from school as often as possible, once getting as far as Gibraltar after joining the crew of a naval ship; his inoculation scars are said to have been used to prove his identity. As an adult, he lived mostly abroad at his parents' insistence. He nevertheless begged money as often as he could, even while spouting lies that outraged his family—such as announcing that he was a bastard son of Sultan Achmet III. He died in 1776.

Mary Wortley, on the other hand, was prim and proper. She married John Stuart, earl of Bute, thereby becoming a countess; her husband later became one of King George III's early prime ministers, and remained one of his closest advisors even after being forced out in a political contretemps. Lady Bute proved no more eager to have her mother come home to Britain than Lady Mary was to live there. Lucky for the rest of us: their correspondence is one of the treasures of eighteenth-century British literature. Unluckily for the rest of us, her children calmed Lady Bute on her deathbed in 1794 by burning Lady Mary's diaries, which she had cherished up till that point.

Charles Maitland returned to Aberdeen in 1726; he died a much-respected bachelor there in 1748, at the age of eighty.

Sir Hans Sloane became president of the Royal Society following Newton's death in 1727. Sloane himself died in 1753, age ninety-two, still poking his fingers into almost every corner of British science. Having collected knowledge all his life, upon his death he willed the material remains of it—nearly eighty thousand objects—to the nation, so long as his daughters were paid £20,000. Parliament agreed that it was a collection fit for a king and footed the bill—and thus was born the British Museum. It would be interesting to know whether a five-and-a-half-pound stone from a gelding's belly formed part of that original collection.

King George I died en route to his beloved Hanover in June 1727.

The Prince and Princess of Wales became King George II and Queen Caroline. For a decade, Caroline is said to have ruled Britain in all but name, managing ministers with discretion and her cantankerous husband with commendable patience. She particularly interested herself in prison reform. Though her husband was famous for scolding her in public, he loved her in his way. Upon her death in 1737, he was heard to say, "I never yet saw a woman who was fit to buckle her shoe." He died in 1760, just shy of seventy-seven.

Their heartily disliked elder son, **Frederick,** died while still Prince of Wales; his son—another George—became Prince of Wales and later King George III. **Prince William** pursued his military passions, making a name for himself as the duke of Cumberland. Far from earning the epithet "the Great," however, after the Jacobite rebellion of 1745 he became known as "the Butcher of Culloden"—though many in England celebrated his ferocity against the Scottish Highlanders.

The princesses lived out their lives in the gilded cages of Hanoverian and continental palaces. Both **Amelia** and **Caroline** remained unmarried. Amelia had many affairs with dashing noblemen; she loved brisk exercise outdoors, and would shock congregations by arriving to church in a riding habit, with a dog under each arm. She became hostess and companion to her younger brother, the duke of Cumberland. Caroline served as devoted companion to her mother; after the queen's death she withdrew from the world, spending her days as an invalid, her fragility increased by hypochondria that exasperated her sisters, especially Emily.

The three others made unhappy marriages. **Anne** was so desperate to escape that she insisted upon accepting the suit of the "grossly deformed" William IV, Prince of Orange, against everyone's wishes, including her father's. When the king warned her of the prince's ugliness, she said she would marry him if he were a baboon; the king shot back that she would "have baboon enough." **Mary** married Prince Frederick of Hesse-Cassel, who abruptly abandoned her and their young children for a former mistress seven years later. **Princess Louisa,** the most like her mother, married the crown prince of Denmark, became that country's queen, and died young as a result of complications from childbirth.

Elizabeth Harrison nursed at least twenty people through smallpox in Hertford in the winter of 1721–22. After that, she dives beneath history's sights: but she looks to have stood a far better chance than most eighteenth-century women with felony records to have wound up on her feet with a reputable career that could support her.

Zabdiel Boylston lived a long, quiet life, apparently never again leaving New England. He practiced medicine into the 1750s, though in 1741 he bought the seventy-five-acre family farm in Brookline, enlarging the house to a fifteen-room, three-story mansion, and moving there from Boston to raise his horses in the country. The house still stands—though it is no longer a country mansion. He worked with rattlesnakes and with the balsam from the white cedar tree. His work with smallpox, he thought, had given him the convulsive asthma that haunted him in later life. It does not seem to have slowed him too much: he was seen in Boston at the age of eighty-four, riding a colt he was breaking.

He died eight days shy of eighty-six, murmuring "my work in this world is done." His tombstone stated, "Dr. Zabdiel Boylston, Esq., physician and F.R.S. who first introduced the practice of inoculation into America. Through a life of extensive benevolence, he was always faithful to his word, just in his dealings, affable in his manners, and after a long sickness, in which he was exemplary for his patience and resignation to his Maker, he quitted this mortal life in a just expectation of a happy immortality, March 1, 1766."

Jerusha lived through most of these quiet years with Zabdiel, dying of cancer two years before him, on April 15, 1764.

Thomas Boylston (Zabdiel and Jerusha's son) became a doctor, training under his father and acquiring enough skill and trust to be sent alone the seventy-two miles down to Newport, Rhode Island, in 1737—at the age of twenty-two—to perform a mastectomy. At the end of that year, he traveled to London for more training at St. Thomas's Hospital, bearing a letter of introduction from his father to Sir Hans Sloane, identifying him as "the first fruit of Inoculation in the American World." Back in Boston, he married in 1744, but died soon afterward in late 1749 or early 1750, only thirty-four years old; he had no children. **John** made himself a wealthy businessman; he remained a bachelor. He moved to London in 1768, and then to Bath. He was a loyalist, but remained concerned for the welfare of his countrymen; during the Revolution, he contributed liberally to the relief of American prisoners-of-war. He died in 1795, age eighty-six, leaving bequests for the orphans and elderly poor of Boston. **Zabdiel junior** went to study in London in 1729 or soon thereafter; by 1733, he had died there of tuberculosis—which had no cure until antibiotics were discovered in the twentieth century. The girls all remained in Boston. Young **Jerusha** married one of Zabdiel's inoculees, Benjamin Fitch, with whom she had eight children. She died a wealthy widow as the eighteenth turned into the nineteenth century. **Mary** died a spinster in 1802, age eighty-nine. **Elizabeth** married Dr. Gillam Taylor, with whom she had three children.

Thomas Boylston (Zabdiel's brother) died in 1739; his widow, **Sarah,** survived to the very eve of the Revolution, in 1774. Painted in later years by John Singleton Copley, she is the only one of the Boylstons who took part in this story to have her image preserved; it is owned by Harvard University.

Jack, Moll, and Jackey disappear from view at the close of the 1721 epidemic. A free black man named John Boylstone and called Jack, however, married one Jane Kennedy at Trinity Church in 1779. As he was born in 1742, he cannot have been this Jack or Jackey: but he could have been Jackey's son—which would mean the family bought or was given its freedom within a generation.

Cotton Mather died one day after his sixty-fifth birthday, on February 13, 1728, believing the Second Coming was imminent: the largest earthquake in New England's history had struck a few months earlier on October 29, 1727, tolling church bells and cracking houses in half. Tremors rolled underfoot through January 1728. As death approached, he called out: "And this is dying! This all? Is this what I feared when I prayed against a hard death? Is it no more than this? O I can bear this! I can bear it, I can bear it!" His last word was a quiet *"Grace!"*

Samuel Mather joined his father as minister of the Old North Church upon the death of his grandfather Increase in 1723; like his father, he possessed strong streaks of both generosity and paranoia. He did not, however, possess his father's breadth of intellect. He came to Boylston's defense in 1730, writing a nitpicking dissection of Douglass's *Dissertation*—anonymously. In 1742, Mather and some of his parishioners seceded to form an independent church that survived until his death in 1785.

Onesimus Mather is last heard of in 1738, assigned to clean streets "pursuant to the Act for the Regulating of Free Negroes."

William Douglass began buying houses and land in January 1723, and never stopped. Between 1736 and 1741, he bought immense acreage in Worcester County, where the town of Douglas was named for him. In 1743, he bought the Green Dragon, complete with cartway, stables, and yard, to serve as his "mansion house" (though it either in part remained or later returned to being an inn). In 1736, he became president of the Scots Charitable Society, an office he held until the year of his death.

Having been thwarted from making his medical reputation with smallpox, he turned to scarlet fever; his medical masterpiece, published in 1736, was the first modern clinical description of a scarlet fever epidemic (then called eruptive military fever). Throughout his life, he kept detailed records of weather patterns and compass variations, collected rare plants, and wrote an important early history of British North America (equally as important for its gossip and hearsay as for its accurate information), as well as an economic tract on the colonies' intractable currency problems: paper money aroused almost as much of his wrath as inoculation once had. He also drew one of the most influential pre-Revolutionary maps of New England. Although he was highly respected for his breadth of learning, his meanness nevertheless made and kept many enemies. Passing through in 1744, Dr. Alexander Hamilton described Douglass as "a man of good learning but mischievously given to criticism and the most complete snarler ever I knew. He is loath to allow learning, merit, or a character to anybody." I have found no record of a marriage, but he had a son, also William Douglass, who was about seven when the doctor died in 1752, about sixty-one years old.

Joshua Cheever rose quickly in both town and church ranks. In 1730, he was elected selectman of Boston, serving as such for three years; in 1732, he joined the artillery company, eventually becoming a captain. By 1733, he is styled "merchant" or "gentleman" in deeds, and soon thereafter began using the term *Esq*. In 1736, he became a ruling elder of the New North Church. He died in 1751, a wealthy merchant in possession of wharves, warehouses, shipyards, many houses, and a great deal of land in Boston's North End, as well as a farm and woodland in Charlestown. **Sarah** died in 1723; the following year he married a widow, Sarah Sears Jenkins, who outlived him by four years. He never had children, but seems to have treated his second wife's son, David Jenkins, as his own; if his will is any indication, he was also close to his many nieces and nephews.

NOTES

Titles

Throughout this book, Lady Mary Wortley Montagu appears as Lady Mary. This isn't undue familiarity; it is correct. Her honorific *Lady* came from her father's title, first as an earl, on up to duke, and was therefore attached to her first name and *only* her first name. She has sometimes appeared in print as Lady Montagu, but that title properly indicates someone else. In the British peerage, a woman uses *Lady* with a title (sometimes but not always the same as the family surname) only when she holds that title in her own right, or, more commonly, when she is married to the man who does. In Lady Mary's circle of friends, there was a duchess of Montagu, but no Lady Montagu—which would have indicated the wife of a baronet, baron, viscount, earl, or marquess whose title was Montagu.

Referring to Lady Mary as plain *Montagu* or *Mrs. Montagu* would have been an unthinkable demotion of rank. Neither she nor her husband much used the surname Montagu in any case. He was known as Wortley; when she wanted to use a surname she usually went by Lady Mary Wortley. However, since she has achieved a minor literary fame as Lady Mary Wortley Montagu, that is the form used here. It is correct, even if more ultracorrect than she usually bothered to be.

In contrast, Caroline of Ansbach held her royal title from her husband, not her father. She was therefore Caroline, Princess of Wales, or the Princess of Wales. She was not Princess Caroline. When her husband ascended the throne as King George II, she became Queen Caroline.

Dates

In 1582 large sections of Europe began adopting the Gregorian calendar (named for Pope Gregory XIII, who first put it into wide use). With some minor adaptations, this calendar is the one we still use today. Although most of Europe had made the transition by 1701, the British Empire, including its American colonies, clung to the old—and less accurate—Julian calendar (named for Julius Caesar) until 1752. As a consequence, during the period covered by this book, British dates (marked O.S., or Old Style) were eleven days behind those on the continent (marked N.S., or New Style). Months and days appear in the British Old Style throughout this book.

Until 1752, the British also held to the old custom of beginning the New Year on March 25 (Lady Day, or the Annunciation), rather than January 1—though they called January 1 New Year's Day. Often, dates from January 1 through March 24 would show up with two years, e.g., March 1, 1715/6. In this book, all years appear in the modern style, changing over at January 1.

Introduction

Lady Mary and Boylston both lamented their exhausting popularity and sometimes terrifying demonization while the inoculation controversy was in full scream. Lady Mary's daughter vividly recalled seeing and hearing servants' reactions to her mother—including the condemnation that she was "unnatural"—when she was a young girl. Boylston's children long remembered him daring insults and assaults to perform inoculations at all hours.

The best popular history of the eradication of smallpox from nature, along with a chilling assessment of its possible future threat, is Jonathan Tucker's *Scourge: The Once and Future Threat of Smallpox,* from which I have drawn the summary presented here. The estimated number of smallpox victims comes from him, as do the comparisons to the bubonic plague and twentieth-century wars, the story of the last sufferer of smallpox "in the wild," and the metaphor of the maximum-security prison.

The odds given of vaccination resulting in death are modern; those of variolation resulting in death are from the early eighteenth century. Serious complications from both vaccination and variolation can result in permanent damage, even when patients survive.

The modern vaccine does not use the cowpox virus, but another virus in the family of "orthopoxviruses." Some have argued that Jenner never used the true cowpox virus, working with horsepox instead; others maintain that the vaccine strain mutated into something new during intensive reduplication in laboratories. In any case, the virus now used for medical purposes is called vaccinia, incorporating the old story of cows and dairymaids right into its name.

Two Marys

When Queen Mary died in Kensington Palace in 1694, doctors had no standard system of classifying the various forms of smallpox. From eyewitness accounts of her symptoms, it is likely that she suffered from what modern doctors would call "late hemorrhagic smallpox, with flat-type lesions." Though rare, it was a death sentence barely less inevitable than the hundred-percent mortality of the "early hemorrhagic" form: about three percent of its victims might survive. The queen was not one of them. I have drawn the story of her suffering and death from contemporary eyewitness accounts and modern biographies, with details on the course of her disease filled in from both eighteenth- and twentieth-century medical treatises.

The resemblance of smallpox to chicken pox remains legendary, but for many years the disease it was most closely linked to (at least in imagination) was the measles. British doctors began differentiating smallpox (especially the hemorrhagic forms) from measles around the end of the seventeenth century and the beginning of the eighteenth (when they began differentiating diseases more generally), but they had by no means reached unanimous agreement on the subject. Well into the eighteenth-century, many still thought smallpox and measles were different forms or degrees of the same illness. At least one of the queen's physicians, Dr. Walter Harris, concluded that she had "smallpox and measles mingled." In their early stages, the two diseases looked enough alike that they were not uncommonly confused until the late twentieth century, when smallpox was removed as a possible diagnosis.

Many years after the queen's death, Harris published a description of her case; from his notes come most of the early details (and much of the imagery) given here, up through the sinking of her blisters and her labored breathing that night. Out of respect for royal dignity, witnesses become vague about many details of the queen's case from this point on, painting the highly unlikely scenario of a comfortable, peaceful, and dignified death. Across the next three centuries, however, their fellow physicians would carefully, even obsessively, catalogue the final horrors endured by more common mortals struck with late hemorrhagic smallpox. I have matched the queen's condition to the main points of this cataloged nightmare.

The rotten-garden imagery appears scattered throughout early descriptions of smallpox; I have put the snappish recognition of its weirdness into the king's mouth, though his general anxiety and near hysteria during his wife's illness is well documented. The letter quoted is his.

Young Gloucester is generally supposed to have died from smallpox, though measles was also diagnosed. The combined diagnosis suggesting a flat reddish rash, his doctors' early declaration that the case was hopeless, and his death on the sixth day of the fever strongly suggests that he suffered specifically from early hemorrhagic smallpox (which invariably kills its victims on or about the sixth day after the onset of fever).

As Lady Mary liked to tell the tale of her visit to the Kit-Cat Club—and as it was recorded in skeletal form by her granddaughter decades after Lady Mary's death—she was not quite eight years old. In the context of her life and the history of the Kit-Cat Club, however, the story makes far more sense set several years later: somewhere between early 1699, when she was not quite ten, to late 1701 or early 1702, when she was twelve. (Other than Lady Mary's dubious timing of this anecdote, the Kit-Cat Club is not known to have existed before 1699 or 1700.) I have set the scene at the beginning of the London social season late in 1701, when she was twelve, expanding her story with contemporary detail.

The men's verses are drawn from a list of Kit-Cat toasts given in 1703. Garth made the verse quoted; I have given Lord Halifax—famous as an extempore versifier—an unattributed toast. Lady Mary must have said something pretty as well, for her father's friends praised her brilliance as well as her beauty. Within a year or two, she wrote a poem to Lord Halifax, praising him for his praise, in turn, of the countess of Sunderland. (One of the four famously beautiful daughters of the duke of Marlborough, Lady Sunderland was the elder sister of Lady Mary's friend, Lady Mary Churchill.) I have drawn Lady Mary's verse exchange with him from this slightly later poem. The first couplet adapts lines from the later poem to the Kit-Cat situation; the second I quote verbatim. Halifax's verse within hers is adapted from another of the 1703 toasts.

Jesting stories as to the origin of the Kit-Cat Club's name became legion soon after its rise to fame. I have accepted the three most common theories. That 1. a tavern owner-cum-pastry chef named Christopher Cat 2. served the mutton pies called Kit-Cats 3. at an establishment under the sign of the Cat and Fiddle makes as much—or more—sense as one combined story than as three separate stories. Sheer—or Shear or Shire—Lane, where the first meeting place stood, has since disappeared beneath the white fairy-tale castle of the Royal Courts of Justice. Soon after Lady Mary's visit, the club moved to larger digs at another tavern under the sign of the Fountain, in the Strand.

Three Rebellions

Lady Mary recorded her girlhood escapades, her clashes with her father, and her courtship with Wortley in detail in letters and in her diary. Her letters often report whole conversations; her diary was lively enough that her granddaughter remembered what she read of it for decades. I have also adapted some dialogue from Lady Mary's more auto-biographical romances and poems.

Lady Mary later recalled that her brother had always been her best friend; every scrap of evidence suggests that she regarded her father with awe and fear. From the beginning, Wortley both intrigued and irritated her.

The garden-wall episode with the Brownlows is true, as was her practice of giving her girlhood friends names out of romances—and listing them in her notebook. Lady Mary did indeed slit twenty pages from her earliest album of poems and stories (dating from 1702–04, when she was twelve to fourteen), and then burn them. She squeezed the poem quoted into a blank space on an earlier page; its content strongly suggests that while it was she who carried out this "burning and blotting," she did not do so voluntarily. The poem's phrasing sounds as if it answers direct accusations: I have reconstructed the book-burning episode from these clues.

The critic who made her mutilate her work remains unknown, however, as does the exact nature of the offense. Very young, she developed a dangerous taste for both reading and writing tales that lightly masked real people's adventures as fiction. Later, this tempta-tion would get her into much worse trouble; I have surmised that her mistake at fourteen may have been an early foray into this habit. Whatever the problem was, it was particular to the excised pages, or the whole book would have burned.

Her tormentor may have been her French governess, Madame Dupont, or her brother's tutor (who possibly also tutored Lady Mary), but the anger-prone authority in her life whose biography was hands down most tale worthy was her father. I have drawn his character from sketches to be found in her diary and romances. He did, in fact, always require from his children the ritual court greeting of bended knee and kissed hand. In 1709 Kneller painted Kingston in a suit of purple velvet; I have drawn his physical de-scription from this painting, and put him in morning dress of the same material.

Lady Mary gave out many different stories about teaching herself Latin in secret. At times she credited Wortley with sparking her desire to learn. She also credited both Wort-ley and Congreve for help along the way.

As an old woman, Lady Mary saw her father in a rakish character from Samuel Richardson's novel *Sir Charles Grandison*; had she survived to read Jane Austen's *Pride and Prejudice*, she would surely have seen Edward Wortley Montagu in Elizabeth Bennett's first disagreeable impressions of Mr. Darcy: but Wortley never transformed into Prince Charming. Lady Mary described him in arch detail in her letters and romances—especially the tale of Princess Docile (herself) and Prince Sombre, clearly a fictionalized alter ego of Wortley. "He had all the qualities of an upright man, and no single quality of an amiable one," she wrote: a line I've adapted as an exchange between Lady Mary and her sister. Wortley's letters to Lady Mary uphold her romance characterizations of him, good, bad, and irritating.

It is not clear when or where they met, though they certainly continued to meet through the convenience of seeing Anne. Why Anne died in February 1710 is uncertain, but at the time typhus—London's other great eighteenth-century scourge—was rampant.

Wortley carefully preserved the squabbling letters that passed back and forth between him and Lady Mary, including the mischief-making note of Betty Laskey, endorsed by

Richard Steele. Nothing is known of Laskey beyond this note and Lady Mary's lamentations about her. In one autobiographical romance, however, Lady Mary made her hero Sebastian (Wortley) incur wrath of the heroine Laetitia (Lady Mary) by falling for just such a trumped-up offer on the part of an orange-woman who had played go-between for the lovers in Hyde Park. I have sketched Betty Laskey from that hint, drawing on contemporary engravings of street hawkers using the cries "Fair Lemons & Oranges" and "Six pence a pound fair Cherryes."

Wortley's anxiety about Lady Mary's possible loss of "colour" or complexion betrays his apprehension about her diagnosis. Given the timing of her illness within the worst smallpox epidemic London had yet known, his fears suggest that he was all too aware of the long-standing confusion between measles and smallpox.

The epidemic of 1710 was at its height from May through July. Using James Jurin's slightly later statistic that one of every five or six Londoners who came down with smallpox died, I have extrapolated the number of people ill in 1710 from the official figure of 3,138 dead of smallpox that year. The quack bills are adapted from Daniel Defoe's *Journal of the Plague-Year*. Defoe's fictionalized history covers London's last great epidemic of the bubonic plague in 1665, but within a year of writing it in 1722, he had been eyewitness to the devastations of another disease: the smallpox epidemic of 1721. Though that more recent epidemic was not near so fearsome as the 1665 outbreak of the plague, it also seems to have progressed through the city from west to east. Other details, too, are general enough to fit London's panic in the face of any epidemic disease.

I have given Wortley encounters with various epidemic scenes, as well as thoughts comparing smallpox to the plague: Creighton documents the general awareness of smallpox as a threat of growing intensity and frequency, such that it began to replace the plague as Britain's most feared disease in the early eighteenth century. (The plague could and did kill far more people than smallpox within the span of a single epidemic. In London, however, its "visitations" were far fewer, and it was virtually absent between epidemics; after 1665, it also belonged to the past. Smallpox remained a steady killer in that city even in "healthy" years right into the twentieth century; at the beginning of the eighteenth century, fearsome smallpox epidemics began appearing with markedly increasing frequency.)

Margaret Brownlow's death is the first known instance of smallpox interfering in Lady Mary's life. Beyond the two facts that Margaret fell ill and died of smallpox while Lady Mary was convalescing from the measles, and that her sister Jane did indeed marry Margaret's intended husband in June 1711, however, I do not know the details. I have given her the nickname of "Meg" and a standard set of smallpox symptoms. Cream applied with a feather was a traditional regimen for preventing smallpox scarring.

Emperor Joseph and the grand dauphin Louis both died of smallpox as stated. The emperor certainly was given the ancient "hot" treatment; given descriptions of the dauphin's rooms just after his death, he may well have endured the "cold" treatment (an innovation of the famous seventeenth-century English doctor Thomas Sydenham). I have made Dorchester and his cronies discuss these regimens; they surely discussed the political consequences.

Lady Mary detailed her longing for her unidentified Paradise and her loathing of Skeffington in her many letters to "Dear Phil." I have condensed and combined a few of them and pulled her dramatic sentence "Limbo is better than Hell" into the place of a conclusion because it crystallizes her tortured choice of Wortley over Skeffington; otherwise, the letters stand as she wrote them, save for modernizing spelling and punctuation.

Lady Mary reported her various interviews with her father, family, and brother on the subject of the match to Skeffington—complete with most of the dialogue presented here—in several detailed letters to Wortley just before the elopement, as she tried to make him see that her father would not easily forgive them and was certainly not going to pony up money. I have added her brother's unhappiness with his own marriage, on the strength of Lady Mary's extreme reactions against it, and his own willingness to help her escape a similar fate. I have divided between Lady Frances and Lady Kingston the reactions Lady Mary reported as generally being those of the family. When she gave her father her "final" answer, she first chose the single life, but relented in a letter following her father's threat to pack her into the country immediately. The threat is Kingston's as Lady Mary later reported it to Wortley; its presentation in a valise is my way of literalizing the cramped life he was offering her. She gave no indication as to the dates or settings of any of these familial encounters; those are my surmise.

The particulars of her aversion to Skeffington are lost, but surviving letters suggest that it was both primarily physical and inexplicable to others (especially her father). Skeffington's family were the proud lords of Castle Antrim and other vast estates in Northern Ireland.

Her long bickering courtship with Wortley was Byzantine in its plotting and spying, and their elopement was worse: a two-months' tangle of aborted attempts, near breakoffs, procrastinations, and terrors. I have streamlined both courtship and elopement, but the general arc of events—including the two major breaks—remains accurate. Whether the lovers actually met in the inn on the way to West Dean is unclear, but they certainly passed a flurry of notes that attest Lady Mary's laughter at Wortley's "highwayman" getup, her indignation at his inability to provide the "decent conveyance" of a coach, Wortley's suggestion that they borrow her family's, and her absolute refusal to implicate her brother—though he was undoubtedly an accomplice.

How Lady Mary received word of her brother's illness is unclear, though the timing is accurate. I have let her learn from Lady Frances, though a face-to-face meeting would have dared their father's wrath. It seems to have been Lady Frances who later took it upon herself to keep Lady Mary informed of Will's progress.

A Destroying Angel

Lady Mary poured her anguish over her brother's death into her diary and letters; her sorrow and rage made a lasting impression on her granddaughter, reading them many years later.

Wortley's vengeance in coyly threatening to consign his wife and child to an infected house is taken directly from their letters, though I have reconstructed his first (*I have taken a house in Duke Street . . .*) from her reply to it.

Pope's readings of his *Iliad* translation before Halifax took place somewhere between October 1714 and May 1715, when Halifax died. I've taken the liberty of including Lady Mary at the second gathering, as she was in town and fast becoming a fixture in the literary crowd that Halifax—an old acquaintance and good friend of her father's—liked to entertain. She was certainly on jesting terms with Pope by the summer of 1715. Pope's illness and reflections on his own appearance are amply documented.

The "ridiculous adventure" with Craggs is one of the few that Lady Mary's granddaughter reported in detail from her reading of Lady Mary's diary. I have supplied Craggs's rebuke to Lady Mary, reported only as "a bitter reproach with a round oath to enforce it." In a polite age that enveloped passion in delicate nettings of euphemism, such frank anger carried the force of a slap across the face.

The real distress evident in Craggs's reaction, as well as the extravagant emphasis that Lady Mary's granddaughter lavished upon the awfulness of her indiscretion, suggest that Craggs was worried about far more than just being revealed as an impetuous young man— which in any case he was already known to be: such pranks were common among the nobility, even if not often run directly under the king's nose. I have opted for rivalry as the most likely undercurrent of danger, given the king's known interest in the lady.

The appearance and habits of King George I, Schulenberg, and Kielmansegg (including their nicknames and La Schulenberg's pastime of snipping caricatures out of scraps of paper), are all attested by their contemporaries.

Details of Lady Mary's bout with smallpox are few but richly suggestive. Gossip revealed that Lady Mary was "very full"—i.e., that she had a case of confluent smallpox— and that she was thought to be fighting for her life for two days around Christmas. From these details, I have given her a classic case of confluent smallpox, following Ricketts's description of "confluent smallpox with severe suppurative fever." The notion that victims looked weirdly old or young is Ricketts's, as is the image of the gray caul. Richard Mead, one of Lady Mary's physicians, wrote a treatise on smallpox published in 1747, though written much closer to the time of Lady Mary's illness. His words, as well as the details of her treatment, come from this book. The statistics are from the World Health Organization.

In eighteenth-century England, surgeons (who learned from apprenticeship and often did not hold any university degree whatever) were properly titled "Mr." rather than "Dr."—the latter being an honorific reserved for physicians (who held medical doctorates). With what is now a bit of reverse snobbery, modern British surgeons retain this ancient distinction of title, going by Mr.—or Miss, Ms., or Mrs.—though they hold medical degrees. In colonial America, where trained doctors were in perennially short supply, strict divisions between physicians, surgeons, and apothecaries collapsed; the title "Dr." was given to those with proven talent and experience, whether their training came from the university or from apprenticeship.

I have dramatized the scene of Lady Mary's first look at her ruined face from her eclogue titled:

Satturday
The Small Pox
Flavia.

According to her granddaughter, "she always said she meant the Flavia of her sixth Town-Eclogue for herself, having expressed in that poem what her own sensations were while slowly recovering under the apprehension of being totally disfigured." From this poem come the details of her reclining on a couch, holding a mirror reversed in her right hand, the identities of her doctors (Mead as Mirmillo with the golden-headed cane, Garth as Machaon wearing a red cloak), Garth's reassurance about her beauty, and her order to have the Kneller removed from her sight. Her granddaughter attested the loss of Lady Mary's "very fine eyelashes." I have supplied the detail of the veiled mirrors; it fits with the general desire to keep her calm, and with her lack of any knowledge about what she looked like well into convalescence.

At the end of this chapter and elsewhere through the book, I have made Lady Townshend stand in for Lady Mary's wide circle of aristocratic friends. Her comment on Lady Mary's loss of beauty is adapted from one recorded by Lady Hertford. Lady Mary's reply comes from her own assessment of her loss of face in "Carabosse"—a personalized version of "Sleeping Beauty," in which the cursed princess is clearly herself. She probably wrote this French fairy tale years later, but the feelings it records about smallpox echo those of Flavia, and were probably of long standing.

Bidding the World Adieu

From her fascination with "Frost Fairs" to her travels to Turkey, Lady Mary's life at times bears an uncanny resemblance to Virginia Woolf's *Orlando*. Whether Lady Mary attended the frost fair of 1716 is uncertain; given her regret for missing the previous one (when she had been trapped up at Thoresby by impassable roads) and Mead's prescription for taking fresh air, it seems likely that she would have done her best to see it, even if only from the window of a coach.

Asses' milk was a standard drink while convalescing from many illnesses; Mead specifically recommended it for smallpox. The scene of Lady Mary and Lady Townshend examining other remedies is my invention; the remedies, however, are drawn from contemporary recipes.

The story of Pope's revenge on Edmund Curll is unfortunately accurate.

Direct evidence that Lady Mary heard about inoculation before leaving London is lacking; circumstantial evidence, however, is very strong: those who were buzzing about the story abroad were among her closest friends and their families. Given Lady Mary's imminent journey to Constantinople, her vested interest in smallpox, and her wide-ranging intellectual curiosity, it beggars imagination to think that none of them should have mentioned the story to her. I have therefore created scenes in which Garth and her other friends who knew the rumors gather to tell her. The timing of these rumors' appearance, however, is accurate.

At some point that spring, Lady Mary satisfied public curiosity and discarded her mask; the particulars are my surmise. Photographs in Ricketts suggest that Lady Mary's face would have recovered significantly during convalescence: the swelling would eventually have disappeared, and the scars faded a great deal. The "nutmeg grater" image comes from the same source. The total disfigurement that Lady Mary feared did not come to pass, said her granddaughter. Lady Mary's famed beauty, however, was gone for good. (Pepys reported a similar outcome for the duchess of Richmond.)

While Maitland cannot be specifically linked to Kennedy, London's learned surgeons were then a tight-knit group; it is far more likely than not that two of their number who were Scottish knew each other at least well enough to discuss such a hot topic, especially when Maitland was soon headed to the source, and Kennedy had been there previously.

Lady Mary wrote an unending stream of letters home about her adventures en route. Wherever possible, I have kept close to her language (or to that of the snippets of gossip about her). Though almost all the originals as well as her own copies have been lost, she later edited these letters into literary gems that run together as an epistolary travel book. As she intended, this was printed after her death. Wortley also kept several pages of her notes recording dates, addressees, and general content lists of her actual letters: these often, but not always, correspond to their edited counterparts.

In Hanover, the king was widely seen to be still fascinated with her, but I have surmised that his interests might have been altered—as hers seem to have been toward him. She had no intention of remaining behind, no matter who might delight in her presence.

Lady Mary's description of her visit to the Baths of Sofia is one of the gems of her *Embassy Letters*. I have dramatized the scene from that description; the dialogue, both direct and indirect, is hers. I have assumed that she used, as she did later, a Greek interpretress.

Lady Mary carefully shaped most of her embassy letters to focus on one Turkish custom at a time: dress, poetry, the baths, inoculation. I have made explicit connections she implies by logic and timing. At the baths, she is quite clear that the ladies' smooth, shining skin is what amazed and delighted her most. Though she does not specifically say that smallpox (or the lack of it) was on her mind, it seems likely that her fascination with their unmarked skin prompted her immediate efforts to figure out how the Ottomans protected themselves from smallpox. Within two weeks, she had ferreted out stories of inoculation and interviewed everyone she could find on the subject. Maitland, it is important to note, was not with her at this point. Whatever she had learned before she left London or along the way, what she discovered at this juncture, she discovered on her own. According to her granddaughter, Lady Mary acknowledged that "former sufferings and mortifications . . . led her to observe the Turkish invention with particular interest."

My Dear Little Son

Lady Mary wrote at length about her sojourn in Turkey; Maitland wrote somewhat more tersely about his inquiries and experiment with smallpox inoculation. Though neither makes much mention of cooperation, much less debate and discussion, with the other, events suggest that all of that was going on. I have woven their accounts together, and given them life as scenes.

Lady Mary wrote about inoculation to many people; her record of letters sent home includes one to her father concerning the smallpox. Sir Hans Sloane later said she also wrote the court and various friends on the subject. The only such letter that survives is the one she included in her *Embassy Letters*—polished and edited for circulation, and addressed to her girlhood friend Sarah Chiswell (who had, by the time of editing, died uninoculated from smallpox). I quote from it, in the place of the lost letter sent to her father, adding a suitable opening; I have also added the word *rendered* where some such word seems to be missing.

She described her Turkish dress in detail to her sister while it was still being made. If her later portraits in it (or a modified version of it) are to be trusted, however, she mixed up a few things. I have followed Lady Mary's written account, "corrected" by what Jean Baptiste Vanmour and Jonathan Richardson seem actually to have seen. (Commissioned by Alexander Pope, Kneller painted another portrait of her in her Turkish robes, but her dress is so shadowed in the reproductions I have seen that it is hard to make out details.)

The disastrous Balm of Mecca experiment comes from a self-mocking letter to the king's half-sister. Lady Mary pointedly lamented her "mortification" at Wortley's reproaches, though the specific reproaches are my inventions.

Wortley engaged Dr. Timonius as the family physician in August, and though Lady Mary seems to have decided earlier to have her son inoculated, she missed the first opportunity to join the regular smallpox parties. I have surmised that the expert Dr. Timonius had a hand in preventing her; though she never gives a reason for missing this opportunity, pregnancy was a very good reason to stay as far away from the smallpox as possible.

I have drawn the conversations between Lady Mary and Maitland from his account of his inquiries into inoculation while in Constantinople, staying as close as possible to his language. That Lady Mary might have had some part in his discoveries or discussions is my supposition; she was certainly investigating the topic for herself during her stay in Constantinople.

The inoculation of young Edward closely follows Maitland's account, save that I have elaborated on the boy's struggles. Mr. Maitland merely remarked that "the good woman went to work; but so awkwardly by the shaking of her hand, and put the child to so much torture with her blunt and rusty needle, that I pitied his cries, who had ever been of such spirit and courage, that hardly any thing of pain could make him cry before; and therefore inoculated the other arm with my own instrument, and with so little pain to him, that he did not in the least complain of it." I find Mr. Maitland's terse explanation suspicious—if understandable, given the need to be complimentary to the Wortley Montagus in print. The Greek woman was far more experienced and almost certainly more capable than he makes out. Given Maitland's extreme reluctance to inoculate later—when he already had firsthand experience of success—his sudden willingness to operate at this point is odd, to the say the least. And while Edward Wortley Montagu, Jr., certainly had spirit and a way-ward courage, he also regularly caused more than his share of mischief and mayhem—even for a scion of the Pierreponts. I have given the boy a minor episode of well-provoked mischief, which goes some way toward *requiring* Maitland to participate.

The boy's course through inoculated smallpox adheres almost word for word with Maitland's account, with some details filled in from modern descriptions of standard symptoms, in particular, Ricketts's descriptions of "modified smallpox"—by which he meant cases seen in people whose protection due to long previous vaccinations had in large part worn out. In many details, these cases resemble those described by inoculators. Nei-ther Lady Mary nor Maitland had much to say about the incisions. Medical paintings of variolation, however, suggest that their development would have been startling.

Rosebuds in Lily Skin

From the Wortleys' return to London in 1719 through the spring of 1721 (including the location of their house, the illness of Princess Anne, the rift in the royal family, and the bursting of the South Sea stock bubble), the events Lady Mary recalls are well docu-mented. Her reverie, however, is my invention. While she certainly knew Dryden through and through, I am responsible for having her ponder this particularly weird poem at this apropos moment.

Some of the tiniest details in this chapter are true: roses and violets did indeed bloom in January 1721, after which the early warmth dissolved into a cold, wet spring. The small-pox house in Swallow Street did exist, serving as both refuge and quarantine, primarily for servants from the great houses of St. James's and Piccadilly.

Lady Mary began to lose friends and family to smallpox in frighteningly large num-bers in February 1721. She does not appear to have considered inoculating her daughter until the beginning of April, however, at which point she was suddenly insistent. This abrupt switch suggests a known exposure; unfortunately, the loss of Lady Mary's diaries has obscured the details. As no particular close friend or family member seems to have succumbed to smallpox right around this time, I have located such an exposure in the nurse. It is at least plausible, in explaining Lady Mary's suddenly sharp fear for her daugh-ter. Furthermore, if she was the same nurse that Mary had had in Constantinople, she was vulnerable: according to Lady Mary, the reason little Mary was not inoculated in Turkey along with her brother was that "her Nurse has not had the smallpox." Presumably, she re-fused to be inoculated as well.

More generally, servants were always a concern as agents of infection. No doubt there was a great deal of class prejudice involved in this fear, but it was not without foundation. Servants worked long and exhausting hours for mere pittances, and even in great houses their rooms could be crowded, cold, damp, and unsanitary. Furthermore, the work of sup-plying their masters with food, drink, fuel, and other necessaries took many into the crowded streets and marketplaces even during epidemics. The living and work conditions of servants, in short, not infrequently made them more vulnerable to disease than their more comfortable masters.

Charles Maitland is the chief source for young Mary's inoculation. He sketches out the bargaining that went on before he would agree to perform the operation, though he does not give details as to the situations in which the negotiations occurred. (I am responsible for making Lady Mary conjure up Constantinople for him.) But he did request witnesses, and Lady Mary at first refused. According to family tradition and her own later writings, she feared that professional jealousy and greed would induce physicians to try and make the inoculation fail. For his part, Maitland appears to have been reluctant to inoculate in London at all. No doubt his stated reason of wanting to increase the operation's credit and reputation in part explains his insistence on witnesses. Self-protection, however, seems also to have been an issue.

Little Mary's long wait of ten days before the outbreak of fever is attested by Maitland, as is the summons of an "ancient apothecary." Neither Maitland nor any of the later witnesses date Mary's inoculation any more precisely than the month of April; I have made the fever coincide with the birth of Prince William Augustus, the future duke of Cumberland, on April 15, 1721, to great (if typical) rejoicing.

Zabdiel and Jerusha

The facts about Zabdiel Boylston's boyhood are nearly as fragmentary as the dream I have given him. Here's what's real: He was born March 9, 1680 in Muddy River, later Brookline, Massachusetts, to Dr. Thomas Boylston and his wife Mary. The only child, of twelve, to follow his father's interest in medicine, he was fifteen when his father died in 1695; there is no record of the cause of death. Judging by Zabdiel's account of the 1721 smallpox epidemic and by his business dealings, of all his siblings, he was closest to his youngest brother, Thomas.

As late as 1700, the hamlet of Muddy River spread across five thousand acres of fields, marshland, and forest; its population was below two hundred. It incorporated as the town of Brookline in 1705.

Family tradition has it that Zabdiel's father had an Oxford M.D., but the university has no record of granting him any degree whatsoever. The Boylstons, however, had apothecary relatives in both Birmingham and London; Zabdiel later visited several of them. I have made his father visit them first. I have found no firm record of Zabdiel's apprenticeship under Cutler: but there seems no reason to doubt this bit of family lore. He certainly completed an apprenticeship with a doctor who trained him well and helped establish him within Boston's medical community.

Zabdiel later wrote that he had nearly died during the 1702 smallpox epidemic. At that time, he was at or near the end of his apprenticeship, possibly already setting up on his own. He may well have deliberately contracted the disease, or have dispensed with any attempt to avoid it. Young doctors sometimes did so: they were otherwise virtually useless in an epidemic. Thomas Dover, one of Sydenham's famous protégés, for example, took notes on his own progress and treatment, just as I have had Zabdiel do. Before the shields of antisepsis and antibiotics, being a doctor was not for the faint of heart: repeatedly risking "putrid" fevers (typhus and typhoid, not then differentiated), dysentery, and various streptococcal infections, to name just a few of the common killers in colonial New England, required no small dose of personal courage. At least smallpox only had to be suffered once.

Zabdiel's father served briefly in the cavalry troop of Captain Thomas Prentice in

King Philip's War, during the Mount Hope campaign against the Narragansetts. This tribe was supposed to be loyal or neutral toward the English, but the women and children were slaughtered anyway, when it became apparent that they were sheltering Wampanoag women and children. The elder Dr. Boylston, who probably served as a surgeon, seems to have removed himself after this first campaign, though the war dragged on. I have found no record that any of his sons ever served against the Indians (though they would have been too young for this war).

Zabdiel Boylston's character and habits as a doctor have to be pieced together from fleeting phrases and tiny shreds of evidence, as well as from his general reputation. Later, he exhibited open-minded interest in Native American medicine, using it, if briefly, as one of his defenses for being open-minded about African medical practice. I have presumed that this attitude was fostered in part by his father. Likewise, Zabdiel's record as a daring and unusually successful surgeon suggests that he was, for his day, unusually clean, quick, and precise, as well as unusually well versed in anatomy.

Jerusha Minot was born in Dorchester on January 28, 1679 (possibly 1680; the genealogies do not specify old or new style dating). Both her parents died of smallpox in Dorchester during the 1690 epidemic—her father on January 26 and her mother on April 6. Three of her brothers—Israel, Josiah, and George—are not traceable after that time, though the Minot family genealogies covering that generation are quite detailed; it is at least plausible that they died unrecorded during the epidemic. In 1702, she lost two young cousins in Boston to the disease. These exposures, plus the fact that Zabdiel never inoculated her, make it all but certain that she herself survived it, either in 1690 or 1702. References to her as "of Boston" suggest she went to live with her closest Bostonian relative, her uncle Stephen Minot—who was, as stated, a wealthy merchant—after she was orphaned in 1690.

I don't know any details of her courtship with Boylston, other than the date of their marriage, and their ages at the time: average for him, a little late for her. Boylston advertised or prescribed everything I have her encounter in his shop, however. Later writings show his interest in Indian remedies for rattlesnake bite, as well as ambergris.

Curiosities of the Smallpox

I have taken Cotton Mather's diary entry from December 16, 1706—the day several men from his parish presented him with the slave he named Onesimus—and a letter he wrote to the Royal Society in July 1716, and reversed them to tell the events from Onesimus's point of view.

Mather repeatedly identified the man as "Guramante," a classical term phonetically close enough to "Coromantee" to make the confusion of the two quite plausible on the part of an eager scholar such as Mather. "Coromantee" was a general and imprecise English (specifically West Indian) term for the Akan-speaking peoples of Africa's Gold Coast, now known as Ghana. The most famous and numerous of these peoples are the Asante or Ashanti. In the early eighteenth century, Coromantees were the most valuable and sought-after slaves among the British; they were also the most feared, thought to be prone to fomenting violent revolt.

The outlines of Onesimus's experience of the Middle Passage on a slave ship, his voyage broken in the West Indies before being sent up to Boston on a ship whose main cargo was not slaves, follows the general pattern of the triangle slave trade in the early eighteenth century. If Onesimus was, as Mather wanted, a young man worth £40–£50 on the slave market—then at or near the top of the pricing—he would have been a relatively unusual figure in Boston: unless specially reserved for a buyer of note, strong, healthy young men were skimmed off for hard labor in the West Indies or the Carolinas. Especially in the early years, Boston tended to get what were called "refuse" slaves: the young, the old, the frail, the troublemakers.

In Boston, unlike on the big plantations far to the south and the farms to the west, most slaveholders had only one or two slaves. Though they did heavy and dangerous chores, they were domestics. They lived in their master's houses, and were often treated as part—though a low-ranking part—of the patriarchal Puritan family.

I have borrowed various wonderings and observations from Olaudah Equiano, also known as Gustavus Vassa (1745–97), another brilliant young African man whose unquenchable curiosity led him to observe in minute detail places, persons, and cultures that he could not yet understand, yet saw with a fine eye; he later wrote one of the earliest slave autobiographies to survive. From him come the interpretations of snow as salt and of books as boxes containing voices.

Mather's letter stands pretty much as he wrote it, though I have abridged and edited it slightly for the sake of readability, and lifted the sentence about "Small-Pox proving a great plague to us poor Americans" to appear higher than it does in the original. His thoughts are closely paraphrased or borrowed outright from his own words.

Mather and others recorded his struggles with a terrible stutter. He overcame it by forcing himself to speak extremely slowly and deliberately, and by learning to sing his words. At points of high stress, however, the stutter would return.

The Beauty of the Sea

The story of Captain John Gore dying from smallpox within sight of home on November 7, 1720, is all documented, save for his wife Rebecca's farewell voyage out to the vicinity of his ship, which is my addition. Gore was eulogized as quoted by the Reverend William Cooper. Through his wife, Gore inherited property in Boylston's neighborhood of Dock Square. He seems, however, to have lived a little farther west, on the slopes of Beacon Hill: a favorite spot for seagoing captains, though well back from the water, because the whole spread of the harbor was visible from these heights. Gore, like Boylston, was a member of the Brattle Street Church; they were close in age. I have taken the liberty of making them friends.

There's plenty of evidence for the general outlines of the smallpox outbreak in Boston at the beginning of May 1721. The fragments are spaced widely enough, though, to allow for connecting the dots into a number of different specific stories. I have told what I think is the most likely tale.

In particular, there is a mystery—and at least one lie—in the matter of identifying the source of the epidemic. Boston's selectmen pointed repeatedly at HMS *Seahorse*, the sixth-rate ship, or frigate, assigned to run convoy with the merchant fleet between Boston and the West Indies. In what remains of the ship's official documentation, her commander, Captain Thomas Durell, never acknowledged his ship as the source of the infection, nor do either the master's log or the ship's paybook note any deaths or sickness due to smallpox. The paybook, however, does list several deaths as well as many desertions and discharges that are consistent with a smallpox outbreak on a ship whose crew was largely, but not entirely, immune through previous survival of the disease.

It would seem that either all six selectmen and Dr. John Clark—their appointed medical examiner as well as a representative to the Massachusetts General Court and at various times the speaker of the House and a member of the Governor's Council—were lying outright, or Captain Durell was lying by omission. I have concluded that one man lying by omission is inherently more likely than a conspiracy of seven lying outright: especially in light of further circumstantial evidence linking *Seahorse* to the Boston outbreak—namely, the Paxton family.

Here's what we know:

I have put an accurate examination of the *Seahorse*'s surviving paybook and master's log into the hands of Dr. John Clark, the physician chosen by the selectmen to inspect the suspect ship; his discoveries and frustrations are those any modern historian might have while sifting through the surviving fragments. Thomas Gibson, ship's surgeon, was in a position to know the answers. Unfortunately, Gibson's log, like most surgeons' logs from eighteenth-century British naval ships, does not appear to have survived. In Clark's case, I have made Gibson (and his log) absent on the cruise after pirates (documented by both Captain Durell and his master, or navigator, though the only man explicitly named on that cruise is Lieutenant Hamilton).

On May 8, 1721, the selectmen asked Dr. Clark to inspect the *Seahorse*, having heard that one of the ship's sailors was sick with the smallpox in town: I have quoted the meeting's minutes in full, save an introductory phrase. The wording is open to several interpretations. It is possible, for instance, that the "certain Negro man" in from the Saltertudas aboard the *Seahorse* was one and the same man as Captain Paxton's servant. No member of the crew stands out as an obvious match, though two are possibilities:

Able seaman Hector Bruce joined the *Seahorse*'s company four days after Charles Paxton. His name directly follows Charles Paxton's in the *Seahorse* paybook. Bruce was a slave owned by Paxton's father; his pay went to Captain Paxton's agent. When Bruce later ran away, the captain ran an advertisement describing him as an Indian, so he is probably not the "certain Negro" in question, however. Furthermore, pockmarks were commonly used identifying markers for runaways; if Bruce had been the sick man, it is unlikely that Paxton would have omitted mention of them in the runaway notice, given that Paxton took pains to describe Bruce's face, stature, and skill as a sailor.

The only other Seahorse with any clear connection to the Paxtons is able seaman Richard Kent. He joined the ship's company the same day as Bruce; his name follows Bruce's in the paybook. Like Bruce, his pay went to Wentworth Paxton's agent: except that the tag, "agent to Wentworth Paxton, agent" has been added, which may indicate that he was a free man, contracted with Paxton as his own agent. He was discharged by request on October 30, 1722. If he is the same Richard Kent to be found in the Thwing archives, he married the year of his discharge and became a shipwright and an innkeeper. He was certainly not a slave, though in 1721 he may have been some kind of servant, possibly indentured; he probably was not black.

The likeliest interpretation of the selectmen's minutes is that the black *Seahorse* sailor was a different man than Captain Paxton's black servant. In this case, that the selectmen did not order the sailor put under guard suggests that they did not know exactly where he was.

By May 12, Clark had reported back that "two or three" men were indeed sick with the smallpox on that ship, that "sundry others" were sick on shore, and that most of the crew had gone off on a cruise to chase pirates. I have written an inspection scene consistent with a discovery of this information.

Possibly, the infection entered the town through a number of ships in the Saltertudas fleet, most of which had probably made some call in Barbados, but the selectmen chose to finger *Seahorse* alone. This still does not explain Durell's reticence.

Able seaman John Dunn of the *Seahorse* died (without explanation) on May 4, 1721.

Gunner's mate Joseph May died (also without explanation) on May 14; I have identified May as the missing black sailor, though beyond the coincidence of timing, there is no evidence that he was.

The lone specifically identified and located man known to be ill with smallpox on May 8—Captain Paxton's black servant—also points, if circumstantially, back to the *Seahorse*. For Captain Paxton's son Charles was, as stated, a sailor on that warship, having been entered into the *Seahorse* paybook, rated "ord" for "ordinary seaman," on December 1, 1720. A note next to his name states that he had shore leave from January 6, 1721 (the day *Seahorse* sailed for Barbados) through April 22, 1721 (when she returned); his pay was duly docked. He is the only sailor to be granted such leave while Durell was in command of HMS *Seahorse;* no reason is supplied. Other sailors appear to have been discharged altogether when they could supply legitimate reasons for leaving the ship, or they were marked as having run, and then later reentered, under different numbers, when they rejoined—or were forced to rejoin—the crew. The two most obvious reasons for young Paxton's leave are illness or some kind of special privilege accruing from an agreement between Captains Paxton and Durell, possibly in light of his age, which was young—though not remarkably so. I have opted for the latter.

Neither of Paxton's two men aboard *Seahorse* seems likely to have been either of the black men sick with smallpox. However, as both hustled (or were hustled) on board directly after the boy, I have tied them into the story of Charles Paxton's shore leave, making them a sort of doubled payment-in-kind for the boy's temporary release from the ship. Given the high desertion rate, Durell seems to have needed men more than money.

Epidemiologically, Paxton's servant's bout with smallpox fits precisely with the arrival of the *Seahorse* on April 22, and a presumed return of young Charles Paxton to the ship on or about the twenty-third. The virus's average incubation period of twelve days following initial infection (anywhere from ten to fourteen being normal), followed by three days of fever before the telltale eruption, dovetails with exposure on April 23, duly followed by the appearance of the rash on May 7 or 8. The man may well have been exposed while returning Charles to the *Seahorse*, or possibly while carousing with sailors ashore. Since the *Seahorse* remained in the relative isolation of a mooring off Castle Island until April 27, when she removed to an anchorage off Boston's Long Wharf, I have opted for the first explanation.

The name of this servant, probably a slave, was never recorded by any of the authorities. Slaves, in particular those newly shipped over from Africa, were named by their masters. While pious Bostonians—like Cotton Mather—tended to opt for Biblical nomenclature, classical names such as Scipio, Caesar, and Pompey were popular among more worldly, self-consciously cultured gentlemen and merchants. I have given Captain Paxton's servant the name of the black slave who was one of Judge Samuel Sewall's most trusted personal servants.

The official records remain silent about whether or not Charles Paxton came down with smallpox at this time. Since he was born in 1707, five years after Boston's last bout with smallpox, he was vulnerable. If indeed the *Seahorse* was infected and Paxton went aboard, odds are vanishing to none that he escaped infection himself; I have assumed that he was one of the "sundry others" from that ship sick on shore, and that his name was kept out of the record. It is notable that both people specifically scapegoated as the first to fall ill were black men.

The young Paxtons' father, Captain Wentworth Paxton, had been the commander of an earlier, smaller *Seahorse* in 1701; he appears to have resigned his naval commission after being refused a larger ship. His proud temper later got him memorialized in Samuel

Sewall's diary, as the judge once fined the captain for beating another gentleman in the street with his cane. After leaving the navy, Captain Paxton married well, gaining the hand and the fortune of the widow Faith Gillam Middleton, who inherited a third of the merchant empire of warehouses, wharves, and houses owned by her father, Captain Benjamin Gillam. Most successful Boston merchants of the period left trails of deeds, buying and selling properties all over the town; Paxton's deeds are almost all sales. Possibly, he wished to consider himself a gentleman unsullied by trade, living off investments; possibly, he was not terribly successful in business, and was gradually forced to sell off his (or his wife's) assets.

Captain Durell would seem to have been well thought of, at least by the Admiralty, who promoted him, giving him larger and larger ships. He had a long and solid navy career. Not surprisingly, his surviving letters from this period are obsessively focused on pirates, mostly in the Caribbean. His work-a-day job was to sail convoy. His letters reveal, though, that he yearned for more daring action, pitting his men, his ship, and his seamanship whenever possible against the wily robbers of the sea. During the spring of 1721, the ship was severely damaged off Barbados during one such chase, by the wind and the sea rather than by enemy fire. From this, I have extrapolated a character of some rashness, zeal, and intense focus.

Durell was indeed enamored of trumpets. He recruited a trumpeter on May 16, 1721 (a sixth-rate ship was allowed one). In 1724, Judge Samuel Sewall visited the captain to request that he not sound the ship's trumpets on Saturday nights, as Bostonians kept the Sabbath from sundown Saturday to sundown Sunday, and found the trumpeting "offensive." Durell promised to comply.

Boston did indeed have laws governing quarantine; they specifically grant to the selectmen and their medical examiners the powers to inspect and quarantine ships. I have not been able to find any description of how such inspections worked day to day, though it seems likely that they would have been based on or even linked to the customs bureaucracy already in place.

Boylston had the personally rough fall and winter described; the Boylstons' eighth child, Josiah, was born on July 11, 1720, but had almost certainly died by the time of the smallpox epidemic, since Boylston never mentions him among his other children at that time. I have deduced the furor over cancer treatments and the mastectomy (the first known in North America) from newspaper advertisements, which appeared as quoted (save for some minor editing for readability) in Boston's two papers, both weeklies appearing on Mondays: the *Boston Gazette* and the *Boston News-Letter*. If the advertised Mrs. Winslow was, as I believe, the Sarah married to Captain (later Major) Edward Winslow of Rochester, then Boylston's operation truly was successful: she survived to the age of eighty-five.

In New England, many adult slave men were trained as highly skilled assistants to their masters. Although we do not know about Jack in particular, there were other black slaves who were physician's assistants. Jack would also have been responsible for such heavy chores as hauling wood and water and mucking out stalls. That he was a slave is clear from Boylston's first reference to him in the *Boston Gazette*.

While I do not know that Tommy Boylston pulled his father away from work to see the ships, it seems reasonable behavior for a six-year-old late on a Saturday afternoon. The names of the ships and their captains are real. On March 31, 1721, the *Seahorse* counted fifty-nine vessels in her convoy. Though a few probably peeled off to other destinations before reaching Boston, the convoy was a spectacularly large one by North American standards of the time.

Caging the Monster

This chapter's anchorholds in fact are the quoted minutes and newspaper articles, as well as entries in Cotton Mather's diary and the master's log and paybook for the HMS *Seahorse*. As with the previous chapter, these fragments reveal a lack of candor and detail, as much as anything else. Here are my reasons for taking the paths I chose from fact to fact:

As their minutes of May 12 show, the freeholders of Boston voted in a full town meeting to require the selectmen to approach the governor about the *Seahorse* going to Spectacle Island. Dr. John Clark, the inspecting physician, seems as likely a person as any to demand that quarantine be complied with to the full letter of the law. The selectmen's minutes record that *Seahorse* was headed for Bird rather than Spectacle Island. Rather than either surprise or dissent with this shift, they record a substantial offer of help to Captain Durell in securing the ship's hasty removal. I have put into the mind of William Hutchinson my own suspicion that somebody somewhere, made a deal.

To a man, in May 1721, the six selectmen of Boston were deeply invested in the mercantile interests of the town, over and against royal and religious concerns. Elisha Cooke was widely recognized as the leader of this pack. (There were supposed to be seven selectmen, but the seventh, Dr. Oliver Noyes, had died just days after being elected in March.) The others were William Clark (of the North End; brother to Dr. John Clark), Ebenezer Clough (of the North End), Thomas Cushing (of Dock Square in the center of town), and John Marion (of the South End). On May 12, Captain Nathaniel Green was chosen to replace Oliver Noyes.

The council room on the upper floor of the Town House, with its three east-facing windows, still exists. The Bunch of Grapes Tavern, once at the head of the Long Wharf, on the corner of King (now State) Street and Mackerel Lane (now Kilby Street), has long since disappeared beneath massive bank towers. The Bunch of Grapes seems to have been one of the favorite haunts among the rich and powerful of Cooke's town (or popular) party, while the Royal Exchange, across King Street and farther up from the wharf, served the same purpose for the governor's (or court) party. This division held into the Revolutionary era.

The early form of billiards the selectmen indulge in had, by 1721, been popular in England for fifty years; it reached Boston by 1730, when public billiards rooms (that is, tables in the large common rooms on a tavern's ground floor) were advertised as drawing points. I have installed a more discreet table in a private upper room in the Bunch of Grapes a few years earlier.

On May 10, two days before these meetings (and two days following the selectmen's request to Dr. John Clark to inspect the ship), Captain Durell discharged three able seamen from his ship, apparently no longer quite able. "Unserviceable" was what he noted in the paybook against the names of two strangers (as Boston called noncitizens): Gilbert Anthony and John Wilkinson. It was not a remark Durell handed out with frequency. Save for one further man, on June 1, 1721, he did not use it again while in command of the *Seahorse* (though in 1723, he discharged several men for "Sickness"). The third man, James Mansell, had joined the ship in Boston and was probably a local. He was discharged by request (Durell's standard, almost unvaried, reason for discharges that were not straight to other navy ships). I have equated these three sailors with the "two or three" men Dr. Clark reported sick aboard the *Seahorse*. Discharging them at this time would have removed the evidence for quarantine, just before Dr. Clark was to make his formal report on May 12.

There were many reasons a man might be discharged as unserviceable: weakness due to scurvy, syphilis, or any of a host of chronic diseases common to sailors, or debilitating injury, for example. Captain Durell did not, however, use this explanation outside the limits of the dates his ship stood in Boston Harbor, suspected of carrying smallpox and admitting nothing. Furthermore, May 10—ten days into a port call and nowhere near departure—seems odd timing for discovering men to be unserviceable. Outside fingers pointing at the ship as the bearer of smallpox make this disease a very strong candidate as the culprit.

The two "strangers" were later warned to leave town—as were all indigents whose welfare Boston did not see it had any responsibility to underwrite. However, Wilkinson was not told to leave until May 19, and Anthony not until May 23: depending on the stage of smallpox they may have reached by May 10, these are dates consistent with recovery and release from quarantine.

On the fourteenth of May, Durell noted Joseph May's death in the paybook, once again giving no explanation. It may have been a coincidence that he died the very day that the ship moved out to an anchorage off Bird Island. However, sheer numbers suggest that May had gone ashore a few days earlier with most of the rest of his shipmates; in that case, he may well have only been discovered to be dead the day that the ship was to leave. Given the town's fears, I have presumed there would have been a dockside search for any and all missing Seahorses.

With nigh on half her complement of men away, the *Seahorse* would have needed some help to weigh anchor and maneuver with precision through the sea lanes and shoals of the inner harbor, even if the remaining half of her sailors had all been hale, hearty, and truly able. Captain Timothy Clark and a body of Boston's civilian mariners helped remove the *Seahorse* to Bird Island in accordance with the selectmen's request, and were duly paid for their help.

The newspaper reported the door-to-door search of the town on May 20. I have added the hogreeves to the list of officers included in the search: mostly because I find the need to elect a body of hog catchers each year both amusing and highly descriptive of Boston's street life.

Cotton Mather's third wife, Lydia, was a strong-willed woman, accustomed to luxury and pampering; it is possible that she was just fed up to the screaming point with Dr. Mather, and he assumed that displeasure with him must stem from madness or possession. However, the fact that he sent his two much-loved daughters to live out of the house in order to escape their stepmother suggests that the problem was not merely sweetness and light gone a little sour in the face of rigid piety. Lizzy, like Sammy, was Mather's child by his second wife, Elizabeth, née Clark, sister of Dr. John Clark and Selectman William Clark. At this time, Lizzy was living with her uncle John and his family. Although Mather did not divulge his source for the information that smallpox was loose in the town by May 26, his daughter is an obvious link to the man most likely to know.

All Mather's trials, his fears of smallpox hovering near, as well as his feelings of triumph and tribulation in communing with angels, are to be found in his diaries, voluminous writings, and Kenneth Silverman's biography. As much as possible, I have kept close to Mather's language in trying to follow his thoughts. In particular, I have dipped into another long diary entry for May 28. Mather himself named the smallpox "a destroying angel," which he imagined looming over the town. For others, this might have been a poetic metaphor. Mather, however, is more likely to have meant it to approximate truth: he believed in angels and demons who could wield fiery swords and golden voices both for good and for ill.

Mather's writings on smallpox across the spring and summer of 1721 present quite a tangle. The clearest unraveling is George Lyman Kittredge's article, "Some Lost Works of Cotton Mather." I have followed his lead with one major exception. Kittredge argues that Mather wrote only one letter to the physicians, while he manifestly wrote two. The first, requesting a meeting, he wrote on June 6. Its dated conclusion was reprinted twice in the ensuing pamphlet wars; that is the piece quoted here, via Isaac Greenwood. Apparently circulated in a single copy, the letter went first to Dr. Nathanael Williams (identified as a schoolmaster/physician) with a specific plea to forward it on to Dr. William Douglass, among others.

Kittredge believed that this letter included a transcript, or at least a lengthy abridgment, of both Timonius and Pylarinus. I think it more likely that this first letter was relatively short, requesting a meeting to read and discuss the articles in question. Mather certainly disseminated such transcripts, but I think he did so much later in the month. See the notes to "Fathers and Sons."

At this point, Dr. Mather canvassed Boston's black population, with a clear interest in people born in Africa. He later claimed there was "an army of Africans" who could attest to the practice of inoculation; Douglass scoffed that there were only six or ten. The unnamed black man's description of the African practice appears in Mather's treatise on smallpox, later included as the twenty-second chapter of his medical magnum opus, *The Angel of Bethesda*. Other men might have produced such broken English as mockery of African ignorance; that kind of humor was beyond Mather's ken. Given his fascination with both the subject and its origins, this quotation is likely to be as close to word for word as he could get: and where language was concerned, Mather could get pretty close.

Some scholars have assumed this description came from Onesimus. I find that unlikely: Mather did not produce it for Dr. Woodward's perusal in his letter of July 1716 to the Royal Society, when Onesimus was his one and only direct source. Furthermore, by 1721 Onesimus had long since bought his freedom and was no longer living under Mather's roof. While I do not know that the reverend interviewed the free black men sent out to clean the streets in late May, they are one obvious source for his queries. (Onesimus was not one of them.)

Demonic Wings

I have drawn Dr. Douglass's attitudes toward Boston, Bostonians, money, smallpox, his fellow physicians, and especially Cotton Mather from his own writings, using his words where possible. Though his knowledge on many topics was encyclopedic, the man was hard pressed to write a single sentence that did not drip with scorn; where his reputation was concerned, he was prone to paranoia.

Douglass was also, however, a superb observer of both nature and human affairs, especially in the fields of medicine and botany; geography, weather, and history were also pet topics. Most of the statistical data about Boston's 1721 outbreak of "natural" smallpox (as opposed to inoculated smallpox) comes from his pen. In particular, he stressed the eighteen-day span from "seizure to seizure" as the disease spread.

For all his richly attested disagreeableness, Douglass seems to have been right about the eighteen days. This time span jibes with what's known about the transmission of smallpox: from one person's "seizure" (by which he probably meant the onset of the first fever) to the appearance of the rash takes about three days. After that, it takes roughly another three days for the pocks inside the nose, mouth, and throat to mature and begin to burst: at which point, the ill person spews thick clouds of smallpox virus with every breath. Anyone vulnerable who breathes in that infection then has about twelve days of symptomless incubation before their own "seizure" or onset of the first fever—for a total of eighteen days. Measured from rash to rash, as I have done here, the span is the same as from fever to fever. All the different stages, of course, can vary somewhat in length. Also, patients remain infectious for a long time beyond day three of their rashes, and they can become infectious earlier. As Douglass himself noted, the pattern of widening rings of infection is easiest to see at the start of an epidemic.

Boylston, Mather, and others wrote that Douglass retrieved from Mather the volumes containing the Timonius and Pylarinus articles, and that he locked them up, refusing to let anyone else, even the governor, so much as peek at them. This must have occurred after June 6, when Mather first spread their contents abroad, and before June 23, when Mather sent his treatise out to the physicians—after which such hoarding would presumably have lost most of its point.

Mather sent his first letter, summoning the physicians to a meeting, to Dr. Nathanael Williams, with a particular request to forward it to Dr. Douglass. (Apparently, it was a single copy meant to circulate among the town's physicians.) Williams's compliance with this request seems the most likely avenue for Douglass's discovery of Mather's meddling. As no one else seems to have seen the letter (other than Mather's later defenders, who likely had access to the author's draft copy), it seems reasonable to suppose that it was Douglass who squelched it, along with stopping the circulation of the books.

Douglass is not known to have possessed a house of his own before 1724. (Possibly, his profits from this epidemic materially helped him toward that purchase.) There are passing references in early histories to him living in rooms in the Green Dragon; later, he bought the entire building, though it seems he did not live there at that time. He mocked Zabdiel Boylston for riding horseback, implying that a carriage was more proper to a physician's status; presumably, therefore, he kept one himself. Given his concern with appearances, and with the appurtenances of rank, I have assumed that he also kept at least one slave, though there are no details; certainly, to keep a coach meant keeping at the very least one servant as driver and groom. Again, his mockery of Boylston and Mather reveals that he had no high opinion of African thought or practices.

In reverse, mockery aimed at Douglass suggests that he spoke with a strong Scottish accent, peppering his sentences with obviously Scottish vocabulary.

A number of witnesses said that the next "parcel" of smallpox rashes appeared in the middle of June; Douglass specified the "change of the moon, middle of June." The new moon occurred on June 13. People then began fleeing the town in droves; Douglass claims that the refugees numbered in the thousands. As with refugee situations throughout history, housing prices in the suddenly desirable areas no doubt saw a significant spike.

The Boylstons' relationship is almost completely hidden from history. Jerusha, however, did leave town with the girls soon after the guards were taken off the houses in mid-June. It would appear that Tommy and John, as well as the young slave Jackey, were left behind in Boston with Zabdiel and his adult slave Jack (Jackey's father). Zabdiel junior seems to have been living outside the house, possibly already at college in Cambridge.

Zabdiel never clearly says where the girls went, or why the boys stayed. I have deduced that the women and girls fled to Roxbury from the following: Tom Boylston's wife Sarah was pregnant when the epidemic broke out, making her a high risk for complications. In October, she gave birth at "her lodgings" in Roxbury; at least two of Zabdiel's and Tom's nieces, the daughters of two different sisters, were present in the same house. Twenty-year-old Mary Lane seems to have been a fellow Bostonian. Rebecca Abbot, eleven, however, lived with her parents (Zabdiel's sister Rebecca and brother-in-law William) in Roxbury. It would seem, then, that many of the female relatives were gathered at one house in Roxbury as far out as October 1721. Since one of these families was resident in

Roxbury, it may well have been their home. I have sent Jerusha and her three daughters to this same household, though it is possible the Boylston women were spread through several homes, or that Jerusha and her girls stayed with Minot relatives in Dorchester.

Until the disease spread from Boston into Roxbury, Zabdiel seems never to have gone there. After that point, however, he spent a great deal of time riding back and forth, as well as to adjacent Dorchester. He sporadically traveled to Charlestown, where his brother Richard lived, and to Cambridge, but his travels to Roxbury curtailed his house visits in these towns. He never, however, seems to have gone as far as his native Brookline (where two more brothers lived). Though he may have gone to Roxbury purely for medical business, it does seem that there was some other draw pulling him there, over and above Boston's other equally panicked neighbors.

Overcrowding in their country retreat seems as likely a reason as any for Jerusha leaving the boys behind. At thirteen, John was of an age to be expected to make himself useful. Six-year-old Tommy and two-and-a-half-year-old Jackey, however, are unlikely to have been held back voluntarily. In the normal pattern of everyday life, boys that young would have spent most their time with the women and other children. Apart from Zabdiel's fears for them, they would have been an unusual burden, just when he had no time to spare. Indeed, Benjamin Colman, whose house looked onto the Boylston garden, noted that the doctor's children were "too much exposed and neglected"—and in fact ran a little wild—due to Zabdiel's long hours away tending the sick.

Apparently, no one else was around to look after them either. From this, it has also seemed reasonable to suppose that Jack was out helping Zabdiel during the day, and that Moll was sent off to Roxbury to do for Jerusha and the girls, as well as to escape contagion herself.

Tommy and Jackey play games they are likely to have played: Jerusha Minot's home had indeed been attacked by a lone Indian and defended by a servant maid in the manner described. No laughing matter now, but it was surely a story the family children knew well and enjoyed the way American children later played cowboys and Indians. In 1721, Captain Bartholomew Roberts was the reigning terror of the seas, already legendary as an order-loving but flamboyant and sometimes heroic king of pirates, as revered by his men as feared by his foes. "Black Bart" was one of his nicknames; "the Great Pirate Roberts" was another. "The Dread Pirate Roberts" is a small bit of homage to William Goldman's *The Princess Bride*. Pirates were all over the Boston newspapers throughout May and June 1721; Roberts made a particular splash in the *Boston News-Letter* of May 15. Not quite a year later, in February 1722, he was killed off West Africa in action against the Royal Navy.

Mather noted his composition of both the smallpox treatise and the second letter in his diary. He also, the day before, noted his intention to help Dr. Perkins to some business. Touting Perkins seems as likely an avenue as any for the minister's discovery that his first letter had run afoul of Douglass, producing, as he later said, a fair amount of talk in the town, as well as his own clear determination that the second letter should not similarly go astray.

Fathers and Sons

Boylston's description of his first three inoculations is a pretty bald statement of what he did to whom, and when. I have brought his sketch to life by adding particulars that fit with what we know of the man, his family, and Boston and its environs at that time.

Almost the only thing we know about him as a man, apart from what can be gleaned from his scientific writings and genealogy, is his extraordinary love for his horses. Even in an age when horses were a regular part of everyday life, he had a reputation as an unusually skilled horseman. I have given him, therefore, a trait of all the true horsemen and -women I have known: he seeks out a favorite horse when troubled and finds that his mind and heart settle to clarity while riding.

The landscape he rides through has almost entirely disappeared. Nineteenth-century Bostonians quite literally moved mountains: Beacon Hill, in Boylston's day mostly covered by fields and woods, has been significantly lowered; the other two peaks of the Tri-mountain or Tremount (from which Tremont Street takes its name) have been leveled, their earth sunk into the tidal basin of the Charles River to create the area now called the Back Bay. Present-day Washington Street follows the line of the old road south out of town (it was then called Orange Street), across the Neck, and into Roxbury.

Boylston agonized over the safety of his children, acutely aware that he would likely bring the infection home from the sickrooms in which he was spending so much time. The fact that none of the boys fell ill until he deliberately infected them, however, strongly suggests that he was scrupulously clean and possibly observed some kind of quarantine himself. Though no one understood how or why, it was well known that infected people and clothing (including wigs) could spread smallpox. I have therefore made him particular about washing up and changing his clothes on coming home.

Mather's letter to Boylston survived long enough to be printed in 1789; I've quoted it in full, altering only some punctuation for readability, and adding the word *Guramantees*. (The letter's editor notes an "illegible" word at the point where similar sentences in both the treatise written two days before and the letter to Dr. Woodward in 1716 have "Gura-mantees" or "Garamantese"—an obscure enough word to merit confusion, over and above messy or cramped writing in what was then already an old sheet of paper.) This letter reads like a form letter, and intimates an enclosure. Dated June 24, 1721, the day after Mather noted in his diary that he was composing a letter to the town's physicians, in turn the day after he noted writing his treatise upon smallpox, I have assumed that these are all related. This date is far more consistent than the first letter's (June 6) with Boylston's claim that he began the experiment "after short consideration."

While it is impossible to know the shape of Mather's smallpox treatise exactly (it grew over time), I have followed Kittredge in supposing that the *Angel of Bethesda*'s smallpox chapter, "Variolae trimphatae," is a fair approximation. It is this that I have Boylston read.

Boylston's relationship to his slaves is unknown. On the one hand, he did not admit discussing inoculation with Jack in any detail. On the other, most of his published writings were composed as defenses of inoculation, and one of the charges he continually had to answer was a too credulous trust in blacks. Nevertheless, he proved the one man in Boston willing to trust African-born blacks' stories of inoculation (reinforced by the Royal Society) to the point of risking his children's lives. Jack is the obvious person for him to have questioned first in whatever investigations he made about African medicine.

We don't know anything about Jack other than his name, age, and inoculation experience. In Boston, domestic slaves generally lived with their masters as a part of the family (which then indicated everyone regularly living together in a household, not just the immediate blood and marriage relations of the patriarch). In the more humane households (Judge Samuel Sewall's, for example), slaves were certainly on familiar terms with the rest of the family and intimately trusted. Many enslaved blacks seem to have known their masters quite well. Indeed, most probably knew their masters far more intimately than anyone else did, except possibly spouses; certainly far better than their masters knew them. This is the sort of relationship I have tried to paint between Zabdiel Boylston and Jack.

Boylston probably spoke to as many African-born blacks as possible between receiving

Mather's letter on June 24 and inoculating Tommy, Jack, and Jackey on the twenty-sixth. Prizing firsthand examination of evidence, Boylston was later extremely frustrated by his fellow physicians' unwillingness to visit his inoculated patients. That attitude strongly suggests that he would have made every effort to consult witnesses and survivors of the operation before trying it. In his section of *Some Account,* he quotes the same black man that Mather does in his smallpox treatise. Boylston almost certainly relied upon Mather's transcription, though he translated it into more standard English. He may have merely taken the quotation from the minister. Boylston's commentary on the story is different from Mather's, however, and it seems equally likely that he heard the same story from the same source.

As much as possible, the thoughts and debates that Boylston holds with himself are based on his own writings.

The scene of the dying woman entering Boylston's shop is based on the defense of his experiment published in the anonymous *Vindication of the Ministers of Boston* (possibly by Cotton Mather):

> He had just reason to apprehend [his family] in danger of being infected the common way: and here I cannot omit to observe the happy juncture of affairs that united to render this his attempt innocent and blameless. The worthy TOWNS-MEN had taken the Guards off the Infected houses, and in effect proclaimed the infection so prevalent, that 'twould be in vain to strive to suppress it. By this act, the nurses were commissioned to air themselves, who had been stifled for a considerable time by a close confinement with the sick: Liberty was declared to them to walk the streets; and now as the necessities of the sick urged, these infected persons might go to our doctors upon any occasion; and any heedless or headstrong neighbours run in to visit their contagious friends; which must necessarily render their families very obnoxious to the distemper. This clearly evinces the eminency of the danger his [i.e., Dr. Boylston's] family was in; and in a great measure vindicates his procedure.

When he actually performed the operation, Zabdiel at first followed Timonius's instructions to the letter, including the bit of walnut shell as a shieldlike dressing—though he soon substituted cabbage leaves. Mather records that the doctor inoculated one of his first three patients in the neck; I have given him reason to do so.

At 6:00 A.M. on June 26, 1721—the very day that Dr. Boylston began inoculating— Captain Durell did indeed gather his guns aboard HMS *Seahorse;* soon after 10:00 A.M. he fired off a fifteen-gun salute in the harbor. The master's log credits a celebration of "the young princesse's [sic] birthday." The birthday of King George I's granddaughter Princess Caroline, at that time his youngest, was June 10 reckoned by Britain's Old Style or June 21 in the Gregorian New Style, as observed in Hanover where she was born. These two dates were often confused by her grandfather's British subjects. By June 26, though, either date would appear to have been more of an excuse for gun practice than anything else.

I cannot say for certain whether Dr. Boylston met Dr. Douglass that day, or whether they ever discussed inoculation in private. However, since Douglass seems to have taken upon himself the job of orchestrating opposition to Mather's story even before he knew it had been put into practice, it seems at least plausible that he canvassed Boylston among Boston's other medical men, only to find he was too late. I've written this scene to illustrate not only the two doctors' incipient antagonism, but other known defining (and mutually antagonistic) attitudes: as noted before, Douglass looked down his nose at Boylston's habit of making rounds on horseback. Conversely, Boston's streets gave Boylston (and anybody else in a real hurry) a cogent reason for choosing to ride, above and beyond sheer love of being on the back of a horse. The origin of Boston's streets in cow-paths is a joke of three centuries' standing; in the early eighteenth century, these famously "crooked and narrow" roads were often cut by open ditches and clogged with wayward traffic. (For those at wit's end over the Big Dig: Nothing changes under the Boston sun. Throughout the eighteenth century, the minutes of both town meetings and selectmen's meetings are strewn with complaints about the state of the roads, as well as notes on permits to dig them up.)

I've drawn the core of Douglass's expressions from a letter he wrote at the end of July, when he gloated over having cured a lady whose case was tricky; her cure, he said, had brought him wide patronage. In the same letter, he used the phrase *Make hay while the sun shines* in regard to Boston's epidemic, along with the Latin phrase *Hoc age*, meaning "Do this! Apply yourself to what is at hand!" I've substituted *carpe diem*—"Seize the day!"—because it is better known nowadays and in this context, at least, means roughly the same thing.

Conversely, Boylston seems to have regarded the epidemic with unremitting horror. Though frustration at times pushed him into mockery of his opponents, there is no comparable instance of him making light of the epidemic itself, much less exulting in it—though he, too, stood to make a great deal of money out of the disaster.

Douglass later bandied about the notion that Boylston had not treated a single case of smallpox when he began inoculation; I've given him at least a dubious basis for making such an unlikely claim. There is no precise record of either the numbers or the timing of Boylston's patients suffering from naturally contracted smallpox. However, Boylston's defenders, Benjamin Colman chief among them, retorted that he had both more experience and more success than any other doctor in town, with the possible exception of John Clark.

Boylston, Mather, and Hutchinson all wrote about the tremendous clamor in the streets as the town discovered what the doctor had done. To judge by his surgical daring and his horsemanship, Boylston was not a timid man. Nevertheless he repeatedly said he was frightened by both his son's uncontrollable fever and "the clamour, or rather rage of the people against" the new practice. Family legend, recorded by Zabdiel's great-nephew, Ward Nicholas Boylston (grandson of Zabdiel's brother Tom), has it that mobs "patrolled the town in parties with halters, threatening to hang him on the nearest tree." Though Ward Nicholas got many of his facts muddled, this one seems a realistic image of outraged clamor that might have shocked even a risk-taking man like his great-uncle.

The analogy between Zabdiel's life and the story of Abraham and Isaac is close enough that it might well have seemed inescapable to anyone, like Zabdiel, who had grown up amid the Puritan exhortations to apply the Bible to one's own experience.

As is so often the case, fact proves at least as quirky as fiction: from his house at the far end of the Boylstons' garden, the Reverend Colman witnessed Tommy trying to cool himself off under the pump, and Lieutenant Hamilton did indeed name a slave Cotton Mather, entering him into the *Seahorse*'s muster as his personal servant on July 2, 1721. The original Cotton Mather did not find out until the following December; he assumed it was meant as an insult.

Salutation Alley

The main events of this chapter—Tommy's recovery, the *Seahorse*'s departure, the various inoculations and warnings, and even Joshua Cheever's firefighting—are all documented. The details, especially the emotional connections, have to be inferred from the silences between Zabdiel Boylston's rather terse lines.

Tommy's temperature did suddenly go down on the morning of July 4, after his father gave him a "gentle" vomit; in all likelihood, the fever's nosedive was due to the natural course of smallpox rather than to Boylston's treatment.

While I do not know that Benjamin Colman took part in whatever celebrations shook the Boylston household after Tommy's fever went off, he did become one of Boylston's earliest and staunchest supporters—as well as his most convincing. Colman's elegance, moderation, and popularity with women have all been richly attested. As the Boylstons were part of his congregation, he would have been responsible for their spiritual welfare during this crisis.

On Tommy and Jackey's course through the smallpox, Boylston wrote only that on the fourth day "a kind and favourable Small-Pox came out, of about an hundred a piece; after which their circumstances became easy, our trouble was over, and they were soon well." It cannot, however, have seemed so carefree before he possessed the rose-colored glasses of hindsight, especially in light of Tommy's extreme first fever. Boylston did not inoculate anyone else until Joshua Cheever on July 12. By count of days through a typical case of discrete smallpox, that was the earliest point at which he might have been all but certain that both Tommy and Jackey would escape the second fever altogether, to survive without permanent damage.

As with Lady Mary, I've drawn details of Tommy's case (especially the timing and the particular look of the rash) from Ricketts, whose in-depth description of a light case of discrete smallpox with no secondary fever closely matches the outlines of Tommy's experience as sketched by Boylston. Even more intriguingly, Ricketts's description of "modified" smallpox—cases suffered by patients still partially shielded by long-past vaccinations whose protective mechanisms had partly to mostly worn off—also closely resemble Boylston's descriptions of inoculated smallpox. Both were marked by unusual speed in the progress of the disease, as well as by light rashes resembling the chicken pox; both rarely exhibited the fearful secondary fever common in cases of "natural" smallpox.

George Stewart was, as noted, a Scottish surgeon who had married the daughter of Boylston's mentor; professional rivalry goes a long way toward explaining their quick drift into loggerheads. Stewart later wrote a letter to Dr. William Wagstaffe of London in defense of his opposition to inoculation, noting that Boylston had privately admitted to him that his son came close to dying during the first fever. His propensity for pessimism, snide gossip, and defamation is made abundantly clear in an anti-inoculation column he later wrote for the *New-England Courant*. I have built the encounter between him and Boylston from these hints.

In his writings on inoculation, Boylston never pointed out Cheever as a friend; however, he did not point out any of his relations, including his brother Tom, as family either. On the other hand, he did include a few more details about Cheever's life (the firefighting, for example) than he did about most other patients. Just as many of the first inoculees in London have traceable connections to Lady Mary or the Princess of Wales, many of Boston's inoculees have connections to Boylston. I've surmised that both Cheever and Helyer belong among this group—as his friends—chiefly because, outside his family, they were the only two people he inoculated before publicly announcing his experiment. Furthermore, both were men close to him in age and socioeconomic status, and so far as can be traced, Cheever appears to have been, like Boylston, more of an active than a contemplative man.

Outside his family, all Boylston's earliest inoculees—with the exception of John Helyer—have clear ties to homes, jobs, or close family in or near Salutation Alley, to the

Salutation Inn at the eastern end of the lane, or to the New North Church at its western end (at Hanover Street). Cheever, for example, lived on the south side of the alley and was a deacon of the New North. Joseph Webb lived one street farther south, on White Bread Alley, and was also a deacon of the New North. His older brother John was the patriarch of the Webb clan (though at sixty-seven, he seems to have been a little frail, and if the opposition was right, may possibly have been senile); his eldest surviving son was the Reverend John Webb, first pastor of the New North.

I have surmised that John Helyer, a member of Mather's Old North Church, was a part of this same close-knit group of people. See the notes to "Signs and Wonders" for more details.

Salutation Alley still exists, though it has long since graduated to the status of "street." The winding dockside road that Boylston knew as Ann, Fish, and Ship Streets (and I have condensed to the single name of Ship Street) is now called North Street; it is considerably farther in from the shore than it once was. The taverns and inns named here are all known to have stretched in this order along the North End's wharfs at this period, or shortly afterward.

The anti-inoculators later insisted that Cheever and Helyer had pressed Boylston to inoculate them out of desperation, presumably stemming from known exposure to the disease. Boylston eventually inoculated both Cheever and his "lad"—a servant, slave, or apprentice, as he had no children—but not his wife. As with Jerusha Boylston, this implies that Sarah Cheever had either already survived smallpox, or had come down with it before Boylston was willing to inoculate anyone beyond the bounds of his own family. The latter possibility reconciles her own failure to be inoculated with her husband's desperate insistence upon it; furthermore, they lived in Salutation Alley, which was particularly hard hit by this epidemic.

In Massachusetts, public days of fasting, prayer, and humiliation were, by 1721, a traditional response to catastrophes ranging from smallpox to fire to menacing weather, dating back to an era when the iron piety of the Puritan ministers ruled the colony of Massachusetts Bay. July 13, 1721, however, was marked as much or more by political infighting as by devotion.

Boylston wrote that he had been given three warnings before appearing at the selectmen's meeting to discuss the dangers of inoculation on July 21. He did not say who delivered the warnings, or how.

The selectmen did meet on July 17, the last day of the brief adjournment the House had granted itself. Though no official discussion of inoculation was entered in the minutes, the three warnings to Boylston, plus the selectmen's well-organized and united resistance suggest strongly that they came to some kind of off-the-record agreement. The meeting that brought Boylston before all seven selectmen, several justices of the peace, and the town's physicians was likewise left out of the minutes for July 21.

No record of Jerusha Boylston's response to her husband's experiment on Tommy survives. The fact that all three of their daughters were home to be inoculated in one day about a month later, however, suggests that she cooperated, and very likely approved of his actions.

Prying Multitudes

Young Mary's rash did indeed erupt after only one night of moderate fever. Lady Mary's dream, however, comes from my own imagination, spun from Dryden's smallpox elegy and the classical tales that she loved.

Maitland identified none of his hard-won witnesses by name, noting only that "Three learned physicians of the college were admitted, one after another, to visit the young lady; they are all gentlemen of honour, and will on all occasions declare, as they have hitherto done, that they saw Miss Wortley playing about the room, cheerful and well, with the small pox rais'd upon her; and that in a few days after she perfectly recovr'd of them."

Dr. Walter Harris later identified himself in his own writing; he also recorded the number of little Mary's pocks. Dr. Keith's identity is clear from Maitland's notes on inoculating the doctor's son Peter, submitted to the Royal Society as a part of James Jurin's later project to apply statistics to the study of inoculation's efficacy. Keith's quick decision was no doubt hurried along by the fact that his family had proved achingly vulnerable to smallpox.

Wortley family tradition said that four physicians served as witnesses; Maitland had three. I have inferred Sir Hans Sloane as the third man and Dr. Steigerthal as the possible fourth. Sir Hans had long been gathering information on inoculation in the form of letters and testimony from abroad; by June if not before, he had become the driving force behind medical and scientific interest in the operation. As the king's personal physician, he was the liaison between the court and the medical profession. As president of the Royal College of Physicians, he certainly fell under Maitland's rubric of "learned physicians of the college." Dr. Steigerthal had followed the king to England from Hanover at royal request; from beginning to end, he was almost as closely involved in the royal consideration of inoculation as Sir Hans.

Dr. Mead had been Lady Mary's family physician since before she had suffered smallpox herself; Dr. Arbuthnot was a good friend. Though she was suspicious of medical men in general, it seems likely that her own familiar doctors would have been on hand as consultants throughout young Mary's bout with inoculated smallpox.

I've drawn the scene of Lady Mary and Mr. Maitland witnessing the witnesses from what is known about the doctors in question, inflected by attitudes that the two speakers displayed in their own writings. That Lady Mary and Mr. Maitland had something of a comfortable relationship is apparent from her long-standing willingness to trust the man with the lives of her children, and by the fact that he could coax her, at least occasionally, from adamant opposition into agreement with his actions and assessments.

As much as possible, Maitland's thoughts follow the paths and even the words he laid out in *Mr. Maitland's Account of Inoculating the Small Pox*, published in 1722.

As for Lady Mary's other visitors at this time, Maitland identified them only as "several ladies, and other persons of distinction." Lord and Lady Townshend, however, are likely candidates, as they were close friends. Lord Townshend was, as later described, the minister who procured legal clearance for the prison experiment. Among the many friends that Lady Mary and the Princess of Wales shared, I have chosen two: Elizabeth Sackville, duchess of Dorset, and Charlotte (Monck) Tichborne were both confidantes of Princess Caroline, and both girlhood friends of Lady Mary.

It is impossible, now, to trace with any accuracy the scheming that went on in the effort to bring the prison experiment into being, though clearly there was more than a little. Genevieve Miller would have it that the physicians, especially Sir Hans Sloane, were almost solely responsible. Contemporary writers in a position to know, including Maitland and Sloane, give much of the credit to Lady Mary and Caroline, Princess of Wales. Lord Townshend and the Whig ministry also had some part in it. I think it most likely that all these people were deeply involved, for many different reasons, ranging from scientific and medical, to personal and familial, to political. I have followed those who were there in giving to the Princess of Wales much of the credit for organizing the concerted push for the experiments.

The process by which the king came to his decision is obscure. It seems likely, though, that he would have asked the two Turks he knew best—Mehemet and Mustafa. By 1721, they had been with him for years (many more years than he had been king, in fact). They went everywhere with him, including driving in the park and attending the opera, and they could and did enter into quasi-familiar conversations with the king and the courtiers who surrounded him.

People who considered inoculation seriously almost all shared two experiences: first, they themselves had suffered a serious bout of smallpox (as had Zabdiel Boylston, Lady Mary, and the Princess of Wales), or had lost or nearly lost a loved one to it (as had Jerusha Boylston, Lady Mary, the Princess of Wales, and Dr. Keith). Second, they also tended to know one of the early inoculators well. I see no reason to think that in this matter King George would have been different from anyone else. In the absence of Lady Mary's diaries, I have no proof that he spoke to her in person about the proposed prison experiment. On balance, though, given the facts that they were on speaking terms, and that interest in inoculation seems to have been driven more strongly by personal relationships and trust than by anything else (except possibly desperation), it would be stranger if the king had not consulted Lady Mary, than if he had.

An Infusion of Malignant Filth

Five years after the fact, this meeting still made Boylston steam under the collar. Though the selectmen called the meeting, they did not record it in their minutes. A close approximation of what went on that day can be gleaned from the writings of both Douglass and Boylston, along with others who rushed to defend one side or the other. For example, on the subject of African inoculation being a common success, Boylston wrote: "I have as full evidence of this, as I have that there are lions in Africa. And I don't know why 'tis more unlawful to learn of Africans how to help against the poison of the Small Pox, than it is to learn of our Indians how to help against the Poison of a Rattle-snake." Piecing together real sneers and points made by Douglass, I have reconstructed a line of argument that culminates in such comments.

Dr. Douglass's arguments are marked by arrogant erudition and gleeful revelry in slander. In contrast, Boylston's arguments and rebuttals are marked by a wry humor as well as frustration, though it is clear that the plague argument made him lose his temper.

Douglass laid out his line of thought in a letter published in the *Boston News-Letter* three days later, on Monday, July 24; the letter, however, is dated July 20, 1721—a day *before* the meeting. This suggests that Dr. Douglass had advance warning in order to plan his attack; the content suggests that he had every expectation of conquest. He was almost certainly the orchestrator of the opposition at this meeting: Within days, and for the remainder of the controversy, he was the acknowledged leader of the anti-inoculators. That he already held this position by the time of this meeting is further attested by the fact that he was the interrogator and translator of Dr. Dalhonde. (Though Douglass did not sign his name to his inoculation publications until decades later, his veil of anonymity was transparent. Both his contemporaries and modern scholars have identified him as the author of the works I cite as his.)

Boylston's rebuttal was not published until a month later, in *Some Account of What Is Said of Innoculating or Transplanting the Small Pox*. In the second section of that pamphlet, he refutes many of Douglass's arguments point by point.

For both men, I've also relied on later writings that elucidate arguments suggested in these earlier pieces, especially when they do so in pungent language.

I present nowhere near all Dr. Douglass's many objections against inoculation, though I have touched upon those he hit hardest (that it amounted to poison, infringed on God's Providence, produced the plague, and was the product of lies and foolish dreams on the part of Africans, "Asiaticks," and women). Many of his arguments, however, quibbled with word choice and editing decisions in Dr. Mather's (slightly) abridged translation of the two papers from the *Philosophical Transactions*. While some of this is interesting if you have side-by-side texts in front of you, mostly it's mind-numbingly petty. I have tried to convey this pettiness in his stance toward Dr. Boylston: in his refusal, for example, to acknowledge Boylston as "Dr." (amply demonstrated in his writings, when he could bring himself to refer to Boylston by name at all; usually he preferred epithets like "the Inoculator," which he clearly regarded as a slur).

In opposing inoculation, Douglass operated at least as much by vicious personal attack as he did by reasoned argument against the procedure. Besides slandering Boylston, he repeatedly defamed the Greek women and the Africans whose testimony Boylston had accepted. The slurs included here are direct quotes or close paraphrases of Douglass's own words. The exceptions are the dismissive references to black Africans as "idiots" who used language blunderingly. These appear in one of Boylston's statements in *Some Account*.

Boylston was no saint; he was a slave-owner throughout his life. I've found no other instance, however, of his unprovoked use of such derogatory language. Furthermore, he alone had credited African experience enough to stake his child's life on it. In the context of the many arguments presented at this meeting and directly afterward, this particular statement reads to me as a mimicking reply to a particular challenge; since Dr. Douglass repeatedly used such language in making similar challenges, I've put this one into his mouth.

George Stewart recorded that the first part of the meeting devolved into a morass of squabbling in which Boylston was repeatedly asked whether inoculation was infallible, or whether people "might not die by it"—to which he repeatedly replied "that persons might die by a vomit or a purge" too. This did not satisfy the doctors, wrote Stewart, so "after a long debate, Mr. Dalohonde was called upon to say what he thought of it." As Dalhonde is said to have been called for at four o'clock and the standard dinner hour of the day was at two, I have made the company break for dinner.

Boylston attached a copy of an official transcript of Dalhonde's testimony to the end of his *Historical Account;* I have followed it, wherever possible, word for word, though I've loosened it up to wind it into the scene at hand, changing expressions that are incomprehensible without a medical dictionary, or that sound stilted to modern ears. From Boylston's later writings, it seems clear that he was blindsided by the plague argument, as well as by the fury of the opposition.

Dr. Douglass's use of the plague argument was entirely disingenuous. Both Mather and Boylston knew that smallpox and plague were unrelated, as did most medical theory of the day. It defies belief that Douglass did not, especially since, outside inoculation, his medical writing stressed the careful differentiation of diseases. Furthermore, Douglass was for the most part careful to use the smallpox-triggers-plague argument by suggestion rather than by direct argument. He carefully excised it from the anti-inoculation tracts he published in London.

While I can't definitely finger him as the source of the plague stories in the *Boston News-Letter* and later in the *New-England Courant,* they all lead up to—and away from—the double dark stars of Dalhonde's testimony (which he seems to have organized) and the letter he published July 24 in the *Boston News-Letter*. The Scots Charitable Society linked the owner of this paper with Douglass and George Stewart, the other leading anti-inoculation physician, also Scottish; its meetings seem a likely means of transmission.

Dr. Douglass's summation speech is a patchwork of actual statements, again edited for modern readability. The physicians' resolution appears in the appendix to Boylston's book along with Dalhonde's testimony. Its style and wording, including the introduction as the resolution of Boston's "medical practitioners" (the highest designation Douglass could bring himself to give Boston's other doctors) suggest that Douglass wrote it.

Cotton Mather wrote that the selectmen threatened Boylston with "indictment for felony." Douglass repeatedly implied that the felony in question was murder, a capital crime. He also claimed that the selectmen's decision had been unanimous.

Cheever began erupting on this day, by Boylston's own count of days from Cheever's inoculation. In giving Sarah Cheever a fierce case of smallpox and contrasting it to her husband's experience, I have given local habitation and names to the general contrasts, made often and with marked frustation, by supporters of inoculation. Boylston, Mather, and Colman all pleaded with their opponents to compare the ease of inoculated smallpox with the horrors of "natural" or "common" cases—as they called smallpox acquired in the natural way (by breathing in the virus, though they didn't know that part).

Finally, Boylston had inoculated Esther Webb's parents and uncle three days earlier, but not her (or her two younger siblings). I don't know that he saw her on this evening, but her fate was surely on his mind. For more on her and the Webbs, see the notes to "Signs and Wonders."

The Castle of Misery

Most of the individual fragments of this chapter are real; I have put them together into a collage that is factual in its pieces, though fictional in many of the precise connections.

Throughout the eighteenth century, Newgate was London's prison for hard-core violent prisoners, as well as burglars and thieves of all sorts. It had a few wards of debtors as well. Originally built in or near one of the principal gatehouses in the city's medieval walls, this "Castle of Misery" served (through several rebuildings) as a prison from 1188 until it was torn down in 1902. Its reputation was once as fearsome as those of the Bastille and Devil's Island.

London's *Weekly Journal or Saturday's Post* recorded that on July 24, 1721, the Prince and Princess of Wales's physicians, surgeons, and apothecary went to Newgate and picked two men and one woman to participate in the inoculation experiment. The chosen prisoners were removed to the Press Yard, "the most airy part of the prison," in preparation. At that time, the Press Yard certainly offered the most pleasant digs available in the prison; in normal circumstances, it was reserved for those who could afford its very steep rent.

I have surmised that Maitland was involved in the selection of prisoners, as he was the surgeon in charge of the experiment; Sir Hans Sloane may also have been there. Maitland recorded the names and ages of the six prisoners (the papers got the number wrong), as well as the fact that Evans had had smallpox earlier. (He was probably chosen as a control.)

Mary North was convicted, as noted, for the capital crime of returning to England after being transported, following a previous conviction for "robbing the shop of Mr. Baylis, a linen draper near Cripplegate." Her particular destination "beyond Sea" is unknown, though Maryland was receiving large numbers of criminal transports at that time. Also as noted, her husband turned her in. John Alcock was probably convicted of horse theft: the newspaper reporting his sentence is torn after the word *horse*. I have given the others capital crimes that often appear in the *Newgate Calendar*—the contemporary collection of "true-crime" stories relating the histories of interesting (or "infamous") prisoners in Newgate. Ann Tompion has been identified as the wife of the famous watchmaker Thomas Tompion. I've accepted this ID, though I have been unable to confirm it. Tompion was an unusual name, and while she was very young to have been his wife (he died, aged seventy-four, in 1713), it is likely that she was in some way related. She may have been the wife of the elder Tompion's nephew by the same name, also a watchmaker.

Elizabeth Harrison drew extra attention and interest from the men orchestrating the experiment, including Maitland and Sloane. I have given her a personality consistent with that interest. I do not know her particular trials and tribulations in prison, but all those mentioned here—the thick layers of lice, the misery of the Stone Hold, the sale of female prisoners to male prisoners, and the hard drinking and gambling in the prison's own tavern—are well attested at this period. Relatively trustworthy (and probably burly) men were indeed made quasi turnkeys, or wardsmen, by jailers who were chronically understaffed and often unwilling to pay for outside labor. There was also, right around this time, an infamous case of a murderer who cut a prostitute's throat while she was providing her services. Whether or not these particulars were part of Lizzy's story, they were certainly part of Newgate's history at this period.

The details of how the prisoners came to be selected have been lost. Most people, however—including prison doctors and chaplains—avoided entering the common side of the prison when they steeled themselves to enter the place at all. Besides the stench of its open sewers, the continual roaring, and a population of vermin so thick that you could hear it scrabbling on the floor, Newgate was a known breeding ground of both smallpox and typhus, then called jail fever (or ship fever). I've surmised that a number of prisoners were hauled out to some "airy" part of the prison for the inspection, and that even then, the inspectors maintained some distance.

One of the attending physicians noted that prisoners who were not part of the experiment tormented those who were with tales that the smallpox experiment was a sham, and that the doctors meant to drain their blood.

Signs and Wonders

Of the first twenty-three people Boylston inoculated, six were family. Of the remaining seventeen, fourteen had demonstrable ties to Salutation Alley: they either belonged to the extended Webb or Langdon clans, or were their neighbors or tenants. Of the last three, John Helyer was Cotton Mather's parishioner at the Old North Church; though I have not located either his workplace (he was a cooper) or his home at this time, he was close enough to Boylston to be one of the only two nonfamily members inoculated before publicly advertising the operation. I strongly suspect, though I cannot prove, that Helyer, like Cheever, was among the regulars at the Salutation Inn, and a close friend of Boylston's. Samuel Mather, of course, was Dr. Mather's son. The sole remaining inoculee was Samuel Valentine, nineteen-year-old son of John Valentine, His Majesty's advocate general of Massachusetts and Rhode Island. The Valentines belonged to King's Chapel, Boston's lone Church of England establishment; they lived in the South End, on Marlborough (now Washington) Street, near the governor's house.

Other than the Boylstons, who belonged to the Brattle Street Church, and Samuel Valentine, who belonged to King's, all these inoculees belonged either to Mather's Old North Church or John Webb's New North Church. In short, inoculation was a family, neighborhood, and congregational affair. (Even after the practice began to spread, almost all the inoculees belonged to the four churches of the ministers who signed the letter in defense of Boylston: Old North, New North, Brattle Street, and Old South. Mr. Cook's First, or "Old" Church provided a conspicuously low number of inoculees, as did King's Chapel.)

Lady Mary's biographer, Isobel Grundy, has presented overwhelming evidence from England showing that two main factors were crucial in convincing people to overcome rampant fears and put themselves or their children under inoculation: significant family losses from smallpox (parents, siblings, or children), and close personal ties to one of the inoculators or patrons of inoculation. So far as I have been able to trace, Boylston's list of inoculees follows suit—with the possible exception of Samuel Valentine, whose inoculation had clear political as well as personal import.

Unfortunately, for different reasons, both Boylston and Mather kept such family and neighborhood ties out of their writings on inoculation. The personal ties and emotional drives pushing early inoculation in Boston have to be reconstructed from what is known of the personalities involved and the intricate webs of family, workplace, and timing. The main sources are Boylston's *Historical Account,* Mather's diary, and various newspaper articles, along with genealogies, official town and province records, and the Thwing and Boston Church Records databases. Luckily, Bostonian Puritans were inveterate record keepers. I have pieced these fragments together into a plausible chain of events and emotions.

Here's what's indisputably historical:

Esther Webb and a servant or slave of the Cheevers were two of the first people Boylston inoculated, when he resumed inoculating. (All the dates and identities of inoculees are accurate; their courses through inoculated smallpox follow Boylston's notes on their cases.) Esther nursed her parents and uncle through their inoculations, but her own came too late; she came down with confluent smallpox, caught in the "natural" way, probably from her patients. (It is virtually impossible that her inoculation could have produced her illness, as she was showing symptoms within twenty-four hours.)

Boylston never said why he did not inoculate Esther Webb with her parents on July 19. Later, however, when a similarly large household in Roxbury begged to be inoculated simultaneously, he refused, dividing them up into two groups five days apart, so that everyone would not reach the spiking heights of the first fever all at the same time. I have given him the same reason in this earlier case. If he had indeed intended to inoculate Esther and her younger siblings three to five days after her parents, the selectmen's threat of a murder charge foiled their plan by a day or two.

Furthermore, if the Webbs' cases of inoculated smallpox followed the timing of Ricketts's "modified smallpox," then August 5 turns out to have been one of the earliest days it would have been possible to feel certain that the parents (the last of his first set of inoculees) would survive unscathed. It looks a lot as if after the meeting, Boylston was not waiting for the selectmen to relent so much as he was waiting until he had his own firm evidence that inoculation at the very least did not harm, before he tried it again. When he did, he immediately inoculated people he might have helped to put in harm's way.

Samuel Mather was the first and last person Boylston inoculated in secret; it was his grandfather Increase Mather who first suggested—and then pressed—for secrecy. His father vacillated for two weeks, finally allowing the operation the very day that Sammy's roommate at Harvard, William Charnock, died. (I follow Mather for the date of August 15, as his diary entry was written that day; Boylston's date of August 12 was printed six years later, from his notes, and is more open to error.) I have surmised that Mather maneuvered his way into the secret inoculation. Sly manipulating was part of his character; he seems to have been adept at disguising his machinations from himself, reading their results as the work of Providence. His inoculation-as-duty argument comes from a later pamphlet; it dovetails with his need to urge Boylston back into inoculating.

We do not know where the inoculation took place, but given Mather's need for secrecy, it may well have taken place on neutral ground, so that neither party would seem to be visiting the other. Boylston did inoculate Edward Langdon that same day. Langdon was soon to become a deacon in Mather's church; a few days before, Mather was privately worrying about his "pious barber"—likely to have been Langdon. Even from this distance in time, a visit to the barber's shop seems a great cover for a surreptitious meeting.

Dr. Mather did indeed let Providence open the Bible for him; he says it fell open to John 4:50, "Go thy way, thy son liveth." As if realizing that others would suspect a little Matherian help, he protested to his diary that Providence had not only not had help, but had had to work against a paper lodged behind the page. Many of Mather's thoughts in this chapter are drawn from diary entries I do not otherwise give; where possible, I stay close to his language. I have, however, put the apropos lamentations of Rachel (Jeremiah 31:15) into his mouth.

I have streamlined the confused and often vicious shouting in the newspaper, but Douglass's insults appear as he wrote them; Colman penned the distressed rebuttal that his fellow ministers signed.

Ben Franklin was, as written, the fifteen-year-old apprentice of his brother James Franklin, and thus responsible for delivering the *Courant*. In his *Autobiography*, he recalled having become a vegetarian when he was about sixteen. He wasn't too precise about dating childhood events, but I may have shifted this one up by six months or a year. By 1722, he was writing (anonymously) the famous set of "Silence Dogood" essays that are by far the best pieces published in the whole run of the *Courant*. I have made him slyly suggest a few bits of phrasing a little earlier. The words of warning he hears whispered in his ear is taken from a much later musing over this period, again in his *Autobiography*.

I don't know precisely how or when the selectmen discovered Samuel Valentine's inoculation; I am fairly certain that their reaction was similar to the one I have given them, in intent and force. Both the squabbling and the fear at the assembly of the General Court out on the Neck in the George Inn are apparent in the House of Representatives' *Journal*.

Newgate

Charles Maitland seems to have been a neat and deliberate man, down to his handwriting; he kept a detailed journal of this experiment, and published it as part of his book, *Mr. Maitland's Account of Inoculating the Small Pox*—one of the chief sources of London's earliest experiments with inoculation (Lady Mary's included). Much of this chapter, especially the sections from Maitland's point of view, quotes or closely paraphrases this journal. Alcock's bout of jail fever, his pricking of his pocks, Mary North's untimely bath, and even the three women's synchronized menstrual cycles all come from the surgeon's notes.

For all his precision and caution, Maitland could also lose his patience and even his temper now and again—just visible in bursts of irritation with John Alcock and Mary North.

According to Sir Hans Sloane, Maitland at first refused to conduct this experiment, and had to be coaxed into it by Sloane himself, after the Princess of Wales had already begged permission for it from the king. As is implied in several sources, I've therefore given Sir Hans supervisory charge of the whole, while delegating day-by-day control to

Maitland. Sir Hans's lecture during the operation itself quotes (with slight editing to fit the situation) from his later essay on inoculation.

About twenty-five men seem to have been present at the inoculation; many more visited in the ensuing weeks. One of these was the German Dr. Boretius, who noted that the prisoners trembled as Mr. Maitland drew out his lancet—as a result of other prisoners' tales that their blood was to be drained.

Dr. Wagstaffe published an anti-inoculation treatise in which he included his own journal of the experiment (he visited the prison almost every other day). Maitland wrote an answering pamphlet. Their exchanges here are based on the arguments and acidic tone of those pamphlets, keeping close to original language where possible.

In Boston, the chief anti-inoculation argument was that the operation spread the distemper—and put patients and others at risk for other diseases, such as the plague. In London, the chief argument of the opposition—at least at this early stage—was that the operation was a sham: that it communicated chicken pox, or something like it, not genuine or "true" smallpox: and therefore did not confer immunity. As in Boston, the participants quickly politicized the controversy, and the newspapers gleefully joined in.

Elizabeth Harrison's thoughts have been lost; along with the nickname Lizzy, I have given her an interest in nursing consistent with her later history.

I do not know the shape of the hall where the inoculation took place, or whether a barrier was erected to separate prisoners and spectators. It is clear, however, from many witnesses, that the prisoners were on display, rather like exotic animals at a zoo, for much of the day. Contemporary mental hospitals put their patients on display (often for a fee) in much the same way.

That Lady Mary was the "Mr. Cook, an eminent Turkey Merchant" whose "very ample testimony" Maitland "cannot forbear mentioning" in his Newgate journal is an intriguing possibility. I have pursued the notion for the fun of it—as Lady Mary certainly did with similar larks at other times in her life. A year later, she wrote a defense of the Turkish practice under the literary disguise of "a Turkey Merchant." (Isaac Massey quickly retorted that the piece was by "a sham Turkey Merchant"—though he did not appear to know who was behind the mask.) In Turkey, she had delighted in the habit of wandering about incognito in Turkish clothing—though usually dressed as a woman. She did maintain, however, that she had once sneaked into the Hagia Sofia disguised as a Turkish man. (She also visited it on an officially sanctioned tour, but that is no reason to discount such an escapade.) There were, however, a few Londoners named Mr. Cook who engaged in trade with Turkey at the time—though even that does not necessarily preclude such an adventure on the part of Lady Mary.

Isaac Massey fumed about hearing Maitland at Child's, boasting of the "success and security" of the Newgate experiments, though they had just begun—"as if," Massey wrote a year later, "he had had twenty years experience without any miscarriage."

Sir Hans Sloane was considering a further experiment to test the protective abilities of inoculation by August 22, when he wrote his friend Dr. Richardson that "We intend to try if carrying in people just up of the small-pox will infect these inoculated people or not." Another letter indicates that he had solidified his plans by September 14.

The sentences I have had Maitland draft for a report to the Princess of Wales appear in *Maitland's Account,* which he dedicated to her. On August 26th, the *Daily Journal* reported that the Newgate physicians had been ordered to lay an account of the progress before the king. As it was officially a royal experiment, it seems reasonable to assume some such order was made.

An Hour of Mourning

In his published account of inoculation, Boylston presented each patient separately, giving the date of his or her inoculation and noting symptoms and interesting developments, placing them in time by the number of days they appeared after inoculation. Into this calendar of hope and woe, I've woven other relevant material from Cotton Mather's and Samuel Sewall's diaries, the newspapers, Boylston family legend, opponents' snickerings, and various genealogies. I have not mentioned every inoculation he performed, though I have covered most of them. In general, I follow Boylston using the surrounding material to fill out the social and emotional implications.

Boylston devoted more space to detailing Mrs. Dixwell's case than he did to any others except Tommy, Jack, and Jackey, right at the beginning. She was, he said, "a fat Gentlewoman of a tender Constitution" who "came frightened into the Practice" after "passing some Days before by a Door wherein lay a Corpse ready for the Grave, which died of the Confluent Small-Pox, the stench whereof greatly offended and surprised her with Fear of being infected."

At least two of her children also had smallpox at that time; I have given it to all four. Boylston only mentions that two were allowed to visit her near the end, when they themselves were recovering from the natural smallpox. I have provided the reasons that the others did not visit. Though I don't know for certain that the infant Mary died of smallpox about this time, that event lies somewhere between possible and probable. She was certainly dead by 1725, when the three older children were mentioned in a deed as their mother's heirs, but little Mary was not. Boylston recorded Mrs. Dixwell's recurrent hysteria near the end; I have linked it to her baby's fate, as well as her own fears of death. Her husband's family history is fact.

Without knowing that Mather's and Boylston's records of Sammy Mather's inoculation were about the same person, it would be hard to guess that was so; I've tried to bring out the drama implied by that discrepancy. The boy's father was frantic with fear. In his eyes, his son's fevers were not merely life threatening, but the worst on record; his account suggests that the boy's distress reached hysteria. I have made him speak words he wrote in his diary. Boylston, on the other hand, tersely noted the second fever as "brisk." He adds the detail of giving Sammy an anodyne—or painkiller, often laudanum (tincture of opium)—along with bleeding him. Laudanum was a common treatment for hysterical nerves.

Boylston kept very close to the chest about his family; we do not know how he and Jerusha came to the decision for her to return, bringing the girls to be inoculated. He doesn't even say when they returned, though I am assuming that he inoculated them immediately. He certainly inoculated Zabdiel junior immediately after learning he had been exposed. The Turkish doctors called for a meatless diet while patients were under inoculation; I've fed the Boylston family such a dinner drawn from contemporary recipes.

The house of glazier Moses Pierce is one of the few from this period still standing in Boston; better yet, it is a museum, part of the Paul Revere House complex. I have surmised that Pierce was not inoculated because he had already survived smallpox. As their youngest child (at that time) was buried in 1721, it is likely that his wife, Elizabeth Parminter Pierce, was inoculated because her children had fallen ill.

Mrs. Bethiah Nichols's case follows Boylston's notes closely. Boylston, however, identified her only as "Mrs. N——s" without even the age that is so often helpful in identifying his patients with particular Bostonians: probably due to the serious and personal nature of her complications. However, he inoculated her at a time when he was still almost exclusively inoculating Salutation Alley folks, most of them belonging to either the

Webb-Adams or Langdon clans. Bethiah Webb Nichols, daughter of old John Webb—
one of Boylston's first inoculees—fits into this situation in every way possible. She was of
childbearing age, she had indeed been in the way of infection for over a month, and she
belonged to the tight-knit group of people most inclined to trust him with their lives.

The selectmen recorded their regulation of funeral bells in their minutes for September 11, 1721; on the twenty-first, they reissued the decree more stridently, suggesting that
their previous directive had been ignored. I do not know whether it was ignored on the
particular occasion of Frances Bromfield Webb's funeral: but that funeral, recorded by
Samuel Sewall, presented ample opportunities for tension between the inoculators and the
anti-inoculators to surface.

Whether or not Boylston was Frances Webb's physician is unclear, though he certainly
served as physician to many others in her family. I have invented her personality (and given
her the common nickname Fanny), but she was certainly much mourned at a very crowded
funeral; Mather did indeed preach the sermon.

The Adams's inoculations follow Boylston's account (and Adams/Webb/Jones genealogies) except that Boylston noted he inoculated "Mr. John Adams, about 35," that day,
along with Mr. Jones's child, Mrs. Adams (apparently Mr. Adams's wife, in context) and her
child. The Mrs. Adams and child were the particular two Marys identified. Boylston's John
Adams, however, would appear to be a mistake, confusing two brothers among the large
and tangled Adams family. Most likely, either "John" was a slip for his brother Samuel,
then thirty-two and husband of the thirty-year-old Mrs. Adams and father of the four-
year-old girl inoculated that day, or Boylston was badly off in estimating the man's age, as
John was then only twenty-eight. What seems likely is that both men were present and
one slipped in for the other in his notes. I have opted for keeping the nuclear family together, and gone with Samuel as the inoculee.

Boylston called Mrs. Margaret Salter "a weakly hysterical woman" who was "often
ill"—an unusually harsh assessment for him. "Tho' she had the Small-Pox very favourably,
as to Number," he added, "yet she complain'd much of Pain in her Head, and Vapours,
which gave me some Trouble; but in a short Time those Symptoms went off, and she soon
was well." I've extrapolated her insistent hypochondria and spoiled selfishness from his
uncharacteristic impatience.

One of Boylston's opponents tells the story of the saddle tarred and feathered on the
wrong horse. I have made Boylston and Cheever present, fitting the prank into a specific
time and place with plausibly high tension. I have also let Boylston once again display his
known horsemanship in calming the horse down. Mobs certainly trailed Boylston; the supposition that the Langdons and Webbs (and Cheever) helped protect him is mine.

With winter approaching, the firewood supply was a serious enough issue that
Mather did indeed consider it, and the selectmen did take up his suggested solution. Finally, while I do not have weather records for individual days of September 1721, it was a
wet enough month that powers as high as the governor worried about widespread crop
failure. Given that their Old Style dates are a week and a half behind our modern calendar dates, they were well into New England's leafy autumn fireworks by the time of Mrs.
Dixwell's death.

The King's Pardon

Elizabeth Harrison's deliberate reexposure as a smallpox nurse closely follows Mr.
Maitland's account. He does not, however, record the details of his offer or her acceptance, only those of her stay in Hertford. I have assumed that her acceptance was to some

degree voluntarily, as the crown seems to have observed its agreement to offer the inoculees full pardons.

She had every reason to be eager to find a place: no easy task for a woman of no training, no connections, and an unspotted reputation, and nearly impossible for a convicted felon. As bad as Newgate was, the descriptions of the Press Yard sound much more inviting than descriptions of London's slums at the same period, which do not seem to have been considerably better than the airless, windowless dungeons on the common side of the prison.

Sloane says that he and Dr. Steigerthal paid out of their own pockets for this extension to the Newgate experiment. I have given Maitland reason to select Elizabeth Harrison for such a nursing position, by giving her an aptitude for caring for the sick.

The Christ's Hospital buildings still exist in Hertford, though the school has moved. The students are still called bluecoats; statues donated in 1721 give a good sense of what they looked like.

Maitland's accounts of the Batt child and servants, and of the Heaths, is based on his *Account*, and remains close to his wording where possible. He told these histories separately; I have woven them back into Lizzy Harrison's story by having him tell her. Going by their difference in status alone, this would be unlikely; shared experiences of such tension as the Newgate experiment, however, can forge otherwise unthinkable bonds.

Maitland's final summation comes almost word for word from his *Account*, though I confess to moving paragraphs and some phrases around, and editing for modern readability: changing the now obscure word *imposthumes* to *abscesses* and shifting the *destroying angel* phrase so as to serve as part of his final word on the subject. The force and the drift of his words, however, remain his.

Raw Head and Bloody Bones

Once again, Boylston himself provides much of the raw data for this story, but the emotional impact has to be inferred by looking at what he did—and did not do—to whom, and when, and putting that together with fragmentary evidence from Mather, Douglass, the House of Representatives, the newspapers, and genealogies.

Dr. Douglass wrote the first of his many anti-inoculation letters to Dr. Alexander Stuart of London on September 25, 1721; it is hard to see how this was not in some way triggered by satisfaction with what he perceived to be proof of inoculation's failure: Mrs. Dixwell's death the evening before. The "one or two" deaths he records seem strangely haphazard for one so nigglingly precise—unless he already had Mrs. N—s in mind as a possible second.

Paxton advertised for his runaway slave in the papers, as noted; his elder son Roger was entered into the *Seahorse* paybook on September 25. The suggestion that the money and place for Roger would have been especially useful at this time is mine, though it is entirely plausible: Boston trade was at a standstill.

Mrs. N—s's complications are drawn from Boylston's notes—including her miscarriage of an eight or nine weeks' pregnancy, accompanied by serious hemorrhage, her delirious talk of floating in "the Waters" (for which I have supplied biblical references), and her loss of an eye. Boylston also recorded his midnight visit and his discovery of the fetus ("a small imperfect substance") in the bed the next morning (though I have added the detail of it being covered in pocks—something Mather claims happened in other circumstances). To the ends of their lives, Boylston's children remembered the whole family trembling whenever Boylston left, fearful that he would never return.

Cotton Mather recorded his daughter Abigail's death—and his reactions to it—in his diary. His *Account* is dated September 7, but is likely to have been the treatise sent over sea at this time. The Boston papers do not record any ships departing for London post–September 25 until Captain Mark Trecothick's *Friendship* was reported on October 2 as having already cleared outward; it is quite possible that this ship carried both Douglass's letter and Mather's treatise.

That Boylston had some kind of crisis of conscience in reaction to Mrs. Dixwell's death and Mrs. N—s's complications is apparent from the fact that from the day before Mrs. Dixwell's death, he ceased inoculating for almost two weeks: the longest gap in his record during the whole epidemic, other than that following his first inoculations of Tommy, Jack, and Jackey, and that following the selectmen's meeting. Furthermore, it would appear that he went on resisting inoculating for another three weeks: after inoculating Eunice Willard on October 6, he operated on no one else until the Fitches and Lorings convinced him to do so on the thirteenth, and then he ceased again until his brother's wife, having newly given birth, begged for his help.

Why he began again with Eunice Willard is unclear. She seems, however, to have been a personality of some force. The Willards were a large and powerful family of the South End; their father (dead by 1721) had been for years the minister of the Old South Church, and an outspoken opponent of the witchcraft trials. Eunice remained a spinster by choice, refusing several suitors and remaining in the family of her older brother Josiah, with whom she was very close. She was both well educated and well off in her own right; her conversation was said to be "entertaining and instructive, without the pedantry which some learned ladies discover too plainly." In 1737, she donated the sum of £5 to the workhouse—equivalent to as much as £500 today. Boylston had already inoculated David and Elizabeth Melvill (also known as Melvin), her nephew and niece by her sister Mary. I have made her give Boylston an invitation to inoculation that a man like him might well not refuse.

According to Boylston, her inoculation was a good one: at the usual time, she had "a kind, distinct sort, and was soon well." I have drawn details from the pictures of ease (including sitting up reading and taking a glass of wine with visitors) that Mather and Colman drew of inoculation while lauding it in distinction to the horrors of the natural smallpox.

The Lorings had their own connections to the Willards, and may have come to him from that direction; however, Loring's wife Susannah was the widow of Jerusha's maternal cousin Edward Breck before marrying Loring, and her children from her first marriage were thus blood relations to Jerusha. I have surmised that the family relationship might have tipped the balance in their favor. Boylston, of course, made no mention of a family connection—as he did not with anyone other than his own children (including his brother and sister-in-law).

Daniel Loring's elder son Daniel did break out in the symptoms of smallpox the night Boylston was supposed to have inoculated him. Boylston does not say what prevented him. He does say, however, that young Loring's death revealed one of the problems with assessing the successes and dangers of inoculation: it was very hard to tell whether people had already been infected (because of the long incubation period after exposure).

While I do not know how or where Boylston came to read the Boston newspaper accounts of the Newgate experiment, it is notable that their appearance coincides closely with his willingness first to inoculate more of his close family, and second, for the floodgates to open in the Boston gentry's desperate patronage of him and his operation. That his account appears together with the second notice (the first one of success) suggests that he had some forewarning of that success; Musgrave is a plausible source.

An advertisement for the camel appears in the same issue of the *Boston Gazette* as the first announcement of the Newgate trials; I have imagined Tommy's fascination with it.

It does not seem likely that Boylston's departure from Boston to inoculate his sister-in-law in Roxbury on the official Day of Thanksgiving was a coincidence: such days were high holy days. I do not know what happened to the newborn infant—but after the case of Esther Webb, Boylston knew inoculated smallpox was catching. It seems likely the infant boy would have been kept out of harm's way until his mother's recovery. He was not inoculated, and infants stood very poor chances in the face of natural smallpox.

Boylston says a coach fitted with a bed was provided for his sister-in-law's return to Boston; I have made Abigail Mather Blague provide it—and Boylston inoculate her young slave girl in return. The girl was definitely inoculated that day, though the reason is my surmise—as is Mrs. Blague's personality. She was a Mather, however, so it seems likely for her to have been both formidable and generous.

Kittredge would have it that Mather wrote *A Faithful Account;* I follow Fitz in sensing that in style, content, and context, this is from the pen of Boylston.

The Massachusetts House of Representatives' *Journals* show both that body's desire to conclude its business quickly in the face of the epidemic, and its inability to do so.

Mather's run-in with Franklin is only attested by Franklin; however, he had another such public shouting match with Samuel Sewall at an earlier point, so while Franklin may have exaggerated, he probably didn't have to exaggerate very much. Franklin quotes him quoting the loin-smiting passage of the Bible.

Just Retribution

The story of the attack on the Boylstons' home is based on family legend; I have tried to disentangle obvious exaggerations from probabilities and plausibilities, and fit the latter into a sensible pattern based on known facts. Boylston family legend has it that "one evening while [Zabdiel's] wife and children were sitting in the parlor, a lighted hand grenade was thrown into the room, but the fuse striking against some furniture fell off before an explosion could take place, and thus providentially their lives were saved." Because the grenade is said to have lost its fuse—as Mather's certainly did—and because Mather made a fuss that left a long, still readable trail while the Boylstons did not, it has sometimes been assumed that the attack on the Boylston home is Ward Nicholas Boylston's confusion of his family's story with the Mathers' story.

Against that, Ward Nicholas knew his great-uncle Zabdiel and his mother's cousins (Zabdiel's children), who were present, as well as his own grandfather (Zabdiel's brother Thomas), who was in a position to know the truth. While Ward Nicholas often exaggerates, I think complete confusion or creation of this attack de novo is unlikely. Thomas Hutchinson (who was ten in 1721, and later became governor of the province) later wrote that Boylston's "family was hardly safe in his house, and he often met with affronts and insults in the streets." Boston had a bad reputation as a town prone to mob violence; it was so bad in 1721 that the General Court had passed a riot act earlier that year. As the dying reached its height—and people began running to be inoculated—street violence certainly picked up. Furthermore, much more of the violence and hatred seems to have been aimed at Boylston than Mather. I think a rain of stones against the Boylston house, possibly topped off by some kind of poorly made grenade or bomb—the same as might have been used against Mather—is not only plausible, but probable.

If the attack on the Boylstons' home took place the same night as that on the Mathers'—which seems likely, given the nature of crowds—Boylston responded by inoculating once more the following morning. Quietly putting his head down and going right ahead with his practice, while refusing to pursue vengeance (legal or otherwise), seems as much a part of Boylston's personality as shouting and demanding justice from the authorities seem a part of Mather's. I do not know that Pierce replaced the broken windows, but it seems plausible for exactly the reason stated.

Ward Nicholas also says that Zabdiel visited patients "only at midnight, and in disguise." Boylston's own notes record visiting Mrs. N——s at midnight, when called on an emergency; no doubt there were others. On such occasions, he may well have wrapped himself in a cloak against weather and recognition—but a false nose and glasses seem as unlikely as the notion of taking *no* precautions in the face of threatening mobs.

As for hiding, Ward Nicholas records that "the only place of refuge" left to Zabdiel "at one time was a private place in the house where he remained secreted fourteen days, unknown to any of his family but his wife." Given Zabdiel's inoculation records, this is not possible. It is possible, however, that he did not go out much in the two weeks following Mrs. Dixwell's death. I have made him hide the one and only time it would have seemed necessary: when a potential lynch mob was actually storming the house. The place is my own invention.

Finally, Ward Nicholas noted that "parties entered his house by day and by night searching for him." Again, this seems an exaggeration—though without a police force, it would be hard to stop mobs from doing so. I have created a search I think more likely: a more calm search on the part of authorities—looking for Boylston ostensibly in order to protect him, and also for the out-of-town inoculees that these authorities had recently declared illegal.

Mather recorded in his diary the 3:00 A.M. attack on his house—along with a description of the "grenado" and the threatening strip of paper wrapped around it. The governor and council convinced the House to offer a £50 reward for information about the culprit (in Britain, this would have meant roughly £5,000 in today's money, though colonial currency was notoriously unstable). Though the reward was handsome, no one came forward.

The Royal Society's minutes reveal that Alexander Stuart read the first of Douglass's letters to him from Boston on November 16, the same day that Sloane reported Maitland's conclusions from Hertford. French and English drafts of this report are extant in Sloane's papers in the British Library; Miller has argued from internal evidence that the French drafts were meant for the Prince and Princess of Wales (who preferred to do their official reading in that language, though they had learned at least some English by this point).

I do not know for sure why Dummer held back from publishing Mather's report, especially since someone—possibly Dummer himself—seems to have leaked news of its positive nature to Sloane; the possibility that they were urging the use of Mather's name seems a plausible reason.

Dr. Douglass's retreat from the public eye and his defensive admission that his own plan of treatment had not gone as well as he hoped are drawn from his own (later) words.

Hutchinson's illness, will making, and death, the consequent panic and proroguing of the General Court, Robie's inoculating, and Boylston's sudden popularity are all documented. I have woven these events together; the connections are more plausible than a sudden cluster of coincidences. I have specifically made Hutchinson's case confluent and have surmised that Robie was his doctor: I do not think it was coincidence that Robie began inoculating the very day that Hutchinson died—and one week after Boylston began inoculating Robie's students and fellow Harvard faculty members en masse. One month earlier, Boylston noted that several people who had refused inoculation then died of the natural smallpox, spending their final breath urging their friends to "hasten into" the operation; I have made Hutchinson one of these people.

Sewall recorded that Hutchinson's funeral was a "great" one. I do not know whether Boylston went or not, nor do I know that he joined the Salutation Inn crowd later. His sentiments there, however, are his own.

In Royal Fashion

Maitland's *Account*, Dummer's belated (and anonymous) release of Mather's *Account*, and the further trials on six genteel subjects all hit London's notice at virtually the same time.

I do not know when precisely the princess became specifically interested in Boylston. She kept close abreast of inoculation publications, however, and Neal was summoned to speak with her soon after his publication. (I have surmised that she also spoke to Dummer.) Neal's suggestion that Boylston be asked for his account is the first I have been able to locate. In the end, it was the princess and Sloane who convinced Boylston to put pen to paper; I have let Neal plant this suggestion in her brain. In the matter of inoculation, I have also deduced some measure of competition arising between the colonies and the capital, along with respect and curiosity—as history showed them to have in so many other matters.

Sloane's conversations with the Princess of Wales and the king are based on his own reports. He does not give locations or specific times, but he does include the most important parts of the dialogue. The princess asked his advice about inoculating the princesses, he refused, and she followed up by asking if he would dissuade her. The king (who was famous for tiring out others on long walks in the park, regardless of the weather) asked whether inoculation would work and, when told accidents might happen, retorted that any physic might at times go wrong. I do not know whether Sunderland (or anyone else) was present, but as Sunderland was certainly close in the king's counsels and suddenly decided to inoculate his son just before the princesses' operation, it's a plausible supposition.

Beyond Amyand, Maitland, Sloane, and Steigerthal, I do not know who was present at the inoculation of the princesses at St. James's. I've drawn this scene from Amyand's and Maitland's reports to the Royal Society of what they did, and from contemporary and modern assessments of the royal family's character and habits. Princess Amelia was called Emily by the family; she took after the king in loving dogs, horses, hunting, and brisk walks outdoors; the prettiest of the three sisters, she was an extrovert and a flirt. Princess Caroline was a shy mother-hen who doted on her oldest sister and her mother. Pierre and Anne-Caroline are my imagination, though they fit in with the princesses' personalities. Princess Anne had become Handel's pupil at age eight, and often played for the family.

The accounts of the Sunderland, Amyand, Bathurst, Berkeley, Townshend, Tichborne, and De La Warr children follow factual reports by their physicians and surgeons. Arbuthnot—one of the attending doctors—provided the best account of the death of Bathurst's servant (though anonymously, in *Mr. Maitland's Account . . . Vindicated*); Dr. Wagstaffe supplied other details. The newspapers reported that the princess spent the evening of April 25 with her daughters, while the king and the prince went to Handel's opera.

Lady Mary's literary masquerade as a Turkey merchant, taking on the physicians, is genuine. It is not clear when she wrote it, though Grundy argues it was well before the edited version appeared in print. Lady Mary's run-in with Sloane is my supposition. She attended, however, many of the inoculations performed under the supervision of Sloane,

Steigerthal, Arbuthnot, and Mead, and by Maitland and Amyand (though she did not give many particular names). Given the level of her ire, it seems improbable that she did not have regular disagreements with these men in person—she certainly knew Sloane, Arbuthnot, Mead, and Maitland well enough to speak her mind frankly before them. That one or several of them faced her with her literary "crime" also seems probable: by the following spring, someone had convinced her that the two deaths she here calls murders were not, in fact, due to inoculation.

Wagstaffe, Edmund Massey, and Isaac Massey were the leading opponents of inoculation in London.

Jurin made his report to the Royal Society at the time stated, later publishing it in the Society's *Philosophical Transactions,* as well as separately in a pamphlet.

As for the princesses' inoculation, I do not know who beyond the medical men attended the inoculation of Prince William at Leicester House—but that, even more than the princesses' operation, was an occasion of state importance: the little prince was third in line for the throne.

Lady Mary gave very few specific names of those who begged her presence and got it—though she said repeatedly that she was run off her feet in complying. The duchess of Ancaster, however, is a very good bet: Jane Brownlow Bertie was a childhood friend who had specific smallpox memories with Lady Mary. I have, however, given her the title of duchess about one month earlier than she acceded to it (by the death of her father-in-law); when her daughter was inoculated on May 11, 1723 (the same day as the prince), she was the marchioness of Lindsey. I have written the scene to bring to life the unbalancing difference between the hooting and jeering of crowds, and the anxious supplications of parents Lady Mary recorded in her diary. Her final words I have borrowed from the closing sentence of her inoculation piece in her *Embassy Letters.*

Meetings and Partings

Whether or not Lady Mary and Zabdiel Boylston met remains one of the great enigmas of this tale. In solving the mystery, I have been more speculative in this chapter than in the others. I have built the story, however, on tantalizing fragments of evidence.

In brief, Boylston embarked for London in December 1724 on Captain Barlow's ship. During his year-and-a-half stay, he did not perform any inoculations, but he was in high demand to attend them. At the time, so was Lady Mary. Many of the same people who welcomed him warmly into the Royal Society were her close friends. So, although I have uncovered no evidence of their meeting, it is hard to imagine that they did not.

Here are the historical details:

Boylston's brief remembering of the end of the epidemic, through the summer of 1723, is accurate in the events, though I have supplied emotions and reactions that make sense. In May he inoculated six people who were soon packed off to Spectacle Island; Robie noted that they had been "forced" there by the "Boston mob." Boylston was hauled before a town meeting. Though Boylston did write the medical excuse that got James Franklin released to the press yard, I do not know if it was Josiah Franklin who asked him to do so. Samuel Adams of Revolutionary fame was born as noted. The grim numbers are drawn from Boylston and Douglass, both quoting official town statistics.

Boylston family legend has it that Sir Hans Sloane invited Boylston to London. While I have found no hard evidence of such an invitation, it seems plausible enough. Sloane certainly chaired the first meeting of the Royal Society that Boylston attended—soon after his arrival in London. Boylston himself intimates that both Sloane and the Princess of

Wales encouraged him to write up his account of inoculation early in the spring, again, quite soon after his arrival.

Additionally, Boylston's submission of a paper to the Royal Society before he took ship suggests that someone was pushing him to bolster his résumé, so to speak—or, as I have surmised, that someone at the Royal Society elicited a paper from him, assuming he would realize that what the Fellows really wanted to know about was inoculation. Both the bolstering (if it was that) and the writing are out of character for Boylston. In contrast to Mather, he took little pleasure in writing papers and letters to the Royal Society once he was a member—and did so only rarely. In no other instance did he write to publish without some kind of duress: self-defense, royal command, or (as is obvious in his few later communications with the Royal Society) a burdensome sense of duty too long neglected.

The instigator might well have been Cotton Mather, who wrote Boylston letters of introduction to Sloane and Jurin, suggesting a royal presentation. Sloane, however, was an even more inveterate collector of knowledge than Mather. He wrote voluminously to many people, and he was also the orchestrator of the English trials of inoculation— certainly at the princess's behest, but also, apparently, to satisfy his own professional curiosity. He may well have taken it upon himself to make such an invitation, or to solicit it through contacts like Mather—especially if it already had royal force behind it.

For the few words Boylston reads from Sloane's "letter," I have used standard phrases of politeness that Boylston later employed in the dedication of his book.

Boylston's report home to Colman confirms that he was in part an emissary to the governor for the moderates of Boston. This may have been another inducement for him to go—though his aloofness from Boston politics make it unlikely that this diplomatic mission was his primary reason for heading to London.

I do not know whether Sloane or anyone else found Boylston's submission of a paper on ambergris funny. The merchant Thomas Hollis certainly thought Boylston "ingenuous" by London's worldly standards. Back in Boston, though, the "ambergrease"/bear's grease confusion was real: though it may have been a deliberate prank rather than a muddleheaded mistake, as the man then in charge of the *Courant* was none other than Benjamin Franklin.

It is not clear whether or not Boylston's family went with him, but the few extant clues suggest that they did not. His son Zabby certainly remained at Harvard, where he got into enough trouble drinking and carousing to be reprimanded by the president. None of the few notices of Boylston in London mention anything about his wife or children being there as well—though Hollis twice found fit to mention Boylston's horses. Furthermore, his advertisements appear to offer to rent part of his garden and the right to sell its produce out of his shop—but not to rent the house, stables, or shop itself. Finally, his first extant letter back to London—to Sir Hans—notes his joyous return to family, friends, and country.

A number of his horses, however, did go and caused something of a stir, at least among the Americans in London. I have assumed that Jack went with him, as servant and groom, and possibly Jackey as well. Curiously, I have found no scrap of evidence indicating whether or not he returned to America with the horses. That he took them at all is intriguing—it cannot have made for a small shipping charge or an easy crossing. Even more intriguing is Hollis's note that he was refusing to part with them even for very handsome sums, coupled with his own later offer (through Jurin) to send the royal children saddle pads, in what sound like surprisingly familiar terms. This suggests the possibility that he intended his horses as princely gifts, and quite possibly presented them—though again, I have turned up no evidence.

Family legend also has Boylston inoculating the first two royal princesses (Emily and Caroline); his great-nephew Ward Nicholas Boylston insisted upon this point, though it is patently impossible (Amyand did it, and Boylston was in Boston at the time, in any case). Dr. Boylston was, however, in London at the time that Princess Mary was inoculated. He may well have been invited to be present, given the royal family's penchant for having all possible experts dancing attendance: he was, after all, far and away the world's most experienced inoculator outside Turkey and western Africa. Sergeant Amyand did the cutting, once again, but Boylston's possible presence as witness seems a likely—and understandable—source for his great-nephew's later insistence that Boylston inoculated a princess or two.

I have drawn his encounters with Prince William and Prince George from their known personalities and interests, matched with Zabdiel's own pride in his horses. That he spoke to William is suggested—though not proven—by a letter he later sent to Dr. Jurin, offering to send "Prince William and the young princesses" saddle pads—a specific kind of American training saddle. In context (it occurs as an afterthought, in a postscript) it reads as if he has met the children—particularly William—and discussed horses with them. This certainly fits in with family legend that he met the royal family—and was given a reward for his work. (The stated sum, £1,000, is likely an exaggeration, however, as that was the lavish sum given by the king to Maitland for traveling to Hanover and inoculating Prince Frederick.)

Lady Mary's encounter with her father as he arrived unannounced in her dressing room was burned into the memory of her daughter, who was present; she in turn, passed the story on to her children. It was the only time that young Mary (later Lady Bute) recalled laying eyes on her grandfather. In the family tale, the visit stands alone, unconnected to any particular event: I have linked it to his decision to inoculate his heirs. In Lady Bute's much later memory, she seems at the time to have been of an age to make this connection plausible.

The letters from Mather to Jurin, Boylston to Colman, Lady Mary to her sister and Boylston's final letter to Sloane are genuine. Jerusha's "Come home to me," however, is supposition, though surely some sort of plea must have been made.

Both Lady Mary and Boylston are hard to trace across the year 1725–26. What little information I've given for Boylston is what can be gleaned from later writings and genealogies. For Lady Mary, I have relied upon Isobel Grundy's biography—though I interpret the Richardson painting (c. 1725) differently. Her clothing comes very close to the Turkish costume described in her *Embassy Letters*—though the décolletage and the waistline have been altered to suit European style. The black boy is often referred to as a "page," which may well have been his job; the disturbing gleam of a silver collar around his neck, however, surely indicates that he was a slave, whether or not he was hers. His identity has never been discovered. The Wortleys are not known to have had a black servant, though he may well have been "borrowed" from friends who did.

Richardson was a regular at the Royal Society's unofficial home at the Grecian, and his closest friends included many of the Society's staunchest advocates of inoculation: Arbuthnot, Cheselden, Mead, Sloane, and Dr. Frederick Slare. Another of the painter's dearest friends was Alexander Pope. (Both Richardson and Cheselden spent time with Pope at his villa in Twickenham; Pope stayed with Richardson when he was in London.) All of these people, with the exception of Cheselden and Slare, were also Lady Mary's good friends. Boylston certainly met all of the Fellows, and may well have crossed the Atlantic in part to learn the new method of lithotomy from Cheselden. Although I cannot finger a time or place when all these people came together, the circumstantial evidence that Boylston circulated among these people is very strong. It lends some credence, too, to the possibility that the painting in question does indeed commemorate the battle against smallpox. Such portraits were often commissioned by patrons other than the sitter; Pope, for one, was known to have commissioned and treasured other portraits of Lady Mary. Small groups of friends gathering to watch an artist at work in his studio was a common and convivial pastime among the leisured classes.

From her letters, Lady Mary appears to have been giddily in love in the summer of 1725; by the spring of 1726, this infatuation had faded, apparently unconsummated and possibly unrequited. Again, her beloved's identity is lost. While she gazed elsewhere, Alexander Pope was gazing at her.

To her family, Lady Mary maintained that the infamous quarrel between her and the poet began when, with ill-chosen timing, he declared his passionate love for her, and she laughed at him. Pope scholars tend to dismiss this event as fiction; Lady Mary scholars tend to accept it as at least a contributory factor.

Smallpox did kill Lady Townshend that spring; with terribly irony, it also took another of Lady Mary's girlhood friends who had refused inoculation. In the latter case, however, I have avoided introducing a new character, but preserved the historical irony by substituting Philippa Mundy in the place of Sarah Chiswell—probably another of the Sisters in Affliction. (As Lady Mary's live-in companion, Chiswell played her own part in the Paradise adventures; presumably because she was present. No letters survive to trace her role.)

Boylston presented his book to the Royal Society to great acclaim. The sentence I have him read is his (though I have edited and abridged it slightly and added the phrase *also called inoculation*). The image of taming the smallpox, in other words, is Boylston's; I am, however, responsible for making him restate that idea more succinctly as "we have tamed the smallpox." The standing ovation is my crystallization of all his other applause— I do not know precisely what went on in that room in Crane Court, though it was clearly highly complimentary.

His ensuing election as a Fellow is recorded fact.

ABBREVIATIONS

BG: *Boston Gazette*
BL: The British Library
BNL: *Boston News-Letter*
BTR: *Boston Town Records*
CM: Cotton Mather
CMA: CM, *Account*
CMD: CM, *Diary*
CMAB: CM, *Angel of Bethesda*
CMSL: CM, *Selected Letters*
DAB: *Dictionary of American Biography*
ELCP: *Early Letters and Classified Paper* (The Royal Society)
EWM: Edward Wortley Montagu
Grundy, LMWM: Isobel Grundy, *Lady Mary Wortley Montagu*
JHRM: *Journals of the House of Representatives of Massachusetts*
LM: Lady Mary Wortley Montagu
LMCL: LM, *Collected Letters*
LMEP: LM, *Essays and Poems*
LMRW: LM, *Romance Writings*
Miller, AIS: Genevieve Miller, *The Adoption of Inoculation for Smallpox*
MMV: *Mr. Maitland's Account . . . Vindicated.*
MS: Manuscript
MSS: Manuscripts
NEC: *New-England Courant*
NEHGR: *New England Historical and Genealogical Register*
NPG: National Portrait Gallery, London
PRO: The Public Record Office, London
PTRS: *Philosophical Transactions of the Royal Society*
RCB: *Records of the Churches of Boston*
RSI: The Royal Society, *Inoculations*
SM: *Selectmen's Minutes*
SSD: Samuel Sewall, *Diary*
Thwing RCN: Reference Code Number, *Inhabitants and Estates* database on the Thwing CD

WD: William Douglass
WDCC: WD, "Letters . . . to Cadwallader Colden"
WDD: WD, *Dissertation*
WDPE: WD, *Practical Essay*
WDS: WD, "A Digression Concerning the Small-Pox"
WHO: Frank Fenner, et. al., *Smallpox and its Eradication* (published by the World Health Organization)
ZB: Zabdiel Boylston
ZBHA: ZB, *An Historical Account*, 2nd (corrected) ed.

SOURCES

This book is indebted throughout to Robert Halsband's and Isobel Grundy's encyclopedic scholarship on Lady Mary's life, and to their meticulous editions of her works. Kenneth Silverman's scholarship on Cotton Mather has proved equally indispensable. Far less scholarship exists on Boylston, but Gerald Marvin Mager's doctoral dissertation, *Zabdiel Boylston: Medical Pioneer of Colonial Boston*, offers a solid starting point. Charles Creighton's 1894 *History of Epidemics in Britain*, Genevieve Miller's *Adoption of Inoculation for Smallpox in England and France*, and John B. Blake's *Public Health in the Town of Boston, 1630–1822* (the latter two both from the 1950s) all remain treasure troves of eighteenth-century descriptions, medical theories, and statistics concerning smallpox.

The finest modern descriptions of the symptoms and course of the disease are Thomas Francis Ricketts's 1908 study *The Diagnosis of Smallpox*, based on his work as medical superintendent of London's smallpox hospitals, and the World Health Organization's justifiably triumphant *Smallpox and its Eradication*, which appeared eighty years after Ricketts's work, coauthored by the international team of crusaders who finally conquered the disease: Frank Fenner, Donald Ainslie Henderson, Isao Arita, Zdeněk Ježek, and Ivan Danilovich Ladnyi.

Biblical quotations are from the King James Version of 1611.

In quoting eighteenth-century writers and speakers, I have updated spelling and pronunciation, and substituted *you were* for *you was* (then standard), and *it's* for *'tis*. My goal has been to allow the speakers to sound natural to modern ears—as they did to each other—rather than quaint and archaic. I have tried, however, to retain their greater sense of formality and decorum (though their distinctly pre-Victorian humor and oaths were often more earthy than is commonly realized today).

References are keyed to the Bibliography. Throughout, I refer to Lady Mary Wortley Montagu as LM, Edward Wortley Montagu as EWM, Zabdiel Boylston as ZB, Cotton Mather as CM, and William Douglass as WD.

Introduction

Reactions to LM: Stuart 36; reactions to ZB: Peter Thacher 777; ZBHA Preface.
Eradication of smallpox from nature: Tucker 1 (prison metaphor), 3 (victim count

and comparisons to bubonic plague and twentieth-century wars), 116–118 (last-known case).

Odds of the vaccine resulting in death: "Vaccinia (Smallpox) Vaccine Recommendations"; odds of variolation resulting in death: Jurin, *Letter to the Learned Caleb Cotesworth* and his 1724–27 series of pamphlets titled *Account of the Success of Inoculating the Small Pox in Great Britain.* Arguments over the origin of vaccinia: Tucker 37–38.

Jenner: see sources for "The Practice."

Two Marys

Queen's illness and death: Contemporary accounts: Creighton 2:459–60; Walter Harris, *De Morbis Acutis Infantum* 158–63. Modern biographies: Chapman 250–60; Elizabeth Hamilton 327–37. Queen's "why are you crying?" and king's letter: Chapman 252.

Hemorrhagic smallpox (early and late): Ricketts 73–103; WHO 37–38; WDPE throughout; WDS 401–403; Mead 236–239. "Like creatures flayed": ZBHA 38. Fatality statistics: WHO 5.

Garden imagery: scattered throughout Mead; Walter Harris, "De Inoculatione Variolarum" and *De Morbis Acutis Infantum;* ZBHA; WDD; WDPE; WDS.

Historical confusion of smallpox with measles: Creighton 1:448–55.

Gloucester's death: Gregg 120–21. Smallpox death statistics for 1694 and 1700: Creighton: 2:456 (death figures from the London Bills of Mortality).

LM's childhood: Grundy, LMWM 5–13; chasing the sun: LMCL 3:132; chasing the steeple of Salisbury Cathedral: LMCL 1:112. Thoresby: John Harris, "Thoresby House" and "Thoresby Concluded."

Kit-Cat visit: LM's recollection: Stuart 9; toasts: *Miscellany Poems* 5: 60–70; LM's verse to Lord Halifax on the Countess of Sunderland: Harrowby MS 250, folio 4. Kit-Cat history and membership: Allen 33–54; Caulfield. "Pleasure was too poor a word . . .": adapted from Stuart 9.

Eighteenth-Century London: Ashton, Besant, George, Picard; Eighteenth-century dress: Buck, Cunnington.

Three Rebellions

LM's girlhood: Grundy, LMWM 14–29; garden-wall escapade with Brownlows: LMCL 1:23. LM's youthful writings (including the book burning): Grundy, LMWM 18–21, and Grundy, "'The Entire Works of Clarinda.'" The two albums: Harrowby MSS Trust MSS 250 and 251. Dorchester's children greeting him on bended knee: Stuart 31; Kneller's portrait of Dorchester, c. 1709: NPG 3213; Dorchester's character: Stuart 8. Secret learning of Latin: Spence, *Observations* 1:303–04, and Grundy, LMWM 15–16.

LM's friendship with Anne Wortley and meeting of EWM: Grundy, LMWM 28–33. EWM's gift of Quintus Curtius with inscribed poem: Stuart 15. Courtship, elopement, and early married life with EWM, generally: Grundy, LMWM 30–65, LMCL 1:4–181. Betty Laskey fiasco: LMCL 1:27–40; LMEP 80; Laroon 138–39, 166–67; Ashton 365–66, 369–70. 1710 Smallpox epidemic: Creighton 1:461 and 2:57; Jurin's later statistics: Miller, AIS 114–18. Quack medicine advertisements: Defoe, *Journal* 30–31. Life and street encounters during an epidemic: Miller, AIS 37–43; Creighton 2:452–53. Margaret Brownlow's death: Grundy, LMWM 23; LMCL 1:34. Recipe for applying cream with a feather *Accomplish'd Lady's Delight* 58. Intensifying fears of smallpox: Creighton 1:463–67, 2:434–45. LM, "Men are vile inconstant toads": LMCL 1:42. EWM, "I know that when you write": LMCL 1:52. LM, "Madam, you are the greatest coquette": LMCL 1:60, 62. LM and Lady Frances, "He has all the qualities of an upright man...": adapted from LMRW 124. EWM, "At last I am ready to confess...": LMCL 1:100 (16 April 1711); LM's response: LMCL 1:102 (17 April 1711).

Deaths of Emperor Joseph I and the grand dauphin Louis: Hopkins 43–45; McKay 132–33; Saint-Simon 2:128–45. Hot and cold regimens: Creighton 1:447–48, 2:445–50; Hopkins 27, 33; Mead 239–40; Miller, AIS 35–39.

LM to Philippa Mundy: "I am glad, dear Phil,...": abridged from LMCL 1:110–111 (2 Nov. 1711); "Your obliging letters...": LMCL 1:111–13 (23 Nov. 1711 and 12 Dec. 1711, combined and condensed); "My adventures are very odd...": LMCL 1:149–50 (Aug. 1712, slightly rearranged).

LM's letter to Dorchester protesting aversion to Skeffington, and ensuing encounters with him and the family, as well as her "final" answer: drawn from LM's letters to EWM in LMCL 1:133–36 (26 July 1712), 1:146–47 (7 Aug. 1712), 1:160–61 (16 Aug. 1712).

EWM to LM, "I have been grieved...": LMCL 1:125 (16 June 1712). LM to EWM: "Were I to choose my destiny...": LMCL 1:129 (17 July 1712); "Come next Sunday...": LMCL 1:150 (12 Aug. 1712); "A pious prude in love": adapted from LMRW 124; "You have not been gone three hours...": LMCL 1:181 (22 June 1713).

Elopement: LMCL 1:164–167 (18–20 Aug. 1712); LMRW 128–36 ("Princess Docile"); Grundy, LMWM 50–56. "I thought to find Limbo...": adapted from LMCL 1:167, n. 1.

EWM as Prince Sombre: LMRW 124. Dorchester as Sir Thomas Grandison (the title character's father) in Samuel Richardson's *Sir Charles Grandison:* LMCL 3:90.

A Destroying Angel

LM's life from her brother's death through her own bout with smallpox: Grundy, LMWM 66–102. Reactions to her brother's death and her consequent relations with EWM: LMCL 1:181–245; "My Brother... is as well as can be": LMCL 1:182 (25 June 1713); "Your absence...": LMCL 1:183 (3 July 1713). Journal entry about her brother: Stuart 21. Lady Frances's marriage: Grundy, LMWM 72–74; Philippa Mundy's marriage: LMCL 1:109, 177–80, 204–207. EWM revenge: LMCL 1:236–45.

Pope's reading before Lord Halifax: Spence, *Observations* 1:87–88 and Mack 271–72. His illness and appearance: Mack 152–58.

Craggs on the stairs: Stuart 28–29. Personalities and habits of King George I, Schulenberg, and Kielmansegg: Hatton, especially 25, 29, 50–51, 133, 137–38. LM's description of the court, including the Prince of Wales: LMEP 82–94.

LM's bout with smallpox: Ricketts's description of "confluent smallpox with severe suppurative fever": Ricketts 4, 26–42; see also WHO 7–22 and Mead. London gossip: Grundy, LMWM 100–103; the earl of Carnarvon (later duke of Chandos), quoted in Sherburn, 204 and 208 n. 1 (pitted/pitied pun); and Lady Loudoun, quoted in Halsband, *Life* 52.

LM's smallpox eclogue: LMEP 201–204; LM's loss of beauty, and her claim that "Flavia" was herself: Stuart 35. Kneller's early painting of LM: Grundy, LMWM 91–92. Pepys on the duchess of Richmond: Pepys 9:134–35, 139.

Lady Hertford on LM's loss of beauty (given here to Lady Townshend): Grundy: LMWM 102. LM's "reply": adapted from "Carabosse" in LMEP 153–55, 383–84. LM's friendship with Lady Townshend, generally: Stuart 22–24; Grundy, LMWM 22, 66, 91, 214.

Bidding the World Adieu

LM's convalescence: Grundy, LMWM 102–115. Preventatives against smallpox and remedies for the scarring: Mead 262; *Accomplish'd Lady's Delight* 53–62; Miller, AIS 40 (Boyle's excrement-in-wine concoction). Pope's revenge on Curll: Grundy, LMWM 109–10; and Mack 296. Early rumors of inoculation heard in London: Miller, AIS 48–69 (including Mr. Townshend's report to the Royal Society); Stearns and Pasti 106–13; Creighton 2:646 (discussing Kennedy). Original sources: Kennedy; Pylarinus; Timonius. LM's mask: LM, "Satturday, the Smallpox, Flavia," line 70, in LMEP 203; Grundy, LMWM 102, 113.

Departure: Grundy, LMWM 117–18; LMRW 74. Street cries: Laroon. Shops like "gilded theaters": contemporary account (1715) reprinted in Besant 239–40.

LM's travels: Grundy, LMWM, 117–42; LMCL 1:248–446.

Vienna: Travels down the Danube and description of Vienna's buildings and furnishings, LMCL 1:259–61; Viennese gown and hairstyle, and visits with the empresses: LMCL 1:265–69; LM's witty war with Viennese ladies: LMCL 1:295, n. 1. London milk-maid sporting the May Day headdress to which LM compared her Viennese hairstyle: Laroon 120–21.

Pope's letters to LM: Pope, *Correspondence* 1:352–58, 363–65, 367–70, 382–85.

To Hanover: LM's dislike of Bohemia and runaway carriage over the River Elbe: LMCL 1:280–82; the cramped Portuguese ambassador: LMCL 1:286; Hanoverian heaters and midwinter fruit: 1:289–91. Viennese fears for LM, her refusal to give up the journey, Prince Eugene as cross-dressed Hercules, the empress's dwarfs, and LM's farewell to her sister: LMCL 1:293–96. Farewell to Pope: LMCL 1:296–97.

Vienna to Adrianople: LMCL 1:297–304; Battle of Peterwaradin, travels through Turkish Balkans, Achmet Bey: LMCL 1:304–308 and 315–321. Battle of Peterwaradin: see also McKay 158–63. Baths of Sofia: LMCL 1:312–15, and Spence, *Observations* 1:311–12. LM's "former sufferings and mortifications" leading her to observe inoculation: Stuart 35.

My Dear Little Son

LM in Turkey: Grundy, LMWM 142–66; LMCL 1:344–415.

LM's smallpox/plague letter (including story of Maitland's arrival with the second cook, LM's amazement at his recovery): LM to Sarah Chiswell, 1 April 1717, LMCL 1:337–40; "Head of Letters" indicating "Small pox" letter sent to LM's father: LMCL 1:346; Sloane's claim that she wrote the court and her friends: Sloane 517.

LM's Turkish dress: LMCL 1:325–30; Vanmour painting reproduced in LM, *Embassy to Constantinople* 38; on these portraits (and the Kneller), see Grundy, LMWM 142, 201–202, 301–303. Turkish dancing and music: LMCL 1:351; Turkish beauty: LMCL 1:327. Balm (or Balsam) of Mecca: LMCL 1:345 (letter heading to Kielmansegg), 368–69; Prescott 119–22. Eighteenth-century Constantinople, generally: Mansel; like a cabinet full of jars: LMCL 1:397.

Inoculation conversations between LM and Maitland: Maitland 4–7.

Pope's letter to LM re "Eloisa to Abelard": Pope 1:407; LM writing verse on Boxing Day: Grundy, LMWM 159; LM's poem: "Constantinople," LMEP 207–10; young Mary's birth: Grundy, LMWM 149.

Edward Wortley junior's inoculation: Maitland 7–8; LMCL 1:391–94.

Experiences she could not replicate in London: official visit to the Hagia Sofia, bazaar and dervishes: LMCL 1:396–403. Sneaking into the Hagia Sofia: Halsband, *Life* 82–83; Grundy, LMWM 166. LM's Arabian horses: LMCL 1:341. Glimpse of the Sultan: LMCL 1:323–34; Sultan's titles: Mansel 8–9, 28. Emerald big as a turkey's egg: LMCL 1:382; mother-of-pearl and emerald room: LMCL 1:414. Murdered woman: LMCL 1: 407–08. *I am almost of the opinion* . . . : LMCL 1: 415.

Rosebuds in Lily Skin

Dryden's poem: "Upon the Death of Lord Hastings" (1649), in Dryden 1–3. Flowers blooming in January 1721: Grundy, LMWM 209. Wortley Montagu home in Covent Garden: Grundy, LMWM 182, 185–86.

Rift in the royal family, and the king's love for his grandchildren: Hatton 206–10, 213–16; Van der Kiste, *King George II* 62–75. Princess Anne's illness, and the king and the Princess of Wales meeting outside her sickchamber: Cowper 139–49; Sloane 517.

LM's part in the South Sea bubble: Grundy, LMWM 203–209.

London's smallpox epidemics of 1719–21, and the deaths of LM's friends: Grundy, LMWM 209–210, Creighton 2:461–63; Social life ceasing: *Applebee's* no. 1996, Saturday, March 4, 1721. Smallpox house in Swallow Street: Rose 18; Amyand, "List," folio 3 (under Lord Bathurst's servant). Young Mary's nurse having previously refused inoculation: LMCL 1:392; Grundy, LMWM 162; Mary's inoculation: Maitland 8–10; Grundy, LMWM 209–210.

Zabdiel and Jerusha

ZB's early years: Mager; Peter Thacher; Winslow. Genealogies: Wyman; William Gray Brooks; *The Booke of the Boylstones*. Thomas Boylston as soldier: Bodge. Lack of Oxford degree: Foster. ZB nearly dying of smallpox in 1702: ZBHA 1; Sydenham's protégé (Dr. Thomas Dover): Creighton 2:446, note 1; Dover 119–20. ZB's shop: Mager 7–10; ZBHA 46–48. ZB's interest in rattlesnake-bite remedies: Mager 184–86; *Some Account* 9. For the widespread British and colonial fascination with rattlesnakes and their bites, see Stearns, *Science*. ZB's interest in ambergris: ZB, "Ambergris"; Mager 173–74.

Minots: Shattuck; Minot; *Boston Marriages* 7.

Curiosities of the Smallpox

Onesimus: CMD Dec. 16, 1706, 1: 579–80; March 20, 1716, 2:342; and July 31, 1716, 2:363 (slightly anachronistic). See also CMD 2:139, 222, 271–72, 282, 446, 456; and CMSL 213–14. "Dying like rotten sheep": CMA 1–2.

The Middle Passage: Mannix, Huggins. Black slaves in New England: Greene, McManus, Wright. Olaudah Equiano: Equiano. Garamantes in classical literature: *Lemprière's Classical Dictionary*.

CM's life and character: Silverman. Letter to Dr. John Woodward, July 12, 1716: CMSL 213–14; further excerpts in Kittredge, "Some Lost Works" 422. (CM's draft of this letter is in the Massachusetts Historical Society; a transcription of the fair copy sent to Woodward exists in BL, Sloane MS 3340.) Doing Good: Silverman 227–37; CMSL 87–92. Stutter: Silverman 15–17, 33–38, 48–49, 172–73. CM's youthful study of medicine: CMAB iv; Beall and Shyrock 8–10; Silverman 21–22. CM's family and domestic life, including relations with Onesimus: Silverman 261–75, 279–94. Katy Mather: Silverman 267–68, 269, 291–92.

Curiosa Americana and the Royal Society: Silverman 247–54, 260; CMSL 107–22; Stearns, *Science* 403–26. Articles in *Philosophical Transactions:* PTRS 29, no. 339 (April–June, 1714): 62–71 (CM), 72–82 (Timonius).

The Beauty of the Sea

Captain John Gore: Cooper, *Sermon;* obituary in BNL no. 876, Dec. 19–26, 1720; and *Acts and Resolves* 10:28; Thwing RCN 21801.

HMS *Seahorse:* documents in Britain's Public Record Office: paybook: ADM 33/316; master's log: ADM 52/482; Durell's letters: ADM 1/1694; Durell's passing certificate for lieutenant: ADM 107/2. Ship description and specifications: Lyon. Life in the eighteenth-century British navy, including health and medicine: Rodger, Marcus. Durell and trumpets: SSD 2:1018, (Aug. 1, 1724 and note). Durell biography: Fergusson.

Names of ships and their captains arriving in the convoy: BNL no. 896, May 1–8, 1721.

Captain Paxton's letters to the Admiralty: PRO MS ADM 1/2277. Charles Paxton: *Seahorse* paybook, PRO MS ADM 33/316, no. 206. Deeds and possessions: Thwing RCN 48823 (Wentworth Paxton), 32739 (Faith Gillam or Gillum), and (22152) Benjamin Gillam.

Hector Bruce: *Seahorse* paybook, PRO MS ADM 33/316, no. 207; BG no. 97, Sept. 25–Oct. 2, 1721. Richard Kent: *Seahorse* paybook, PRO MS ADM 33/316, no. 208; Thwing RCN 41536.

Selectmen's meeting and John Clark's inspection of *Seahorse:* SM 81–82, and BTR 153–54. Spectacle Island and Boston's quarantine laws: Blake 34–36.

ZB's early career and family: Mager 1–27; Wyman. Sharp's advertisement: BG no. 43, Oct. 3–7, 1720; no. 44, Oct. 10–17, 1720; no. 46, Oct. 24–31, 1720; no. 47, Oct. 31–Nov. 7, 1720, and no. 48, Nov. 7–14, 1720; BNL no. 865, Oct. 3–10, 1720, and no. 866, Oct. 10–17, 1720. Winslow's advertisement, dated Oct. 14, 1720: BNL no. 873, Nov 28–Dec 5, 1720 (edited for ease of reading); with slight alterations (including a surgery date of July 28): BG no. 50, Nov 21–28, 1720, and no. 51, Nov. 28–Dec. 5, 1720. Sharp's later whereabouts: BG no. 65, March 6–13, 1721. Winslow genealogy: Paige 71. Black slaves as physicians' assistants: Greene 118–19. Jack as ZB's slave: BG no. 85, July 10–17, 1721.

Boston history, politics, and topography: Bridenbaugh; Hutchinson, vol. 2; Perry Miller; Thwing, *Crooked and Narrow Streets;* Whitehill and Kennedy.

Caging the Monster

Town meeting, May 12, 1721: BTR 153–54. Payments to Captain Clark and his men: JHRM 3:75, 107–108, *Acts and Resolves* 10:105.

Selectmen's meeting, May 12, 1721: SM 82. William Hutchinson: Thwing RCN 39747; Thomas Hutchinson 2:188. Lion in the South End: BG no. 70, April 10–17, 1721; no. 83, June 27–July 3, 1721. The Bunch of Grapes tavern and billiards: Bridenbaugh 265–66, 428–29, 436–37; Samuel Adams Drake, Elisha Cooke, and John Clark versus the governor: Thomas Hutchinson 2:174–96.

Seahorse: Discharged and dead sailors: paybook, PRO MS ADM 33/316; Ship's movements and Boston weather: master's log, PRO MS ADM 52/482; two sailors warned out of town: SM 86.

Door-to-door search of town: BNL, no. 898, May 15–22, 1721; street cleaning: SM 82–83; Smallpox aboard the captured pirate ship: Captain Durell's letter to the Admiralty from Boston, June 27, 1721, PRO MS ADM 1/1694.

CM, Lydia, Lizzy, Creasy, smallpox, and the angels: Silverman 127–28, 173–86, 292–94, 307–40; CMD May 26 and 28, 1721, 2:620–21.

Thomas Newton obituary and report of eight people ill: BG no. 77, May 22–29, 1721.

Unnamed black man's description of African inoculation: CMAB 107; CM's "army of Africans": "Sentiments on the Small Pox Inoculated," printed anonymously at the end of Increase Mather, *Several Reasons*. WD's "half a dozen or half a score Africans, by others called Negroe Slaves": WD, *Inoculation* 6–7. Colman's interview with a slave: Colman, *Some Observations* 15–16.

General Court adjourning to Cambridge: Hutchinson 2:189; Selectmen moving the school: SM 83; CM's further dithering: CMD May 30, June 2 and 5, 1721, 2:622–24; Obadiah's terror of smallpox: CMD June 6, 1721, 2:624; CM's first letter to the physicians, June 6, 1721: excerpt quoted in *Vindication* 7–8 and Greenwood 5–6.

Demonic Wings

WD's personality and attitudes: BNL no. 912, July 17–24, 1721; Bullock; "Douglass, William" in DAB; WDD throughout, especially 2, 5, 7–8; WDCC 164–71; "Douglass, William, M.D." in James Thacher; Thwing RCN 24444; Stearns, *Science* 480–84; Kittredge, "Some Lost Works" 423–27. I have not been able to look at Muse. Eighteen days: WDCC 168; WDPE 9. Mockery of ZB on horseback: NEC no. 2, Aug. 7–14, 1721; Locking the books away: *Some Account* 10; ZBHA 3; CMA 9; Greenwood 9. Scottish accent (and a mocking view of WD in general): Greenwood. Smallpox studies: WDPE (management of smallpox cases, with special attention to cases of hemorrhagic smallpox in 1721 epidemic), WDD (mostly a rant against early inoculators); WDS (statistical reviews of 1721, 1730, and 1752 epidemics).

CM's library: Silverman 262–63 (an earlier house), 289.

Boylston girls in Roxbury: ZBHA 16–17. Rebecca Abbot and Mary Lane: William Gray Brooks 3, 9. Failing to get to Cambridge, due to Boston-Roxbury travel: ZBHA 23–24. Boys at home: ZBHA ii (where he refers to plural children), 1–3 (Tommy), 6–7 (John); Colman, *Some Observations* 3 (also referring to plural children). Indian attack on the Minot home: NEHGR 15 (1861): 267. This story's truth has been questioned; whether or not it was true, it was certainly a widely told tale. The pirate Roberts: BNL no. 897, May 8–15, 1721.

CM's smallpox treatise and second letter to the physicians: CMD June 22–23, 1721, 2:627–28. Copy sent to WD: *Some Account* 10.

Dr. John Perkins: CMD Aug. 7, 1711, 2:93; March 22, 1721, 2:609; April 5, 1721, 2:611; May 24, 1721, 2:620; June 21, 1721, 2:627; Mager 78; Silverman 246.

Fathers and Sons

ZB's horses: ZB, letter to Benjamin Colman, Feb. 26, 1724/5; Hollis 533, 551; "Boylston, Dr. Zabdiel, FRS." in James Thacher 1:191. The countryside he rides through: Thwing, *Crooked and Narrow Streets;* Whitehill and Kennedy. Hanging of Joseph Hanno or Hono: BG no. 74, May 1–8, 1721, and no. 77, May 22–29, 1721; BNL no. 899, May 22–29, 1721; CMD May 13, 1721, 2:618; May 25, 1721, 2:620; May 31, 1721, 2:623.

CM's letter to ZB/the physicians: Peter Thacher 778. No copy of the original appears to have survived. CM's treatise: CMAB. WD as "complete snarler": Alexander Hamilton 116–17. Death "terrible in all its shapes": ZBHA iii, 38.

Enslaved blacks in colonial Boston: Greene. ZB quoting black man on inoculation:

Some Account 9; smallpox in Africa, and African inoculation practices: Herbert; Hopkins 164–80; WHO 233–35.

The sick woman in the shop: *Vindication* 8–9.

"Make hay while the sun shines": WDCC July 28, 1721, 166–67. *Seahorse* firing her guns: master's log, PRO MS ADM 52/482. Boston's "crooked and narrow streets": Thwing, *Crooked and Narrow Streets* 7–8. WD's claim that ZB had not seen one case of natural small-pox: BNL no. 912, July 17–24, 1721. Colman's defense of ZB: "Letter to the Reverend Mr.————of Boston," July 25, 1721 (MS draft of letter to unnamed minister), printed in Fitz 327. A much-cut version of this letter was printed in BG no. 88, July 27–31, 1721.

Descriptions of inoculation and clamor in the streets: ZBHA Preface, 1–3, 42–50; BG no. 85, July 10–27, 1721; CMA 9–10, 15–18; CMD June 30, 1721, 2:628, and July 16, 1721, 2:632; Hutchinson 2:206; "Boylston, Dr. Zabdiel, FRS" in James Thacher 1:187–90 (incorporating Ward Nicholas Boylston's account of the noose-bearing crowds). More of ZB's thoughts: *Some Account* 8–17.

Tommy at the pump: Colman, *Some Observations* 3. Hamilton's slave named Cotton Mather: HMS *Seahorse* paybook, PRO MS ADM 33/316, no. 266; CMD Dec. 10, 1721, 2:663.

Salutation Alley

ZB's treatment of his son: ZBHA 2, 44–47. Tommy's course through smallpox: Rick-etts 1: 26–28, 43–50, and 64 (chart of a case of discrete smallpox without secondary fever). Colman: Silverman 146–49, 151–56; Turell.

Salutation Inn, and other early Boston taverns: Samuel Adams Drake 45–46, 119; Thwing, *Crooked and Narrow Streets;* Bonner's map of 1722. Cheever: ZBHA 5–6; Thwing RCN 15679. Stewart (variously spelled Steward and Stuart): Stewart; Thwing RCN 56280; NEC Aug 7–14, 1721, "To the Author of the *New-England Courant*" (Ben Franklin identified the anonymous writer as "Dr. Steward" on his own copy, now in the British Li-brary).

BNL's "pestilential contagion" issues: no. 910, July 6–10, 1721; no. 911, July 10–17, 1721. ZB's letter to the *Boston Gazette:* BG no. 85; July 10–17, 1721.

Departure of HMS *Seahorse:* Master's log, PRO MS ADM 52/482; paybook, PRO MS ADM 33/316, especially no. 207; Hector Bruce: letter from Durell to the Admiralty, 27 June 1721, PRO MS ADM 1/1694. Charles, infant son of Thomas and Ann Durell, was baptized on August 2, 1721, at King's Chapel, then Boston's lone Church of England es-tablishment: RCB.

Inoculations of Helyer, Moll, John, Webbs: ZBHA 6–7. Helyer: Thwing RCN 39797. Joseph Webb: Thwing RCN 60405, Vinton 499.

CM: CMD, July 7–20, 1721, 2: 629–33.

Squabbles between the House of Representatives and Governor Shute: Hutchinson 2: 188–96; JHRM 3: 72–78. Governor's proclamation: BNL no. 908, June 29–July 3, 1721.

Identities of early inoculees, and denizens of Salutation Alley: ZBHA, cross-referenced with entries in Thwing's *Inhabitants and Estates*, and RCB. Webb/Adams clan: Vinton.

Prying Multitudes

Mary Wortley's progress through inoculated smallpox: Maitland 9–10.

Physician witnesses of her inoculation, generally: Maitland 10; Stuart 36. Dr. James

Keith (and the loss of his two elder sons): Maitland 11; Henderson 56–61, 141. Dr. Walter Harris (witness, and pock counter): Walter Harris, "De Inoculatione Variolarum" (for Mary's twelve pocks, see page 45). An abridged translation appears in Increase Mather's *Some Further Account*. Sir Hans Sloane: Sloane 516–17; de Beer 70, 74–77. Dr. Johann Georg Steigerthal: Miller, AIS 81, 84, note 54; Amyand, "List," folio 2.

Social witnesses: Lord and Lady Townshend: Stuart 22–23; Grundy, LMWM 66, 91; Charlotte Tichborne and the duchess of Dorset: Grundy, LMWM 218; *www.ihrinfo.ac.uk/office/caroline.html*; LM and the Princess of Wales's shared friends more generally: Grundy, "Medical Advance" 19.

Peter Keith's inoculation: Maitland 11–12; "Persons Inoculated by Mr. Charles Maitland," RSI, Part 2, folio 219.

Princess Caroline's scarlet fever: *The Weekly Journal: or, British Gazetteer*, May 6, 1721, p. 1913; *Applebee's*, May 13, 1721, p. 2057, qtd. in Miller, AIS 80.

Maneuvering toward the prison experiment: Maitland, folio A2^v, Sloane 517; Grundy, LMWM 209–13. For further evidence, along with a different argument (supporting Sir Hans Sloane and the physicians, and more or less dismissing both LM and the Princess of Wales), see Miller, AIS 70–91. LM's distrust of doctors: Stuart 35–36; Grundy, LMWM 217–18. Lord Townshend's legal query and the answer: qtd. in Miller, AIS 75–6. See also Grundy, "Medical Advance" 20. Mehemet and Mustafa: Hatton 99–100.

Personal connections driving inoculation. See sources for "Signs and Wonders."

An Infusion of Malignant Filth

WD: W. Philanthropos (i.e., WD), "To the Author of the Boston News Letter," BNL no. 912, July 17–24, 1721; WDD; WD, *Inoculation* 7 ("There is not a Race of Men on Earth more False Lyars"); WD (anonymous, but later identified by Benjamin Franklin), "A Continuation of the History of Inoculation in Boston," NEC no. 1, August 7, 1721 (unanimous agreement of selectmen).

ZB: ZBHA; *Some Account* 8–17 (for "lions in Africa," "we are yet but learners," inoculation "a great blessing to mankind," "a mighty bustle," and plague argument rebuttals including "excessively ridiculous.")

Stewart: Stewart.

CM's testimony (probably gleaned from ZB): CMA 10–14.

General contrasts between inoculated and natural smallpox: ZBHA; CMA; Colman, *Some Observations*.

Army of Africans: Increase Mather, *Several Reasons* (ZB and CM seemed to share many phrases and conversations on the subject). ZB wrote "a considerable number": *Some Account* 9.

The Castle of Misery

Newgate's history and description, and life inside its walls: Babington; *Complete Newgate Calendar*; Defoe, *Moll Flanders* (first published in January 1722; Defoe did time in Newgate and his descriptions of the prison in this novel are presumed to record personal experience).

Date of the selection and removal of the prisoners to the Press Yard: *The Weekly Journal or Saturday's Post*, July 29, 1721, p. 832, qtd. and paraphrased in Miller, AIS 83. Prisoners' names and ages: Maitland 21. Indictments and convictions: Mary North: *Applebee's*, Saturday March 4, 1721, p. 1996; March 11, 1721, p. 2002. John Alcock: *Applebee's*,

Saturday, May 27, 1721, p. 2069. Elizabeth Harrison: *Applebee's*, April 22, 1721, p. 2039. Ann Tompion as wife of Thomas Tompion: Grundy, LMWM 213, note 36; "Tompion, Thomas (1639–1713)" in the *Dictionary of National Biography*. Richard Evans having had smallpox in September 1720: Maitland 22.

The tale of the prisoners' blood being drained: Dr. Matthias Ernest Boretius, retold (in translation) by Miller, AIS 84–85.

The "Castle of Misery": Babington.

Lizzy's room, and the Press Yard more generally: closely modeled on descriptions by an anonymous Jacobite prisoner held there in 1715: *The History of the Press Yard* (London, 1717), qtd. in Babington 70–80.

Signs and Wonders

Individual inoculees: ZBHA; Thwing, *Inhabitants and Estates*; RCB. Personal connections driving inoculation: Grundy, "Medical Advance" 18–19, 26–28.

CM's thoughts at the library window: CMD 2:633–4, July 21, 23, and 27, 1721. "Distress about Sammy" and secrecy: CMD 3:635–36, Aug. 1, 1721. Diary entries (and thoughts while writing in the diary): CMD 2:635–43, August 1–30, 1721.

WD's newspaper writings: BNL, no. 912, July 17–24, 1721; NEC nos. 1–3, August 7, 14, and 21, 1721. He was shut out of issue no. 4, for August 28: Lemay, "Printer, 1657–1730," 1721, 28 Aug. (a). Colman's rebuttal: Colman, Letter to the Reverend Mr. ———of Boston, MS in the Countway Library of Medicine; printed in Fitz, 326–27 (signed by Colman alone); edited newspaper version: BG no. 88, July 27–31, 1721.

CM as manipulator: Silverman 254–60; his argument that inoculation was not only lawful, but a duty: Increase Mather, *Several Reasons*.

Ben Franklin: Franklin, *Benjamin Franklin's Memoirs* 18–52 (34, for his thoughts about the pitfalls of being argumentative).

Defense of ZB by Cheever, Helyer, and the two Webbs: presumably BG no. 90, August 7–14, 1721. I've found no extant copy, but WD describes it in NEC no. 3, August 21, 1721.

NEC and James Franklin, BNL and John Campbell, BG and Philip Musgrave: Clark 77–140.

William Charnock: Shipton vol. 7, under "William Charnock"; Thwing RCN 15071 (for his father, John Charnock).

General Court at the George Inn: JHRM 3: 84–93.

Newgate

Maitland's "Journal of the Experiment at Newgate": Maitland 20–26; Maitland's note to Sloane: BL, Sloane MS 4076, folio 96. Witnesses of the inoculation: Miller, AIS 84, quoting contemporary newspapers. Sloane's description of the Newgate experiment: Sloane. Wagstaffe's opposition observations (along with identification of Dr. John Freind as one of the witnesses): Wagstaffe. Additional details and modern scholarly accounts: Miller, AIS 84–86; Grundy, "Medical Advance."

Applebee's opposition: *Applebee's*, August 12, 1721, qtd. in Grundy, "Medical Advance" 21 (prisoners pretending not to have had the smallpox); *Applebee's*, August 19, 1721, p. 2139, qtd. in Miller, AIS 86–87 (a way for the guilty to escape). Political implications of the experiments: Wilson; Grundy, LMWM 212.

Mead's experiment with the Chinese method (up the nose): Mead 257; *The Post-Boy*, no. 5005, 19–22 August, 1721, and *The Weekly Journal: or, British Gazetteer,* Aug. 26, 1721, p. 2011 (for the claim that it had been done while the girl was asleep).

LM's summer: LMCL 2: 12–13, Letter to Lady Mar, 6 September 1721 (including "thread-satin beauty" and melting time "in almost perpetual concerts"); Grundy, LMWM 211 (quoting LM's lost diary on the Princess of Wales's "unquailing" support); Grundy, "Medical Advance" 28 (reasons for LM's concealment).

LM/Mr. Cook: Maitland 25; story of sneaking into the Hagia Sofia: Halsband, *Life* 82–83; Spence, *Grand Tour* 359–60 (LMCL 1: 398–99 for officially sanctioned tours of Hagia Sofia and Sultan Suleiman's mosque, the Suleymaniye). Second cook and the plague: LMCL 1: 338. LM's delight in going incognito in Turkish veils: LMCL 1: 328–30, 354–55, 405–12; Grundy, LMWM. Isaac Massey fuming at Child's: Isaac Massey, *Short and Plain Account* 3–4.

Sir Hans on a further experiment: Sir Hans Sloane, Letter to Dr. Richardson, 22 August 1721, in Nichols 1: 277–78.

An Hour of Mourning

ZB's inoculations through the period covered by this chapter: ZBHA 9–15. Mrs. Dixwell: ZBHA 9–10; John Williams, *Several Arguments* 8–9. John Dixwell: Thwing RCN 24202; "Notes and Queries," NEHGR 32 (1878): 93; RCB, New North Church records. Dixwell children: see deeds noted in Thwing RCN 62626 and 62624 (Hannah and John Wormall) and 50805 (their maternal grandfather, John Prout). Sammy Mather: CMD August 30, 1721, 2: 643; ZBHA 8. Mrs. Dodge: ZBHA 11; her father: Thwing RCN 24264 and 24265 (likely the same person). Judge Lynde's young black man: ZBHA 11.

Boylstons' dinner: Gibson 12, 23, 42.

Moses Pierce House: *www.paulreverehouse.org/history3.html*; Moses Pierce: Thwing RCN 49812 (also recording the death of their daughter); Elizabeth Parminter Pierce: Thwing RCN 48596, for John Parminter (her father), recording a birthdate of September 3, 1688, which identifies her with ZB's "Mrs. Pierce, about thirty-two years old." William Clark house: Whitehill and Kennedy 27.

Bethiah Nichols/Mrs. N—s: ZBHA 12–13; Thwing RCN 46997 (for her husband William Nichols); Vinton 500.

Selectmen's meeting to regulate funerals: SM 87. Frances Webb's funeral: SSD 2:982; CMD 2:646. Adams family: ZBHA 14–15, Vinton 499–503 (for relations to Webbs). Samuel Adams: Thwing RCN 212; "Adams Family Bible" 283–84. Samuel Jones: Thwing RCN 41168; RCB, records of New North Church (for marriage to Mary Adams, and baptism of daughter Mary); *Boston Births* 106 (for birth of daughter Mary).

Mrs. Margaret Salter: ZBHA 13–14; Thwing RCN 53516 (her husband), 4210 (her father, Jonathan Balston), and 4209 (her grandfather, also Jonathan Balston, recording the marriage of her aunt Prudence Balston Turner, to John Marion).

The wrong saddle tarred and feathered: John Williams, *Answer* 12–13 (noted in Mager 96).

Firewood: CMD Sept. 16, 1721, 2:646; SM 88–89, September 23, 1721.

The King's Pardon

Lizzy in Hertford: Maitland 19–20, 33; Sloane 517–18; Royal Society *Journal-Book* 12, entry for Nov. 16, 1721. Maitland's other inoculations in Hertford: Maitland 26–35. Christ's Hospital, Hertford: *www.hertford.net/bluecoats.htm; www.christs-hospital.org.uk*

Raw Head and Bloody Bones

WD's letter to Dr. Alexander Stuart: adapted from Stewart and from WD's later published version of his several letters to Stuart. See also Stearns and Pasti 116, and Miller, AIS 93–94.

Paxton's runaway slave, Hector: BG no. 97, Sept. 25–Oct. 2, 1721, and no. 98, Oct. 2–9, 1721; Roger Paxton: *Seahorse* paybook, PRO MS ADM 33/316, no. 280.

Mrs. N—s's (Bethiah Nichols) miscarriage and loss of eye: ZBHA 12–13.

Family's fears for ZB: Peter Thacher 776.

Biblical references: *Thou shalt not kill:* Exodus 20:13, and Deuteronomy 5:17; Waters of God: Genesis 1:2, Ezekial 47:1–5; Isaiah 43:2; Revelation 17:1.

Epidemic statistics: BNL no. 923, Oct. 2–9, 1721; CMD 2: 652, Oct. 7–8, 1721; Stewart (for number of patients visited by doctors daily).

Eunice Willard's inoculation: ZBHA 16. For patients' relative comfort: CM's anonymous "Way of Proceeding" 33–35; Colman, *Some Observations*. Her life and character: Willard 370–71. Loring/Breck and Fitch inoculations: ZBHA 16.

Deaths of Madam Checkley and Martha Cotes: SSD 2:983. Bronsdon children: Thwing RCN 7358 for their father, Benjamin Bronsdon, and genealogy in NEHGR 35 (1881): 362 (Selectman William Clark was married to Benjamin's sister Sarah) Merchant children: Thwing RCN 45446 for their father, William Merchant.

Boston newspaper reports of Newgate: BG no. 100, October 16–23, 1721 (also containing camel and lion advertisements); BG no. 101, October 23–30, 1721. ZB's family inoculations: ZBHA 16–17.

Shute's proclamation for Day of Thanksgiving: BG no. 98, October 2–9, 1721; CM falling ill: CMD 2:654. Loring's death: SSD 2:984, October 27, 1721 (recording the burial). *Faithful Account:* BG no. 101, October 23–30, 1721; arguments re authorship: Kittredge, "Some Lost Works" 460; Fitz. Governor's speech: JHRM 3:137.

Inoculees, Oct. 30–Dec. 2, 1721: ZBHA 17–29.

CM's encounter with James Franklin: NEC no. 18, Nov. 27–Dec 4, 1721.

Just Retribution

Attack on Boylston household: James Thacher 1:187 (account provided by ZB's great-nephew, Ward Nicholas Boylston—grandson of Zabdiel's brother Thomas); Hutchinson 2:206. Boston's reputation for rioting: Bridenbaugh 382–83. Attack on Mather household: CMD 2:657–58, November 14, 1721; Hutchinson 2:207. Reward: JHRM 3:150, 15 Nov. 1721. House's measure to help those in "reduced straits" due to the epidemic: JHRM 3:147, 13 Nov. 1721.

Royal Society's discussions of inoculation on Nov. 16: Royal Society, *Journal-Book* 12:163 (1720–26), under Nov. 16, 1721 (with summary of letter from WD to Alexander Stuart). Crane Court: *www.royalsoc.ac.uk/library/index.html*. Sloane's French translation of Maitland's account of his Hertford experiments: BL Sloane MSS 4034, folio 17, qtd. in Miller, AIS 88, note 68; see also p. 89, note 74. London's Nov. 18 newspaper reports of experiments on charity children: Miller, AIS 88, note 69.

William Hutchinson's illness, death, and funeral: Thomas Hutchinson 2:188, 204; SSD 2:985 for 30 Nov. and 2 Dec. 1721; Thwing RCN 39747; B6 no. 106, Nov. 27–Dec. 4, 1721. Active in the House of Representatives through Nov. 15, 1721: JHRM 3 149–154. Dr. Thomas Robie: Kilgour; Robie; Stearns, *Science* 426–35. Nicholas Sever's inoculation: Robie, Nov. 30–Dec. 18, 1721, cross-referenced with *Historical Register of Harvard*.

WD's withdrawal: Preface to WDPE ii; failure of his cold treatment: WDS 394.
Zabdiel's final thoughts: ZBHA 32 (slightly edited for altered context).

In Royal Fashion

Applebee's poor report of Boston inoculations: *Applebee's*, Feb. 3, 1722, p. 2285, qtd. in Miller, AIS 94. Inoculations of "Noble Duke in Hanover Square" and Charlotte Tichborne: *St. James Evening Post*, Dec. 7, 1721, and *The Weekly Journal or British Gazetteer*, Dec. 9, 1721, respectively, both qtd. in Grundy, "Medical Advance" 37, note 25. Maitland's Feb. 23 inoculations: *The London Gazette* no. 6040, March 6–10, 1722, qtd. in Miller, AIS 88–89. Jeremiah Dummer: CMA Preface (by Dummer). Daniel Neal: Neal 17; Miller, AIS 96 (Princess Caroline's summons).

St. James's orphans: Amyand, Letter to Sir Hans Sloane; Miller, AIS 88–89. Sloane's meetings with the princess and the king: Sloane 518–19.

Earl of Sunderland's family history with smallpox: Grundy, "Medical Advance" 22. Judith (Tichborne) Spencer, countess of Sunderland: Grundy, "Medical Advance" 26–27. Inoculation and death of William Spencer, Sunderland's son: MMV; "Persons Inoculated by Mr. Charles Maitland," RSI, Part 1, no. 27, folio 220; Grundy, "Medical Advance" 22 (for quotation of newspaper articles).

The princesses' inoculations: Amyand, "List," folio 2. Maitland pointing: "Persons Inoculated by Mr. Charles Maitland," RSI, Part 1, no. 27, folio 220. See also Miller, AIS 96–99. Princesses' characters: Van Der Kiste, *King George II* 129–30. Amyand's method: Amyand, Letter to Jurin, Jan. 16, 1723/4, in RSI, Part 1, folio 9, no. 2.

LM's letter to Lady Mar, April, 1721: LMCL 2:15–16.

Townshend inoculations: "Persons Inoculated by Mr. Charles Maitland," RSI, Part 1, no. 27, folios 219–21. Tichborne/De La Warr inoculations: Grundy, "Medical Advance" 27.

LM's Turkey-merchant letter: LMEP 95–97; Halsband, "New Light" 400–403. Opposition: Wagstaffe; Edmund Massey, *Sermon* (on Job 2:7); Grundy, "Medical Advance" 23 (about Massey). Arbuthnot and mathematical analyses: Miller, AIS 106–07, 111–23. Prejudice versus paranoia: Grundy, LMWM 217.

Inoculations of Prince William, Lady Albinia Bertie, Lady Louisa Bertie, and Miss Selwyn, May 11, 1723: Amyand, "List," folio 4; "vexation, persecution and obloquy": adapted from Stuart 35; "Admire the heroism in the heart of your friend": LMCL 1:340.

Meetings and Partings

Sloane's invitation to ZB: Fitz 324–25, Mager 170, James Thacher, 1:189–90. Five more deaths; admission of poor doctoring; "who was he to refuse"; waning urgency to inoculate: ZBHA 20–33.

House of Representatives' attempts to outlaw inoculation: Hutchinson 2: 208; JHRM 3: 178, March 15, 1722, and 3:181 and 184, March 20, 1722. Country fears of smallpox returning to Boston: NEC no. 42, May 14–21, 1722. Town meeting on ZB's last six inoculees: BTR, May 15, 1723. Mob forcing inoculees to Spectacle Island: Robie, May 17, 1722. WD's slurs comparing inoculation to witchcraft and serpents: NEC no. 42, May 14–21, 1722 (first column, see Lemay for Ben Franklin's identification of Douglass as author). More rants: WD, *Abuses and Scandals* and *Postscript to Abuses*. WD's grudging admission that inoculation worked: WDCC, May 1, 1722, p. 143.

Grim numbers: ZBHA; WDS 2:396

Rescue of James Franklin: Mager; Lemay: "Printer, 1657–1730" then "1721," June 12–July 7, especially June 20. Governor Shute's departure: Mager 174.

Advertisements related to ZB's departure (and describing garden): BG no. 193, July 29–August 5, 1723; BG no. 221, February 10–17, 1724; NEC no. 133, February 10–17, 1724; qtd. in Mager 170–71. Ambergris: ZB, "Ambergris found in Whales." "Bear's grease" advertisement: NEC no. 172, Nov. 9–16.

Prince Frederick's inoculation: Miller, AIS 176; "Persons Inoculated by Mr. Charles Maitland, 1724," RSI, Part 1, no. 29, folio 223.

Dispute over CM's FRS: Stearns, *Science* 408–409, 419–21; Kittredge, "Cotton Mather's Election" and "Further Notes." CM's letter of introduction for ZB to Dr. Jurin: CMSL, 402–03; CM's letter to Sloane: BL Sloane MS 4048, folio 241. Colman's letters to Neal and Hollis: Mager 174.

WD's charge that ZB went to London to inoculate: WDD 7.

LM praised for "protecting beauty and inspiring wit": Aaron Hill's line (1724), qtd. in Halsband, "New Light" 404; see also Grundy, LMWM 221. LM to Lady Mar (*des amis choisies;* rat eating the cheese): LMCL 2:45–6, Jan. and Feb. 1725 (two letters condensed and abridged).

ZB's arrival in London with horses: Hollis 533. ZB's introduction to the Royal Society: Royal Society *Journal-Book* 12:532–34, for February 11, 1725.

LM's encounter with duke of Kingston: Stuart 31.

ZB's letter home to Colman: ZB, Letter to Benjamin Colman, February 26, 1724/5.

Pierrepont inoculations: "Persons Inoculated by Mr. Charles Maitland, 1725," RSI, Part 1, no. 30, folio 224; LMCL 2:49; *Daily Post,* March 3, 1725.

Princess Mary's inoculation: "Persons Inoculated by Claude Amyand, 1725," RSI, Part 1, no. 9, folio 19.

Hollis's gossip about ZB's horses: Hollis 551. Prince and Princess of Wales's summer retreat to Richmond: LMCL 2:54, n.4. LM's letters to Lady Mar about horses: LMCL 2:53–55 (July and Aug. 1725).

LM writing up the *Embassy Letters:* Grundy, LMWM 199–201.

Richardson's painting: Grundy, LMWM 301–303. Richardson's friends: Gibson-Wood 74–86. Richardson's studio: Gibson-Wood, 65–72.

LM's son as runaway: LMCL 2:69. Duke of Kingston's death: Grundy, LMWM 250–53. Lady Townshend's and Sarah Chiswell's deaths from smallpox: Grundy, LMWM 248, 253.

ZB presenting book to Royal Society, and being asked to join: Mager 176–77. "It is and shall be acknowledged . . .": ZBHA 40. ZB's departure: Mager 180.

LM's mention of America in romance: "Mademoiselle de Condé," LMRW 39.

ZB's letter to Sloane, upon arriving home: ZB to Sir Hans Sloane, Dec. 14, 1726.

The Practice

Boston's 1730 and 1752 epidemics: Blake 75–77; WDS 394–99; Hopkins 256–57; Mager 204. WD quotations: WDD 8–9, 10. ZB's and WD's 1730 publications: Blake 75.

Benjamin Franklin: Franklin, *Benjamin Franklin's Autobiographical Writings* 38; Mager 178–79; Hopkins 243, 254–56; Duffy 34. John Adams: Fenn 33–35; Ferling 32–33; Mc-Cullough 56. Continental Congress: Hopkins 243. Washington and the inoculation of the Continental Army: Fenn, 88–103; Hopkins 257–261; Tucker 20–22. Inoculation's popularity among Revolutionary women: Hopkins 255, 260; McCullough 142–44

Later history of inoculation in London: Miller, AIS 134–71; Razzell. On the Continent:

Miller, AIS 172–240. Physicians' "improvements" making the procedure "dangerous": Grundy, "Medical Advance" 34. King George III and his son: Hopkins 61.

Jenner: Fisher; Tucker 23–27; Hopkins 77–81; *www.jennermuseum.com* (for quotation from Napoleon). Jenner "I was astonished," Royal Society's rejection, "angel's trumpet": Hopkins 79.

Inoculation chief contribution of Enlightenment: Miller, AIS 195.

Eradication of smallpox: Tucker, WHO. Indian resister: Tucker 106–107. Jenner on vaccination annihilating smallpox: Hopkins 80.

The People

LM and her children: Grundy, LMWM; Halsband, "New Anecdotes"; Spence, *Grand Tour* 346–46. Maitland: Bulloch. Sloane: de Beer. George I: Hatton. George II, Queen Caroline, and their children: Van der Kiste, *Georgian Princesses* and *King George II*. Harrison: Maitland, MMV.

ZB and family: "Boylston, Dr. Zabdiel, FRS" in James Thacher; Mager; Thwing RCN 6727; William Gray Brooks; Wyman; *Booke of the Boylstones*. Thomas (Tommy): Thwing RCN 6725; mastectomy and St. Thomas's Hospital, London: ZB letter to Dr. Mortimer, Dec. 17, 1737, Royal Society MM.20.7; "first fruit": ZB letter to Sloane, Dec. 19, 1737, BL Sloane MS 4055, folio 248–49, qtd. in Mager 187. John: Parsons. Zabdiel junior: Shipton 317–18. Young Jerusha: Thwing RCN 6709; Mary: Thwing RCN 6716; Elizabeth: Thwing RCN 6708 and 57192. Jack, Moll, and Jackey: Thwing RCN 9395, 9441, 40077, 40068, 40084, 40086, 40258, 40330.

CM: Silverman. Samuel Mather: Thwing RCN 45053; Silverman; Samuel Mather. Onesimus: Thwing RCN 30145.

WD: Thwing RCN 24422; DAB; Alexander Hamilton 116–17; "Douglass, William, M.D." in James Thacher 1:255–57; Bullock.

Cheever: Thwing RCN 15679.

BIBLIOGRAPHY

Manuscript and Rare Book Collections:

The American Antiquarian Society, Worcester, Massachusetts
The British Library, London
The Francis A. Countway Library of Medicine, Harvard University, Boston Massachusetts
The John Carter Brown Library, Brown University, Providence, Rhode Island
Harrowby MSS Trust, Sandon Hall, Sandon, England
The Houghton Library, Harvard University, Cambridge, Massachusetts
Massachusetts Historical Society, Boston, Massachusetts
New England Historic Genealogical Society, Boston, Massachusetts
Public Records Office, London
The Royal Society, London

Newspapers:

Applebee's Original Weekly Journal (London)
The Boston Gazette
The Boston News-Letter
Daily Post (London)
The London Gazette
The New-England Courant (Boston)
The Post-Boy (London)
St. James Evening Post (London)
The Weekly Journal: or, British Gazetteer (London)
The Weekly Journal or Saturday's Post (London)

Books and Articles:

The Accomplish'd Lady's Delight in Preserving Physick, Beautifying and Cookery. 10th ed. London: printed for Daniel Prat, 1719.

Acts and Resolves, Public and Private, of the Province of the Massachusetts Bay. 21 vols. Boston: Wright & Potter, printers to the state, 1869–1922.

"Adams Family Bible." *New England Historical and Genealogical Register* 8 (1854): 283–85.

Allen, Robert J. *The Clubs of Augustan London*. Cambridge: Harvard University Press, 1933.

Amyand, Claude. Letter to Sir Hans Sloane, March 14, 1721/2. Sloane MS 4076, folio 33, British Library.

———. "A List of Persons Inoculated by Claude Amyand, Principall & Serjeant Surgeon in Ordinary to His Majesty." *Inoculations*. Part 1, no. 1, folios 2–6. The Royal Society. *Early Letters and Classified Papers* 23.

Ashton, John. *Social Life in the Reign of Queen Anne*. London: Chatto & Windus, 1904.

Babington, Anthony. *The English Bastille*. London: Macdonald, 1971.

Beall, Otho T., Jr., and Richard H. Shyrock. *Cotton Mather: First Significant Figure in American Medicine*. Baltimore: Johns Hopkins University Press, 1954.

Besant, Walter, Sir. *London in the Eighteenth Century*. London: A. & C. Black Ltd., 1925.

Blake, John B. *Public Health in the Town of Boston, 1630–1822*. Cambridge: Harvard University Press, 1959.

Bodge, George M. *Soldiers in King Philip's War*. 3rd ed. 1906. Baltimore: Genealogical Publishing Co., 1976.

Bonner, John. *The Town of Boston in New-England, 1722*. Boston, 1722.

Booke of the Boylstones. MS, New England Historic Genealogical Society.

Boston Births From A.D. 1700 to A.D. 1800. Report of the Record Commissioners of the City of Boston. Vol. 24. Boston: Rockwell & Churchill, 1894.

Boston Marriages From 1700 to 1751. Report of the Record Commissioners of the City of Boston. Vol. 28. Boston: Municipal Printing Office, 1898.

Boston Town Records 1700–1728. Report of the Record Commissioners of the City of Boston. Vol. 8. Boston: Municipal Printing Office, 1883.

Boylston, Zabdiel. [Anonymous.] "A Faithful Account of What Has Occur'd Under the Late Experiments of Small-Pox Managed and Governed in the Way of Inoculation." *Boston Gazette*. No. 101, Oct. 23–30, 1721.

———. "Ambergris Found in Whales." *Philosophical Transactions of the Royal Society* 33 (Oct–Dec., 1724): 193.

———. *An Historical Account of the Small-Pox Inoculated in New England, Upon all Sorts of Persons, Whites, Blacks, and all Ages and Constitutions. With some Account of the Nature of the Infection in the Natural and Inoculated Way, and their Different Effects on Human Bodies. With some short Directions to the Unexperienced in this Method of Practice*. London: for S. Chandler, 1726. Facsimile rpt. in *Smallpox in Colonial America*. New York: Arno Press, 1977.

———. *An Historical Account of the Small-Pox Inoculated in New England, Upon all Sorts of Persons, Whites, Blacks, and all Ages and Constitutions. With some Account of the Nature of the Infection in the Natural and Inoculated Way, and their Different Effects on Human Bodies. With some short Directions to the Unexperienced in this Method of Practice*. 2nd ed. Boston: Reprinted for S. Gerrish, 1730.

———. Letter to Benjamin Colman, February 26, 1724/5. Benjamin Colman Papers, Massachusetts Historical Society.

———. Letter to Sir Hans Sloane, December 14, 1726. Sloane MS 4048, folio 238, British Library.

Bridenbaugh, Carl. *Cities in the Wilderness: The First Century of Urban Life in America, 1625–1742*. New York: Alfred A. Knopf, 1955.

Brooks, William Gray. *Genealogical Record of the Boylston, Walter, and Cotton Families*. Minns fam. MS, Massachusetts Historical Society.

Buck, Anne. *Dress in Eighteenth-Century England*. London: B.T. Batsford, 1979.

Bulloch, John Malcolm. *A Pioneer of Inoculation—Charles Maitland*. Aberdeen: The University Press, 1930.

Bullock, Charles J. "Life and Writings of William Douglass." *Economic Studies* 2 (1897): 265–90.

Caplan, Neil. "Some Unpublished Letters of Benjamin Colman, 1717–1725." *Proceedings of the Massachusetts Historical Society* 77 (1965).

Caulfield, James. *Memoirs of the Celebrated Persons Composing the Kit-Cat Club; With a Prefatory Account of the Origin of the Association*. London: Hurst Robinson, 1821.

Chapman, Hester W. *Mary II, Queen of England*. London: Jonathan Cape, 1953.

Clark, Charles E. *The Public Prints: The Newspaper in Anglo-American Culture, 1665–1740*. New York: Oxford University Press, 1994.

Cohen, I. Bernard, ed. *Cotton Mather and American Science and Medicine: With Studies and Documents Concerning the Introduction of Inoculation or Variolation*. 2 vols. New York: Arno, 1980.

Colman, Benjamin. *Some Observations on the New Method of Receiving the Smallpox by Engrafting or Inoculation, in New England*. Boston: B. Green for Samuel Gerrish, 1721.

———. Letter to the Reverend Mr.———of Boston, July 25, 1721. MS in the Francis A. Countway Library of Medicine, Harvard University.

The Complete Newgate Calendar. Ed. G.T. Crook. 5 vols. London: Printed for the Navarre Society, 1926.

Cooper, William. *A Letter to a Friend in the Country, Attempting a Solution of the Scruples & Objections of a Conscientious or Religious Nature, Commonly Made against the New Way of Receiving the Small-pox*. Boston: S. Kneeland for S. Gerrish, 1721.

———. *A Sermon concerning the laying the Deaths of others to heart. Occasioned by the lamented Death of that ingenious and religious gentleman John Gore, M.A., of Harvard College in Cambridge, N.E., who died of the Small Pox, Nov. 7, 1720*. Boston, 1720 [i.e., January 1721].

Cowper, Mary Clavering Cowper, Countess. *Diary of Mary Countess Cowper, Lady of the Bedchamber to the Princess of Wales, 1714–1720*. London, J. Murray, 1864.

Creighton, Charles. *A History of Epidemics in Britain*. 2 vols. 1894. 2nd ed. London: Frank Cass & Co. Ltd., 1965.

Cunnington, C. Willis and Phyllis. *A Handbook of English Costume in the 18C*. Rev. ed. London: Faber & Faber, 1972.

de Beer, Gavin, Sir. *Sir Hans Sloane and the British Museum*. London, New York: Published for the Trustees of the British Museum by Oxford University Press, 1953.

Defoe, Daniel. *A Journal of the Plague Year*. 1722. Intro. Jason Goodwin. Notes by Ernelle Fife. New York: The Modern Library, 2001.

———. *Moll Flanders*. 1722. Oxford and New York: Oxford University Press, 1998.

Douglass, William. *The Abuses and Scandals of Some Late Pamphlets in Favour of Inoculation of the Small Pox, Modestly Obviated, and Inoculation Further Consider'd in a Letter to A** S** M.D. & F.R.S. in London*. London, 1722. Rpt. Boston: J. Franklin, 1722.

———. "A Digression Concerning the Small-Pox." In *A Summary, Historical and Political, of the first Planting, Progressive Improvements, and Present state of the British Settlements in North America*. 2 vols. Boston: Printed and sold by Rogers and Fowle in Queen-Street, 1749–52. 2: 392–414.

———. *A Dissertation Concerning Inoculation of the Small-Pox. Giving Some Account of the Rise, Progress, Success, Advantages and Disadvantages of Receiving the Small Pox by Incisions: Illustrated by Sundry Cases of the Inoculated*. Boston: D. Henchman and T. Hancock, 1730.

———. *Inoculation of the Small Pox as Practised in Boston, Consider'd in a Letter to A——S——M.D. & F.R.S. in London*. Boston: J. Franklin, 1722.

———. "Letters from Dr. William Douglass to Cadwallader Colden of New York." *Collections of the Massachusetts Historical Society* 4th ser. 2 (1854): 164–89.

———. *Postscript to Abuses, &c. Obviated. Being a Short and Modest Answer to Matters of Fact Maliciously Misrepresented in a Late Doggrel Dialogue*. Boston: J. Franklin, 1722.

———. *A Practical Essay Concerning the Small Pox*. Boston, 1730.

Dover, Thomas. *The Ancient Physician's Legacy to His Country*. 1732. Ed. Kenneth Dewhurst. Metuchen, N.J.: Scarecrow Press, 1974.

Drake, Samuel Adams. *Old Boston Taverns and Tavern Clubs*. Boston: W.A. Butterfield, 1917.

Dryden, John. *Selected Poems*. Ed. Steven N. Zwicker and David Bywaters. London and New York: Penguin, 2001.

Duffy, John. *Epidemics in Colonial America*. Baton Rouge: Louisiana State University Press, 1953.

Equiano, Olaudah. *The Interesting Narrative of the Life of Olaudah Equiano, or Gustavus Vassa, the African, Written by Himself: Authoritative Text, Contexts, Criticism*. Ed. Werner Sollors. New York; London: Norton, 2001.

Fenn, Elizabeth A. *Pox Americana: The Great Smallpox Epidemic of 1775–82*. New York: Hill and Wang, 2001.

Fenner, Frank, Donald Ainslie Henderson, Isao Arita, Zdeněk Ježek, and Ivan Danilovich Ladnyi. *Smallpox and its Eradication*. Geneva: World Health Organization, 1988.

Fergusson, C. Bruce. "Durells in 18th century Canadian History." *Dalhousie Review* 35 (1955): 16–30.

Ferling, John. *John Adams: A Life*. Knoxville: University of Tennessee Press, 1992.

Fisher, Richard B. *Edward Jenner 1749–1823*. London: André Deutsch, 1991.

Fitz, Reginald H. "Zabdiel Boylston, Inoculator, and the Epidemic of Smallpox in Boston in 1721." *Bulletin of the Johns Hopkins Hospital* 22 (1911): 315–27.

Foster, Joseph, ed. *Alumni Oxonienses; The Members of the University of Oxford, 1500–1714*. 1891–92. Nendeln, Liechtenstein: Kraus Reprint, 1968.

Franklin, Benjamin. *Benjamin Franklin's Autobiographical Writings*. Ed. Carl Van Doren. New York: Viking, 1945.

———. *Benjamin Franklin's Memoirs*. Parallel text edition. Ed. Max Farrand. Berkeley and Los Angeles: University of California Press, 1949.

George, M. Dorothy. *London Life in the Eighteenth Century*. 1925. New York: Harper & Row, 1965.

Gibson, Elizabeth Stuart. *The Compleat New England Huswife*. Wenham, Massachusetts: Albion Press, 1992.

Gibson-Wood, Carol. *Jonathan Richardson: Art Theorist of the English Enlightenment*. New Haven and London: published for the Paul Mellon Centre for Studies in British Art by Yale University Press, 2000.

Greene, Lorenzo Johnston. *The Negro in Colonial New England, 1620–1776*. New York: Columbia University Press, 1942.

[Greenwood, Isaac.] *A Friendly Debate; or a Dialogue, between Academicus; and Sawny & Mundungus, Two Eminent Physicians, about Some of their Late Performances*. Boston: n.p., 1722.

Gregg, Edward. *Queen Anne*. London: Routledge & Kegan Paul, 1980.

Grundy, Isobel. "'The Entire Works of Clarinda': Unpublished Juvenile Verse by Lady Mary Wortley Montagu." *Yearbook in English Studies* 7 (1977): 91–107.

———. *Lady Mary Wortley Montagu*. Oxford: Oxford University Press, 1999.

———. "Medical Advance and Female Fame; Inoculation and its After-Effects." *Lumen* 13 (1994).

Halsband, Robert. *The Life of Lady Mary Wortley Montagu.* Oxford: Clarendon Press, 1956.

———. "New Anecdotes of Lady Mary Wortley Montagu." *Literary Scholarship: Essays in Memory of James Marshall Osborn.* Ed. René Wellek and Alvara Ribeiro. Oxford: Clarendon Press; New York: Oxford University Press, 1979. 241–46.

———. "New Light on Lady Mary Wortley Montagu's Contribution to Inoculation." *Journal of the History of Medicine* 8 (1953): 390–405.

Hamilton, Alexander. *Gentleman's Progress: The Itinerarium of Dr. Alexander Hamilton, 1744.* Ed. Carl Bridenbaugh. Chapel Hill: University North Carolina Press, 1948.

Hamilton, Elizabeth. *William's Mary: A Biography of Mary II.* New York: Taplinger Publishing, 1972.

Harris, John. "Thoresby House, Nottinghamshire." *Architectural History* 4 (1961): 11–19.

———. "Thoresby Concluded." *Architectural History* 6 (1963): 103–105.

Harris, Walter. "De Inoculatione Variolarum." Appendix to *De Peste Dissertatio Habita Apr. 17. 1721 in Amphitheatro Collegii Regalis Medicorum Londinensium. Cui accessit Descriptio Inoculationis Variolarum.* London: Printed for William & John Innys, 1721. 40–48.

———. *De Morbis Acutis Infantum. Cui accessit Liber Observationes de Morbis aliquot Gravioribus Medicas Complectens.* 3rd ed. London: William & John Innys, 1720.

Hatton, Ragnhild. *George I: Elector and King.* London: Thames & Hudson, 1978.

Henderson, G.D. *Mystics of the North-East.* Aberdeen: Printed for the Third Spalding Club, 1934.

Herbert, Eugenia W. "Smallpox Inoculation in Africa." *Journal of African History* 16 (1975): 539–59.

Historical Register of Harvard University, 1636–1936. Cambridge: Harvard University, 1937.

Hollis, Thomas. Letters. *Documents from the Harvard University Archives, 1638–1750. Collections of the Colonial Society of Massachusetts* Vol. 50. Boston: Colonial Society of Massachusetts, 1975.

Hopkins, Donald R. *Princes and Peasants: Smallpox in History.* Chicago: University of Chicago Press, 1983.

Huggins, Nathan. *Black Odyssey: The Afro-American Ordeal in Slavery.* New York: Pantheon, 1977.

Hutchinson, Thomas. *The History of the Colony and Province of Massachusetts Bay.* 1774–75. 2 vols. Ed. Lawrence S. Mayo. Cambridge: Harvard University Press, 1936.

Journals of the House of Representatives of Massachusetts. Vol. 3, 1721–22. Boston: Massachusetts Historical Society, 1922.

Jurin, James. *An Account of the Success of Inoculating the Small Pox in Great Britain. With a Comparison Between the Miscarriages in that Practice, and the Mortality of the Natural Small-pox.* London: J. Peele, 1724.

———. *An Account of the Success of Inoculating the Small Pox in Great Britain, for the year 1724.* London: J. Peele, 1725.

———. *An Account of the Success of Inoculating the Small Pox in Great Britain, for the Year 1725.* London: J. Peele, 1726.

———. *An Account of the Success of Inoculating the Small-pox in Great-Britain, for the year 1726.* London: For J. Peele, 1727.

———. *A Letter to the Learned Caleb Cotesworth, M.D. Fellow of the Royal Society, of the College of Physicians, and Physician to St. Thomas's Hospital. Containing, a Comparison Between the Mortality of the Natural Small Pox, and That Given by Inoculation.* London: Printed for W. and J. Innys, 1723.

Kennedy, Peter. *An Essay on External Remedies*. London: Printed for Andrew Bell, 1715.

Kilgour, Frederick G. "Thomas Robie (1689–1729), Colonial Scientist and Physician." *Isis* 30 (1939): 473–490.

Kittredge, George Lyman. "Cotton Mather's Election into the Royal Society." *Publications of the Colonial Society of Massachusetts* 14 (1912): 81–114.

———. "Further Notes on Cotton Mather and the Royal Society." *Publications of the Colonial Society of Massachusetts* 14 (1913): 281–92.

———. "Some Lost Works of Cotton Mather." *Proceedings of the Massachusetts Historical Society* 45 (1912): 418–79. Reprinted in Cohen, vol. 1.

Laroon, Marcellus. *The Criers and Hawkers of London: Engravings and Drawings*. Ed. Sean Shesgreen. Stanford: Stanford University Press, 1990.

Lemay, J.A. Leo. *Benjamin Franklin: A Documentary History*. 1997. Web site: *www.english.udel.edu/lemay/franklin/*

Lemprière's Classical Dictionary of Proper Names mentioned in Ancient Authors Writ Large. 3rd ed. London: Routledge & Kegan Paul, 1984.

Lyon, David. *The Sailing Navy List: All the Ships of the Royal Navy—Built, Purchased and Captured—1688–1860*. London: Conway Maritime Press, 1993.

Mack, Maynard. *Alexander Pope: A Life*. New Haven: Yale University Press, 1985.

Mager, Gerald Marvin. *Zabdiel Boylston: Medical Pioneer of Colonial Boston*. PhD Diss.: University of Illinois at Urbana-Champaign, 1975.

Maitland, Charles. *Mr. Maitland's Account of Inoculating the Small Pox*. London, 1722.

Mannix, Daniel P., with Malcolm Cowley. *Black Cargoes: A History of the Atlantic Slave Trade, 1518–1865*. 1962. New York and Harmondsworth, England: Penguin, 1977.

Mansel, Philip. *Constantinople: City of the World's Desire 1453–1924*. London: John Murray, 1995.

Marcus, Geoffrey Jules. *Heart of Oak: A Survey of British Seapower in the Georgian Era*. London and New York: Oxford University Press, 1975.

Massey, Edmund. *A Sermon Against the Dangerous and Sinful Practice of Inoculation. Preach'd at St. Andrew's Holborn, on Sunday, July the 8th, 1722*. London, 1722. Reprinted in Boston: for Benjamin Indicott, 1730.

Massey, Isaac. *A Short and Plain Account of Inoculation with Some Remarks on the Main Arguments Made Use of to Recommend that Practice, by Mr. Maitland and Others*. 1722. 2nd ed. London: W. Meadows, 1723.

Mather, Cotton. [Anonymous.] *An Account of the Method and Success of Inoculating the Small-Pox, in Boston in New-England. In a Letter from a Gentleman there, to his Friend in London*. London: J. Peele, 1722. Reprinted in *Smallpox in Colonial America*. New York: Arno, 1977.

———. *The Angel of Bethesda*. New London: Timothy Green, 1722. Rpt. Barre, Mass.: American Antiquarian Society, 1972.

———. *Diary of Cotton Mather*. Ed. Worthington Chauncey Ford. 2 vols. New York: Frederick Ungar Publishing Co., 1957.

———. Letter to Zabdiel Boylston, June 24, 1721. *The Massachusetts Magazine; or, Monthly Museum* 1 (1789): 778.

———. *Selected Letters of Cotton Mather*. Ed. Kenneth Silverman. Baton Rouge: Louisiana State University Press, 1971.

———. [Anonymous.] "The Way of Proceeding in the Small Pox Inoculated in New England." *Philosophical Transactions of the Royal Society of London* 32, no. 370 (Jan.–Mar., 1722): 33–35.

Mather, Increase. *Several Reasons Proving that Inoculating or Transplanting the Small Pox, is a*

Lawful Practice, and That it Has Been Blessed by God for the Saving of Many a Life. With Cotton Mather's [anonymous] *Sentiments on the Small-pox Inoculated*. Boston: S. Kneeland for J. Edwards, 1721.

———. *Some Further Account, of the Smallpox Inoculated*. Boston: J. Edwards, 1721 (i.e., 1722). Rpt. from the *Boston Gazette*, no. 115, January 29–February 5, 1722.

McCullough, David. *John Adams*. New York: Simon & Schuster, 2001.

McKay, Derek. *Prince Eugene of Savoy*. London: Thames and Hudson, 1977.

McManus, Edgar J. *Black Bondage in the North*. Syracuse: Syracuse University Press, 1973.

Mead, Richard. *A Discourse on the Small-Pox and Measles*. 1747. In *The Medical Works of Richard Mead, M.D.* New edition. Edinburgh, 1775. Rpt. New York: AMS Press, 1978. 223–95.

Miller, Genevieve. *The Adoption of Inoculation for Smallpox in England and France*. Philadelphia: University of Pennsylvania Press, 1957.

Miller, Perry. *The New England Mind: From Colony to Province*. Cambridge: Harvard University Press, 1953.

Minot, Joseph Grafton. *A Genealogical Record of the Minot Family in America and England*. Boston, 1897.

Miscellany Poems. 6 vols. London: Jacob Tonson, 1716.

Montagu, Mary Wortley, Lady. *Complete Letters of Lady Mary Wortley Montagu*. Ed. Robert Halsband. 3 vols. Oxford: Clarendon Press, 1965–67.

———. *Embassy to Constantinople: The Travels of Lady Mary Wortley Montagu*. Intro. Dervla Murphy. Ed. Christopher Pick. London: Century, 1988.

———. *Essays and Poems* and *Simplicity, a Comedy*. Ed. Robert Halsband and Isobel Grundy. Oxford: Clarendon Press, 1977.

———. *Romance Writings*. Ed. Isobel Grundy. Oxford: Clarendon Press, 1996.

Mr. Maitland's Account of Inoculating the Small Pox Vindicated, from Dr. Wagstaffe's Misrepresentations of That Practice, with Some Remarks on Mr. Massey's Sermon. London: J. Peele, 1722.

Muse, Raymond. *William Douglass: Man of the American Enlightenment*. PhD. Diss. Stanford University, 1948.

Neal, Daniel. "Introduction." *A Narrative of the Method and Success of Inoculating the Small Pox in New England. By Mr. Benj. Colman . . . to Which is Now Prefixed, an Historical Introduction*. London, 1722. Rpt. in Cohen.

Nichols, John. *Illustrations of the Literary History of the Eighteenth Century*. London, 1817; New York: Kraus Reprint, 1966. 1:278–79.

Paige, Lucius R. "The Winslow Family." *New England Historical and Genealogical Register* 25 (1871): 355–58 and 26 (1872): 71–75.

Parsons, Charles W. "Zabdiel and John Boylston." *New England Historical and Genealogical Register* 35 (1881): 150–52.

Pepys, Samuel. *The Diary of Samuel Pepys*. Ed. Robert Latham and William Matthews. 10 vols. Berkeley and Los Angeles: University of California Press, 1970–1983.

Picard, Liza. *Dr. Johnson's London*. 2000. New York: St. Martin's Press, 2001.

Pope, Alexander. *The Correspondence*. Ed. George Wiley Sherburn. 5 vols. Oxford: Clarendon Press, 1956.

Prescott, Hilda F.M. *Once to Sinai*. London: Eyre & Spottiswoode, 1957.

Pylarinus, Jacob. "Nova et tuta Variolas excitandi per Transplantationem Methodus, nuper inventa et in usum tracta." *Philosophical Transactions of the Royal Society of London* 29, no. 347 (1714–16, printed 1717): 393–99.

Razzell, Peter (P. E.). *The Conquest of Smallpox: The Impact of Inoculation on Smallpox Mortality in Eighteenth-Century Britain.* Firle, Sussex: Caliban, 1977.

Records of the Churches of Boston. Transcribed by Robert J. Dunkle and Ann S. Lainhart. Compact Disc. Boston: New England Historic Genealogical Society, 2002.

Ricketts, Thomas Francis. *The Diagnosis of Smallpox.* 2 vols. London, 1908. Rpt. Washington, DC: U.S. Department of Health, Education and Welfare, 1966.

Robie, Thomas. MS Smallpox Diary, 1721–22, Massachusetts Historical Society.

Rodger, N.A.M. *The Wooden World: An Anatomy of the Georgian Navy.* London: Collins, 1986.

Rose, Philip. *An Essay on the Small-Pox.* London: for E. Curll, 1724.

Royal Society. *The Early Letters and Classified Papers, 1660–1740.* MSS in the Royal Society Library, London; Microfilm ed. Paul L. Kesaris. Frederick, MD: University Publications of America, 1990. 23 microfilm reels.

Royal Society. *Inoculations.* 2 parts. Vol. 23. of *The Early Letters and Classified Papers, 1660–1740.* MSS in the Royal Society Library, London; Microfilm ed. Paul L. Kesaris. Frederick, MD: University Publications of America, 1990. 23 reels.

Royal Society. *Journal-Book* 12 (1720–26). MS in the Royal Society Library.

Saint-Simon, Louis de Rouvroy, duc de. *Historical Memoirs of the Duc de Saint-Simon.* Ed. and trans. Lucy Norton. 3 vols. New York: McGraw-Hill, 1967–72.

Selectmen's Minutes, 1716–1736. Report of the Record Commissioners of the City of Boston. Vol. 13. Boston: Rockwell and Churchill, 1885.

Sewall, Samuel. *The Diary of Samuel Sewall, 1674–1729.* Ed. Milton Halsey Thomas. 2 vols. New York: Farrar, Straus & Giroux, 1973.

Shattuck, Lemuel. "The Minot Family." *New England Historical and Genealogical Register* 1 (1847): 171–78.

Sherburn, George. *The Early Career of Alexander Pope.* Oxford: Clarendon Press, 1934.

Shipton, Clifford K. *Biographical Sketches of Those Who Attended Harvard College in the Classes 1722–1725.* Vol. 7 of *Sibley's Harvard Graduates.* Boston: Massachusetts Historical Society, 1945.

Silverman, Kenneth. *Life and Times of Cotton Mather.* New York: Harper & Row, 1984.

Sloane, Hans, Sir. "An Account of Inoculation." *Philosophical Transactions of the Royal Society of London* 49 (1756): 516–20.

Smallpox in Colonial America. New York: Arno, 1977.

Some Account of What is Said of Innoculating or Transplanting the Small Pox. By the Learned Dr. Emanuel Timonius, and Jacobus Pylarinus. With Some Remarks Thereon. To which are added, a few queries in answer to the scruples of many about the lawfulness of this method. Published by Dr. Zabdiel Bolyston. Boston: S. Gerrish, 1721. [Probable authorship: Parts 1 and 3 by Cotton Mather; Part 2 by Zabdiel Boylston]

Spence, Joseph. *Letters from the Grand Tour.* Ed. Slava Klima. Montreal and London: McGill—Queen's University Press, 1975.

———. *Observations, Anecdotes, and Characters of Books and Men, Collected from Conversation.* Ed. Joseph M. Osborn. 2 vols. Oxford: Clarendon Press, 1966.

Stearns, Raymond Phineas. *Science in the British Colonies of America.* Urbana, Ill.: University of Illinois Press, 1970.

Stearns, Raymond Phineas, and George Pasti, Jr. "Remarks Upon the Introduction of Inoculation For Smallpox in England." *Bulletin of the History of Medicine* 24, no. 2 (1950): 103–122.

Stewart, George. Letter to Dr. William Wagstaffe, Nov. 8, 1722. In the Royal Society's

Early Letters and Classified Papers, 1660–1740. Vol. 23. *Inoculations.* Part 2. No. 67, folios 310–11.

Stuart, Louisa, Lady. *Biographical Anecdotes of Lady M.W. Montagu.* In Lady Mary Wortley Montagu. *Essays and Poems.* Ed. Robert Halsband and Isobel Grundy. Oxford: Clarendon Press, 1977. 6–61.

Thacher, James. *American Medical Biography; Or, Memoirs Of Eminent Physicians Who Have Flourished In America.* 1828. 2 vols. in 1 Rpt. New York: Milford House, 1967.

Thacher, Peter [Signed P.T.] "To the Editors." *Massachusetts Magazine* 1(1789): 776–79.

Thwing, Annie Haven. *Inhabitants and Estates of the Town of Boston, 1630–1800, and The Crooked and Narrow Streets of Boston, 1630–1822.* Compact disc. Boston: New England Historic Genealogical Society; Massachusetts Historical Society, 2001.

Timonius, Emanuel. "An Account, of History, of the Procuring the Small Pox by Incision, Or Inoculation; as it has for some time been practiced at Constantinople." *Philosophical Transactions of the Royal Society of London* 29, no. 339 (1714–16, printed 1717): 72–82.

Tucker, Jonathan B. *Scourge: The Once and Future Threat of Smallpox.* New York: Atlantic Monthly Press, 2001.

Turell, Ebenezer. *The Life and Character of the Reverend Benjamin Colman, D.D.* 1749. Facsimile reproduction w. intro. by Christopher R. Reaske. Delmar, New York: Scholars' Facsimiles & Reprints, 1972.

"Vaccinia (Smallpox) Vaccine Recommendations of the Advisory Committee on Immunizations Practices (ACIP), 2001." Centers for Disease Control and Prevention MMWR Recommendations and Reports 50, no. RR-10 (June 22, 2001): 11. On the CDC Web site at *www.cdc.gov.*

Van der Kiste, John. *The Georgian Princesses.* Stroud, Gloucestershire: Sutton, 2000.

———. *King George II and Queen Caroline.* Stroud, Gloucestershire: Sutton, 1997.

A Vindication of the Ministers of Boston, from the Abuses & Scandals, Lately Cast upon Them, in Diverse Printed Papers. Boston: B. Green for Samuel Gerrish, Feb. 5, 1722.

Vinton, John Adams. *The Giles Memorial: Genealogical Memoirs of the families bearing the names of Giles, Gould, Holmes, Jennison, Leonard, Lindall, Curwen, Marshall, Robinson, Sampson, and Webb.* Boston: Henry W. Dutton & Son, 1864.

Wagstaffe, William. *A Letter to Dr. Freind, Shewing the Danger and Uncertainty of Inoculating the Small Pox.* London: S. Butler, 1722.

Whitehill, Walter Muir, and Lawrence W. Kennedy. *Boston: A Topographical History.* Cambridge, Mass. and London: Harvard University Press, 2000.

Willard, Joseph. *Willard Memoir; or, Life and Times of Major Simon Willard.* Boston: Phillips, Sampson, and Company, 1858.

Williams, John. *An Answer to a Late Pamphlet, Intitled, A Letter to a Friend in the Country, Attempting a Solution of the Scruples and Objections of a Consciencious or Religious Nature, Commonly Made Against the New Way of Receiving the Small Pox.* Boston, James Franklin, 1722.

———. *Several Arguments, Proving that Inoculating the Small Pox is not Contained in the Law of Physick, Either Natural or Divine, and Therefore Unlawful.* Boston: James Franklin, 1721.

Williams, Nathanael. *The Method of Practice in the Small-Pox, with Observations on the Way of Inoculation.* Boston, S. Kneeland, 1752.

Wilson, Adrian. "Politics of Medical Improvement in Early Hanoverian London." In *The Medical Enlightenment of the Eighteenth Century.* Ed. Andrew Cunningham and R.K. French. Cambridge, England and New York: Cambridge University Press, 1990. 4–59.

Winslow, Ola Elizabeth. *A Destroying Angel: The Conquest of Smallpox in Colonial Boston.* Boston: Houghton Mifflin, 1974.

Wright, Donald R. *African-Americans in the Colonial Era: From African Origins through the American Revolution.* Arlington Heights, Illinois: Harlan Davidson, 1990.

Wyman, Thomas B., Jr. "Pedigree of the Family of Boylston." *New England Historical and Genealogical Register* 7 (1853): 145–50.

Note on the authorship of *Some Account of What is Said of Innoculating or Transplanting the Small Pox* (Boston, 1721)

This pamphlet was Boston's first separately printed defense of inoculation; it was printed after August 25, 1721, when Mather notes an intention to publish it in his diary, and before September 4 of that year, when the *New England Courant* announced plans to publish a rebuttal.

The title page gives no author but does identify Dr. Zabdiel Boylston as its publisher. The pamphlet has three parts: first, a lengthy abridgement of the two articles by Timonius and Pylarinus; second, a series of defenses of inoculation given in answer to particular arguments voiced against it; and third, some theological reflections on the lawfulness of protecting oneself against disease. The first and third parts are undoubtedly by Cotton Mather. The first is the long abridgment or loose transcription of the Royal Society's inoculation papers that he sent to the town's physicians, and which later shows up in his *Angel of Bethesda*. The third part, as George Lyman Kittredge notes in "Lost Works of Cotton Mather," addresses Mather's subject of expertise (Puritan theology) in his inimitable style.

Kittredge also claimed the second part for Mather, on the grounds that it quotes the same unnamed black man's story of African inoculation that is to be found in Mather's smallpox treatise (later incorporated into *Angel of Bethesda*). Zabdiel Boylston, however, is far more likely to have been the primary author of the second section—though he may have been collaborating with Mather at some level. First, it is written in the first person by someone who pointedly distinguishes himself from the author of the preceding abridgement, i.e., Mather. Named on the title page as the publisher, Boylston is the person most likely to be the "I" of this writing. Second, it appears to have been written by someone with firsthand experience of inoculation. Third, Mather later quoted two paragraphs from this section and identified them as by the inoculating doctor, i.e. Boylston (CMA, pages 25–26). Finally, the reasoning, the frustration, and the sarcastic humor in this section are all echoed elsewhere by Boylston.

As for quoting the same black man, I think it likeliest that Boylston heard the same story from the same source, and then later relied on Mather's transcription when he came to putting it into print. Mather was fascinated by the Creole-influenced English; Boylston smoothed it over into something more like standard English. He also surrounded the passage with different observations and arguments than Mather did. Furthermore, Boylston prized firsthand examination of witnesses and evidence, as his frustration with the doctors who refused to visit his inoculated patients makes clear. It seems far-fetched that he would not have made the same examination of surviving witnesses, before attempting the operation on his own son. It is possible, however, that he merely lifted the quotation from Mather. Either way, its use does not argue convincingly against Boylston's authorship of this section.

I have regarded this second section as the work of Zabdiel Boylston.